Paraplegia

Edited by José Juan Antonio Ibarra Arias
and Carlos Alberto Cuellar Ramos

Published in London, United Kingdom

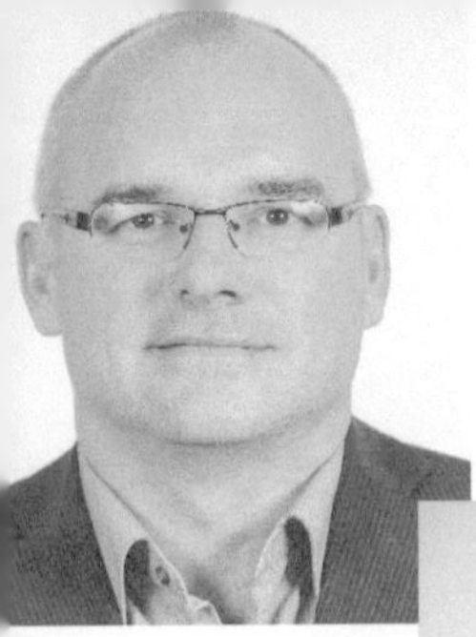
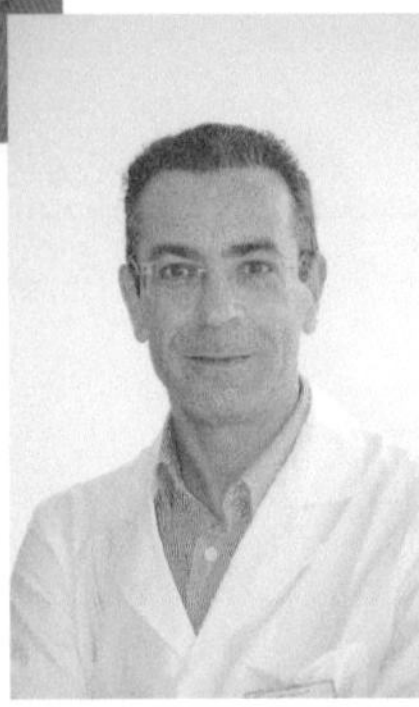
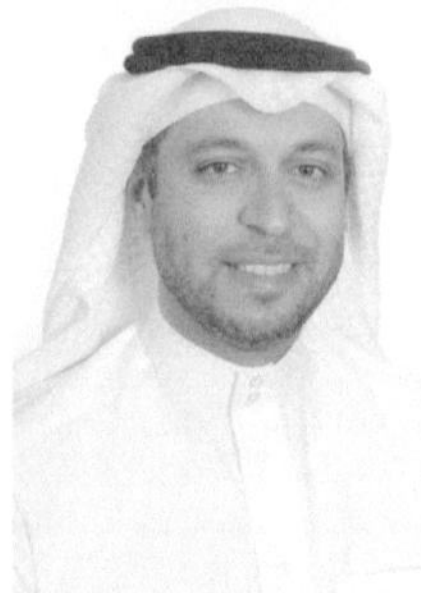
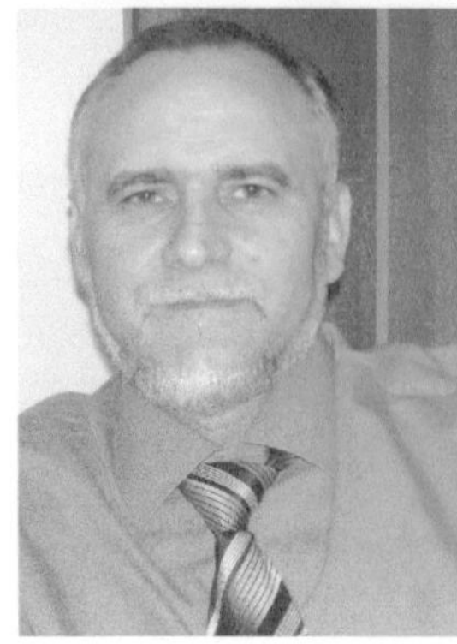
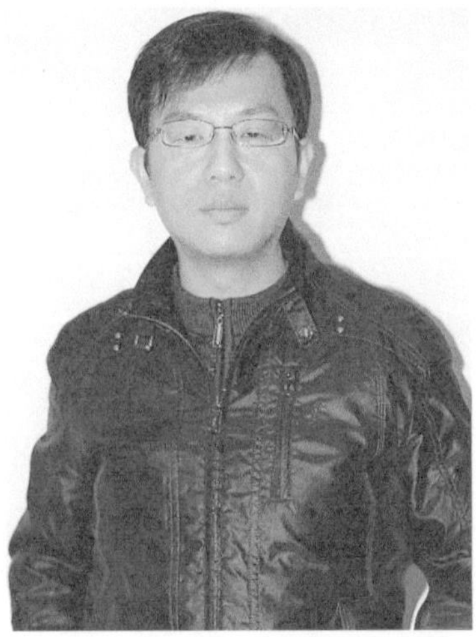
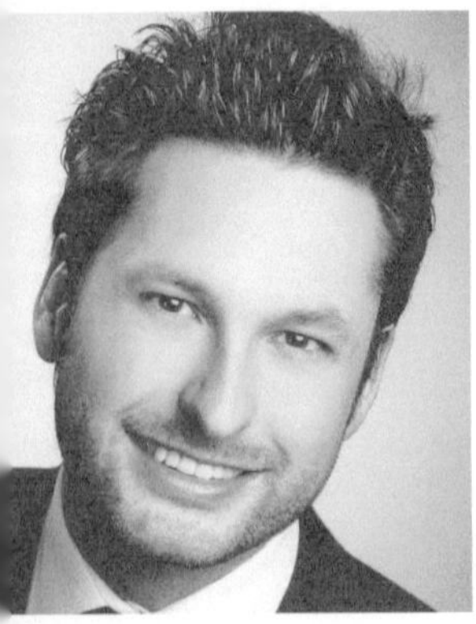
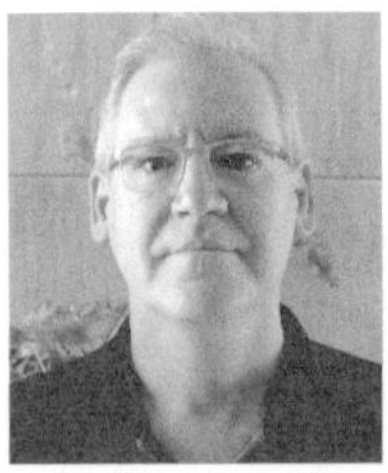

IntechOpen

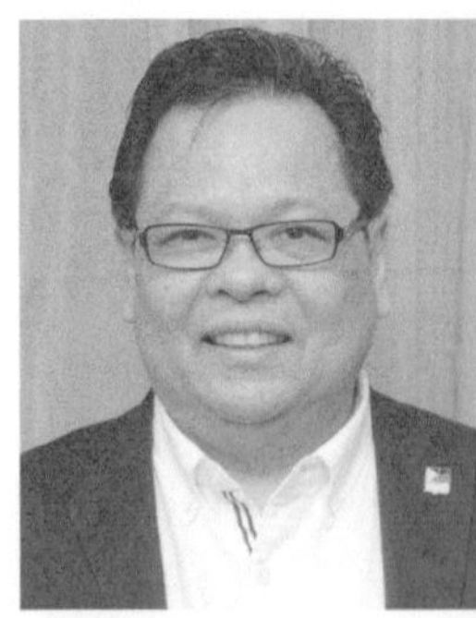
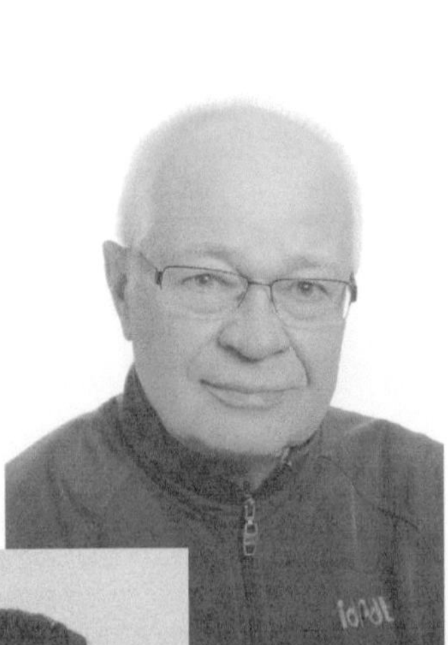
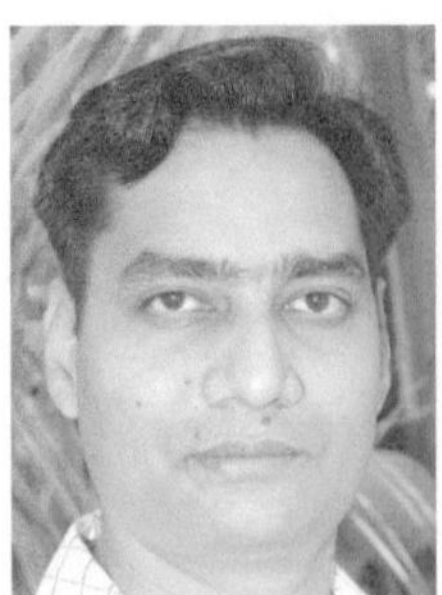
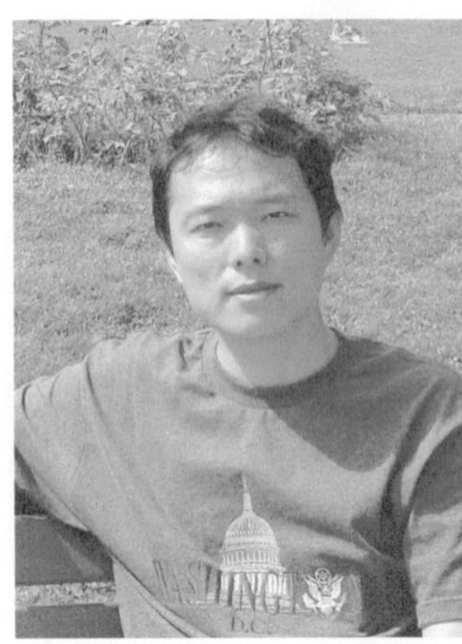
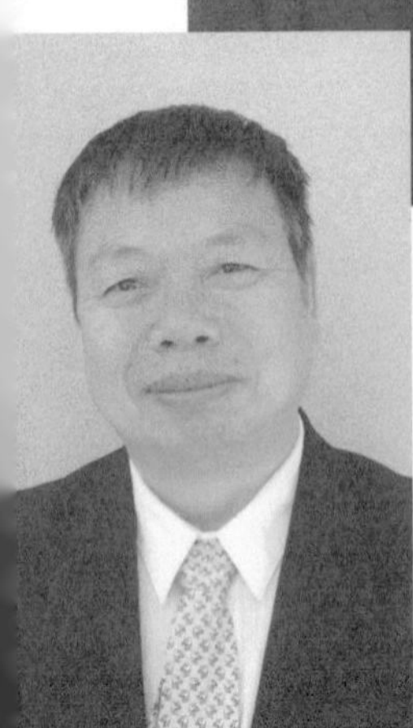
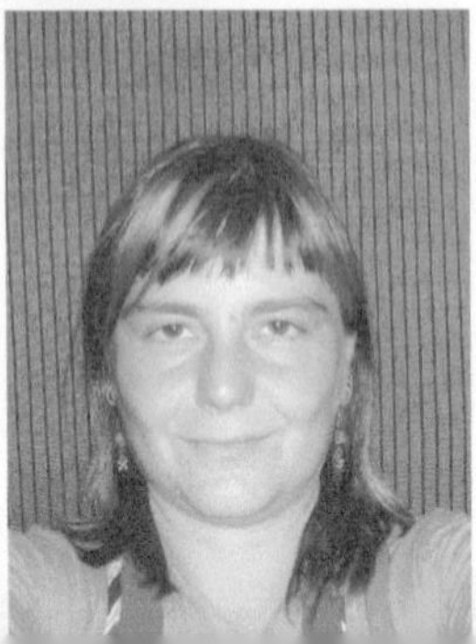

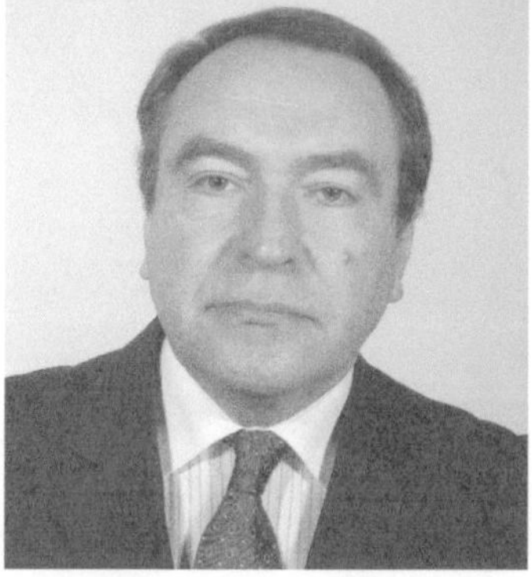

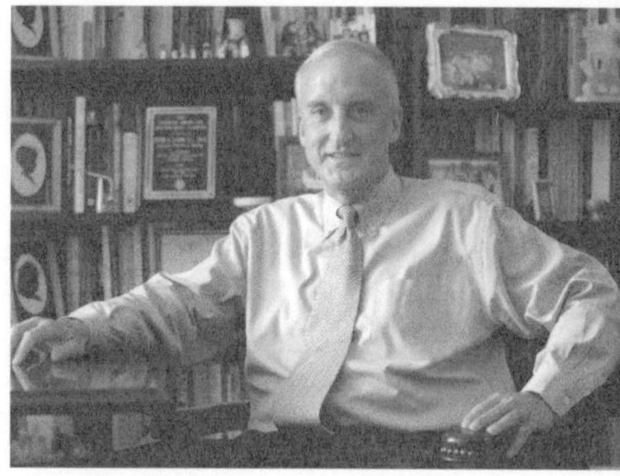

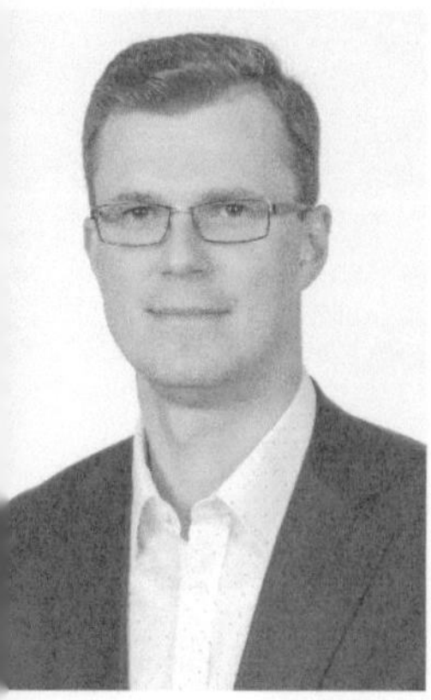

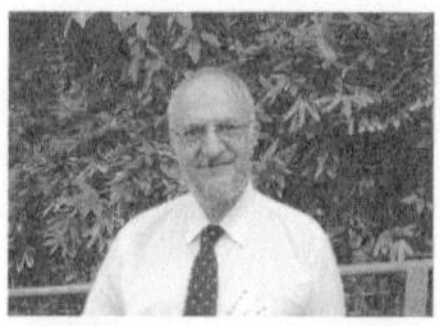

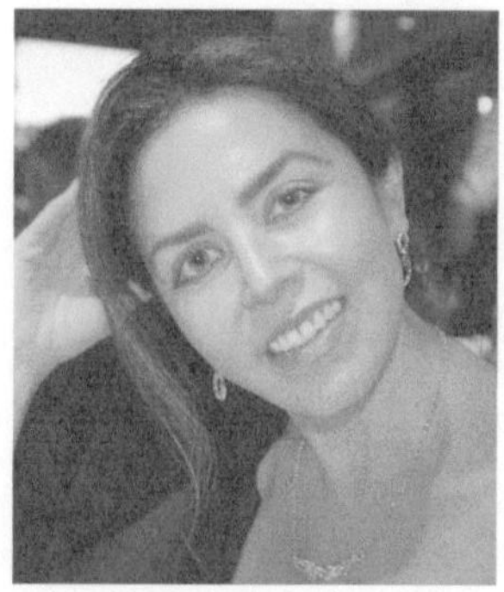

Supporting open minds since 2005

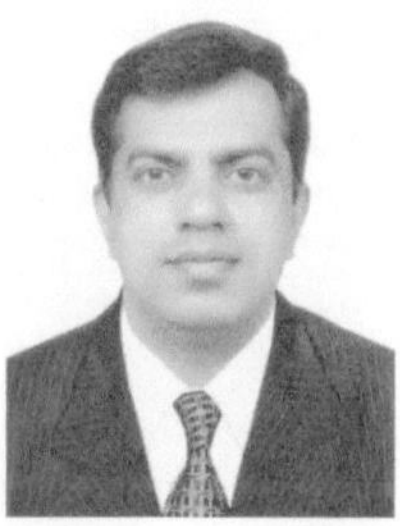

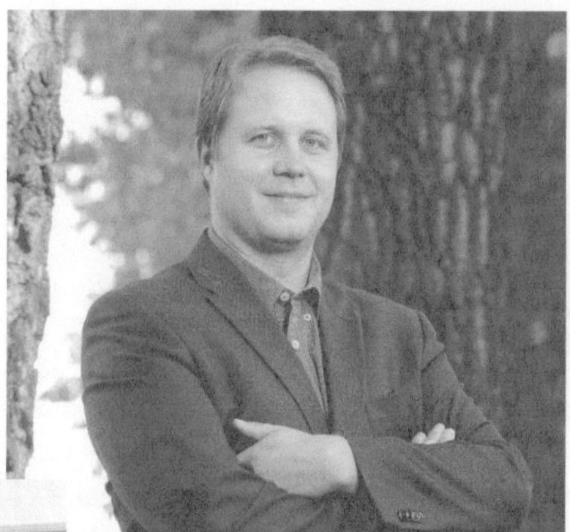

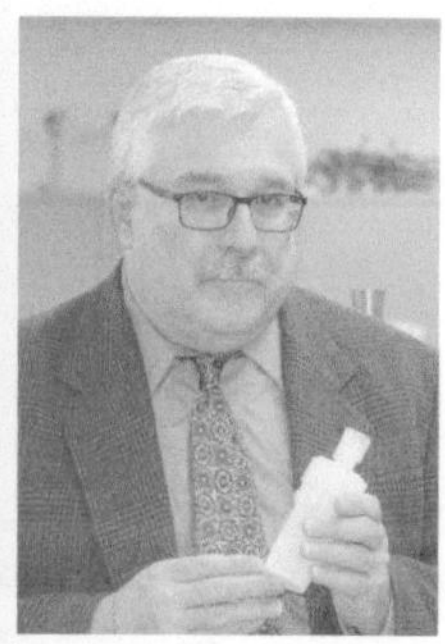

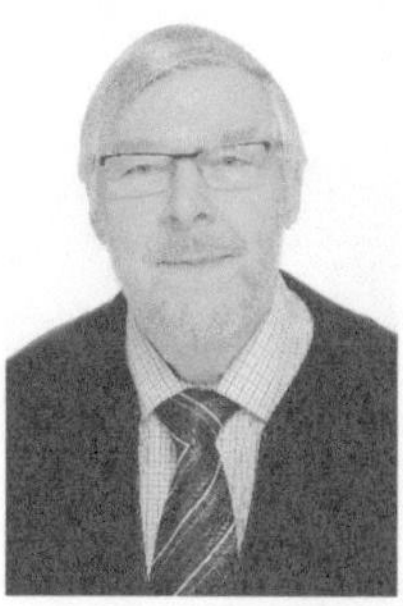

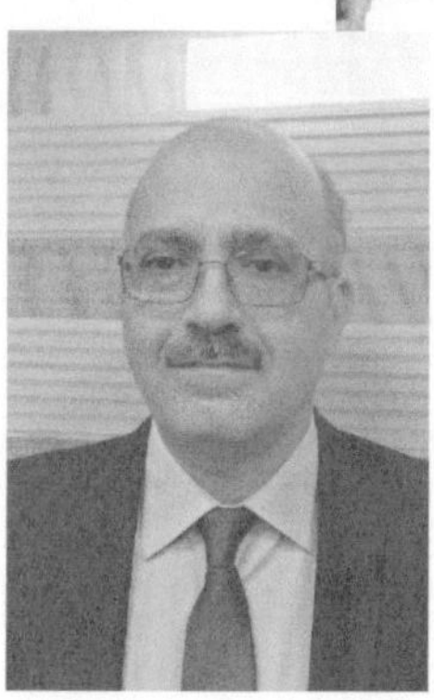

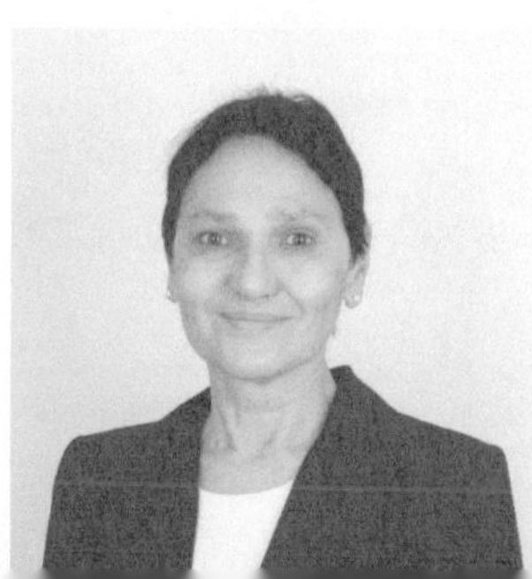

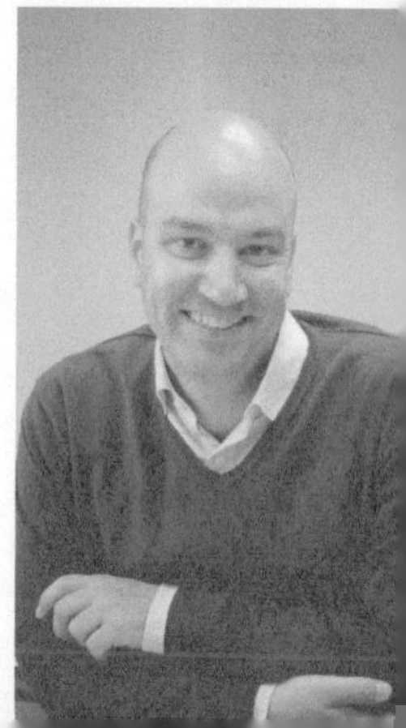

Paraplegia
http://dx.doi.org/10.5772/intechopen.87608
Edited by José Juan Antonio Ibarra Arias and Carlos Alberto Cuellar Ramos

Contributors
Estefanía de la Cruz Castillo, Elisa García-Vences, Fereshteh Azedi, Mohammad Taghi Joghataei, Kazem Mousavizadeh, Stefano Federici, Francesco Artegiani, Daniele Diotallevi, Alessandra Castellani Mencarelli, Giovanna Caruso, Roxana Rodríguez-Barrera, Karla Soria-Zavala, Julián García-Sánchez, Laura Paulina Osuna-Carrasco, Braniff De La Torre-Valdovinos, Carlos Alberto Cuellar Ramos, Susana Martiñón, Ricardo Hernández-Miramontes, Brenda Rodríguez-Mendoza, Paola A. Santiago-Tovar, Marco A. Guerrero- Godinez, Hugo Guerrero-Cazares, Rachel Sarabia Estrada, Gunel Guliyeva, Ricardo A. Torres Guzman, Francisco R. Avila Verduzco, Oluwasen O. Akinduro, Paola Suarez Meade, Antonio J. Forte, Alfredo Quinones-Hinojosa, Ismael Jiménez, Vinnitsa Buzoianu Anguiano, Ignatio Madanhire, Tawanda Mushiri, Panganai Musariri, José Juan Antonio Ibarra Arias, Diego Incontri-Abraham

First published in London, United Kingdom, 2021 by IntechOpen
IntechOpen is the global imprint of INTECHOPEN LIMITED, registered in England and Wales, registration number: 11086078, 5 Princes Gate Court, London, SW7 2QJ, United Kingdom
Printed in Croatia

British Library Cataloguing-in-Publication Data
A catalogue record for this book is available from the British Library

Additional hard and PDF copies can be obtained from orders@intechopen.com

Paraplegia
Edited by José Juan Antonio Ibarra Arias and Carlos Alberto Cuellar Ramos
p. cm.
Print ISBN 978-1-78985-541-8
Online ISBN 978-1-78985-542-5
eBook (PDF) ISBN 978-1-83962-749-1

Meet the editors

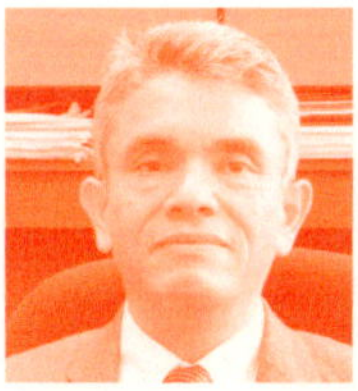

Dr. Antonio Ibarra is Professor and Research Coordinator of the Health Sciences Research Center (CICSA), Faculty of Health Sciences, Anáhuac University, Mexico. As Coordinator, Dr. Ibarra funded the CICSA and developed scientific programs, agreements, and regulations for undergraduate/graduate students and researchers. As a scientist, Dr. Ibarra has studied the development of neuroprotective and neurorestorative therapies for spinal cord injury and cerebral ischemia. Recently, he investigated therapies for cognitive impairment. Dr. Ibarra has numerous scientific publications and has received national and international awards. His research findings led him to lecture at different international meetings. He holds advisory appointments at the National Autonomous University of Mexico (UNAM) and CONACYT (National Council of Science and Technology).

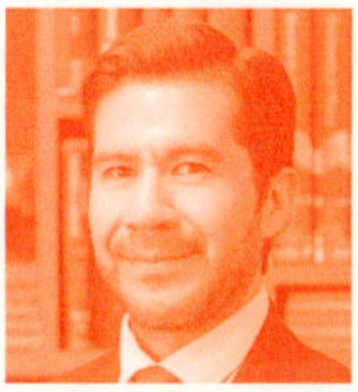

Dr. Carlos Cuellar is a researcher at the School of Sport Sciences, Anáhuac University, México. He received his Ph.D. in Cellular and Molecular Neurobiology from the Center for Research and Advanced Studies, Mexico City. As a research fellow at the Neurological Surgery and Neurology Departments at the Mayo Clinic in Rochester, MN, USA, Dr. Cuellar studied neuromodulation strategies aimed at restoring motor function after spinal cord injury in animal models. His scientific publications include classic electrophysiological techniques and novel approaches to understanding the physiological mechanisms of sensory and motor integration in the spinal cord. His research interests also cover neurodegeneration and plastic changes after an insult to the peripheral and central nervous system.

Contents

Preface

Paraplegia affects mobility after a spinal cord injury (SCI), and it is usually accompanied by sensory and autonomic dysfunction occurring below the spinal level of the lesion. Despite recent progress in the biological sciences, SCI has no cure, and unfortunately, available clinical treatments are limited. Sequelae of this chronic condition include mental health impairments, diminished quality of life, and economic costs related to health care. This book is divided into four sections. The first section presents an introduction, while the second section, "Therapeutic Approaches," addresses the state-of-the-art advances in the use of mesenchymal stem cells from preclinical and clinical studies, as recent discoveries have shown promising results. The section also examines diverse strategies aimed at repairing the spinal cord. The third section, "Rehabilitation Approaches," covers a wide spectrum of strategies for restoring motor, sexual, and bowel dysfunctions. The final section, "Technological Approaches," provides an overview of some of the most recent advancements in devices for motor control (exoskeletons and wheelchairs) and electrical stimulation delivered below and above the SCI.

Paraplegia presents a multidisciplinary perspective in ten chapters that objectively review and address novel potential treatments for the restoration of loss functions below the SCI. For those who are familiar with SCI research, this book is a concise and up-to-date reference. For those interested in this complex pathology, this book presents the latest research targeted to improve daily life activities of paraplegic patients.

The editors express their gratitude to all the contributors to this book and thank them for their efforts and extraordinary work.

Dr. José Juan Antonio Ibarra Arias
Research Coordinator,
Health Sciences Research Center (CICSA),
Universidad Anáhuac México,
Campus Norte Huixquilucan, Estado de México, México

Dr. Carlos Alberto Cuellar Ramos
School of Sport Sciences,
Universidad Anáhuac México,
Campus Norte Huixquilucan, Estado de México, México

Section 1

Introduction

Chapter 1

Introductory Chapter: Clinical Approaches for Treating Paraplegia

Diego Incontri-Abraham and José Juan Antonio Ibarra Arias

1. Introduction to spinal cord injury: epidemiology and biopsychosocial impact

Spinal cord injury (SCI), either traumatic or non-traumatic in origin, is a devastating condition that produces long-term effects that persist throughout life and are associated with severe disability and handicap. Reported traumatic SCI annual incidence rates ranges from 12.1 to 57.8 cases per million. Motor vehicle collisions, falls, violence, and sports represent the leading causes. In comparison to traumatic SCI, there is little literature on non-traumatic SCI epidemiology. The etiologies of this type of SCI include vertebral spondylosis (spinal stenosis), tumorous compression, vascular ischemia, congenital diseases and inflammatory conditions [1, 2].

Depending on the level of SCI, patients experience paraplegia or tetraplegia. Paraplegia is defined as the impairment of sensory and/or motor function in lower extremities. Patients with incomplete paraplegia generally have a good prognosis in regaining locomotor ability (around 76% of patients) within a year. Complete paraplegic patients experience limited recovery of lower limb function if their neurological level of injury (NLI) is above T9. An NLI below T9 is associated with 38% chance of regaining some lower extremity function and only 4% chance of recovery to an incomplete status. On the other hand, tetraplegia is defined as partial or total loss of sensory and/or motor function in all four limbs and has a worse prognosis than paraplegia [3].

Spinal cord injury is a leading cause of disability, particularly in young adults. The highest incidences of SCI occur in persons between 20 and 40 years of age [4], being more common in males (82.8%) than females [5]. However, recent reports indicate an increase in SCI prevalence among older people and females. On the other hand, when classifying the types of disabilities caused by SCI, tetraplegia represents around 60%, while paraplegia represents approximately 40% [6]. Among all secondary complications following SCI, pressure ulcers, neurogenic bladder, urinary tract infections, pain, autonomic dysreflexia, osteoporosis, and muscle atrophy represent the majority. Currently, SCI complications management is challenging, and the outcomes are unsatisfactory [5, 7–10]. Moreover, having SCI may increase the risk of developing a health condition that is an indirect consequence of the impairment itself, such as increasing sedentary behaviors that contribute to the development of obesity and diabetes. Psychological factors (depression, anxiety, drug and substance dependency, post-traumatic stress disorders, etc.) may also complicate these chronic health conditions [11]. In addition, SCI leads to an abrupt change in the professional life and future plans of the patients [12] due to the irreversible restriction of functional movement, affecting not only quality of life but also the ability to live independently. Furthermore, not only economic, educational and social conditions can affect SCI patients. Sexual relationships as well as marriage may be affected in patients who develop a severe disability following SCI [13–15]. These issues have been the most important motivation for the implementation of studies over the last decades that look for novel strategies for SCI. Despite all the progress in both preclinical and clinical studies, new therapies are still needed in order to improve both functional recovery and quality of life following SCI.

Lastly, it is important to mention that disparities between the developing and developed countries capacity to deliver emergency and acute care are evident immediately after a SCI. In many low-resource regions, these disparities can lead to further neurological compromise and poorer first year survival [16]. On the other hand, developed countries have significantly improved survival compared with developing countries. For example, tetraplegics have lower survival rates than paraplegics; however, in developed countries, this gap has narrowed considerably over the last 40 years. Developing countries still have the highest 1-year mortality rates [17].

2. The current understanding of the SCI pathophysiology and management

The immediate event arising from the primary injury consists in a mechanical disruption of tissue. Vascular changes, edema, hemorrhage, inflammation, neuronal, and myelin changes represent the acute phase (hours to 1–2 days). The edema may be vasogenic, defined as a breakdown of the blood–brain barrier (BBB) leading to the leakage of plasma fluid into the extracellular space. This may result in pressure-induced ischemia caused by reduced blood flow to the site of injury. Cytotoxic edema (intracellular swelling) also occur, particularly in astrocytes. Such edema is caused by pro-inflammatory factors, excitotoxicity, oxidative stress, lipid peroxidation, electrolyte imbalances, among others. In regard to neurons, the mode of death appears to be necrosis; however, neuronal apoptosis has been reported as well but only in experimental animals. Myelin breakdown occurs early following SCI and is characterized initially by swelling and ultimately by its fragmentation. During the intermediate phase (days to weeks), there will be several glial responses, necrotic debris will be eliminated, edema will resolve, and there will be revascularization of the tissue associated with a restoration of the BBB. Finally, the late phase of the SCI (weeks to months/years) is characterized by Wallerian degeneration, astroglial scar formation, development of cysts and syrinx, and schwannosis (aberrant intra- and extramedullary proliferation of Schwann cells with associated axons). The Wallerian degeneration is a process that consists in the anterograde disintegration of axons and their myelin sheaths that have been transected following injury. Eventually, an astroglial scar replaces the destroyed myelinated axons; however, this astroglial scar represents an impediment to regeneration [18].

SCI can be categorized also into primary and secondary phases. The primary SCI phase involves the initial mechanical injury (compression, shearing, laceration/transection, and acute stretch) in which the physical force is directly imparted to the spinal cord, disrupting axons, blood vessels, and neural-cell membranes. After the primary injury, a cascade of secondary injury events is initiated which expands the zone of neural tissue damage and exacerbate neurological deficits and outcomes. Secondary injury is a progressive condition characterized by pro-inflammatory cytokines, reactive oxygen species, DNA/protein/lipid oxidative damage, excitatory aminoacids such as glutamate, loss of ionic homeostasis, mitochondrial dysfunction and cell death [19–21]. As mentioned before, mechanical compression of the spinal cord following injury can impair blood flow causing ischemia and an expanded zone of neural tissue injury. Therefore, early surgical decompression is used after SCI to improve vascular supply to the injured area as well as neurobehavioral deficits [22]. Methylprednisolone (MP), a potent synthetic glucocorticoid which upregulates anti-inflammatory cytokine release, has been widely used for SCI management. However, infections are a devastating side effect that may lead to severe pneumonia and sepsis, outweighing the potential neurological benefits [23]. Lastly, blood pressure augmentation is a current strategy in the SCI field. This strategy has emerged to neuroprotect damaged tissue by enhancing perfussion. In addition to these strategies, several neuroprotective therapies targeting key components of the secondary injury phase have emerged in the SCI field. Furthermore, due to the widely recognized difficult regeneration of the adult mammalian central nervous system (CNS), including the spinal cord, the primary and secondary phases of the SCI lead to a progressive loss of neurological function overtime. However, recent progress in the field of SCI research has demonstrated that the CNS has an inherent regenerative capacity. Consequently, while neuroprotective interventions might have a great benefit in the acute phase of injury, the vast majority of SCI patients are in the chronic stage. Neuroregenerative strategies have emerged to facilitate neuronal regrowth in the chronic stage of injury [24].

3. Neuroprotective strategies

Neuroprotective agents aim to reduce secondary insults to the injured spinal cord. Multiple approaches have been studied, and many others are currently under investigation [25]. In fact, the ability of pharmacological agents to limit secondary biochemical damage and cell death has been well established not only in SCI models but also in stroke and head injury [26].

3.1 Pharmacological therapies

3.1.1 Methylprednisolone

MP is one of the most commonly used pharmacological agents due to its anti-inflammatory effects [27]. However, the beneficial effects of MP administration in the setting of acute SCI are outweighed by the risk of significant complications associated to steroids [28].

3.1.2 Riluzole

Riluzole is a benzothiazole sodium channel blocker that protects against excitotoxic cell death by restricting the presynaptic release of glutamate [29]. It is currently approved by the US Food and Drug Administration (FDA) for the treatment of amyotrophic lateral sclerosis [30]. Clinical trials are currently ongoing for investigating riluzole in the setting of acute SCI [31].

3.1.3 Minocycline

Minocycline is a tetracycline-class antibiotic that has demonstrated neuroprotective properties in preclinical models of SCI [32]. A phase II clinical trial demonstrated that early minocycline administration may improve motor recovery in patients with acute SCI [33].

3.1.4 GM-1 ganglioside

GM-1 is a glycosphingolipid found in cell membranes with the ability to enhance neurite growth and nerve regeneration [34]. However, clinical trials in SCI patients found no statistically significant improvement with GM-1 [35].

3.1.5 Fibroblast growth factor-analogue

Fibroblast growth factor (FGF) is a protein found to be neuroprotective against excitotoxicity [36]. A FGF analogue called SUN 13837 was evaluated in a phase I/II clinical trial with results pending publication [25].

3.1.6 Granulocyte colony-stimulating factor

Granulocyte colony-stimulating factor (G-CSF) is found to promote cell survival and inhibit inflammatory cytokine expression [37]. Two recent nonrandomized phase I/IIa clinical trials showed great results in SCI outcomes [38, 39]; however, randomized clinical trials are required to establish the efficacy of G-CSF for SCI.

3.1.7 Hepatocyte growth factor

Hepatocyte growth factor (HGF) increases neuronal survival in SCI models [40]. A phase I/II randomized clinical trial is now underway with results pending publication [41].

3.2 Non-pharmacological therapies

3.2.1 Therapeutic hypothermia

Therapeutic hypothermia (TH; 32°-34° C) reduces the basal metabolic rate and energy demands of the CNS [42]. TH is effective in reducing the extent of CNS injury in neonatal hypoxic ischemic encephalopathy as well as after cardiac arrest [43, 44]. Small studies in SCI patients exposed to TH showed a trend towards neurological recovery [45, 46]. Therefore, these promising results led to a phase II/III clinical trial named "The Acute Rapid Cooling Therapy for Injuries of the Spinal Cord", which has been planned to assess efficacy [25].

3.2.2 Cerebrospinal fluid drainage

Cerebrospinal fluid drainage objective is to prevent spinal cord hypoperfusion in the postinjury period by lowering the intrathecal pressure [47]. A phase IIb clinical trial evaluating mean arterial pressure elevation with cerebrospinal drainage in SCI has been completed with results pending publication.

4. Neuroregenerative strategies

Neuroregenerative strategies aim to restore neurological function [48]. Chronic SCI sets an excellent example because there are currently no interventions to restore body functions after injury. However, due to the inherent and limited ability of the CNS to regenerate, chronic SCI involves a great challenge for regenerative medicine [49].

4.1 Pharmacological therapies

4.1.1 Rho-ROCK inhibitor

Cethrin/VX-210 is a direct Rho inhibitor applied intraoperatively using a fibrin carrier to the epidural space [50]. A phase I/IIa clinical trial of patients with cervical or thoracic acute SCI found a significant improvement in long-term motor recovery for cervical patients [51].

4.1.2 Anti-NOGO antibody

Anti-NOGO is a recombinant human antibody against NOGO-A, one of the best-known inhibitors of neurite growth and plasticity in adult CNS. Intrathecal application is well tolerated in humans; however, efficacy trials are still needed to consider anti-NOGO antibodies for SCI patients [52].

4.2 Non-pharmacological therapies

4.2.1 Spinal cord stimulation

Spinal cord stimulation (SCS) involves the application of electrical stimulus to generate muscle contractions that allows for functional limb use. SCS has been successfully applied to improve ambulatory ability in patients with incomplete SCI [31]. Moreover, a small human study has shown that SCS combined with rehabilitation provides functional recovery of voluntary lower extremity movement in the chronic phase of SCI [53].

4.3 Cell therapies

Stem cell-based regenerative therapy has many roles in SCI recovery, including modulating the inflammatory response, providing trophic support, and regenerating axons into lost neural circuits [54]. Early research in this field used embryonic stem cells (ESCs), however, ethical concerns led to the introduction of other types of stem cell populations. In fact, adult tissue-derived stem cells, specifically bone marrow-derived cells, have emerged as a leading transplantable cell type for many CNS disorders [55]. Mesenchymal stem cells, olfactory ensheathing cells, Schwann cells, neural stem cells, and oligodendrocyte progenitor cells have been evaluated in phase I/II clinical trials of SCI and have shown promising results [31].

4.4 Biomaterials

The cascade of secondary events following acute injury to the spinal cord results in demyelination, axonal degeneration, and cavitation formation. Therefore, regeneration is hindered by the lack of substrate to support cell migration and axonal growth [56, 57]. The development of tissue engineering technology has opened up new avenues for treating SCI. The main strategy of tissue engineering is to inoculate living cells on extracellular matrix substitutes (biomaterial scaffolds) that can provide a physical structure for cell growth and differentiation, as well as to guide the growth of transplanted cells and promote axonal regeneration of residual neurons [58].

The Neuro-Spinal Scaffold (InVivo Therapeutics Corp, Cambridge, Massachusetts) is a proprietary bioresorbable polymer scaffold that promotes appositional healing, spares white matter, decreases post-traumatic cyst formation, and improves functional recovery in animal models of SCI. A pilot study evaluating the safety of Neuro-Spinal Scaffold implantation has completed recruitment and is currently in the follow-up phase. Moreover, a case report of the first patient to undergo implantation of the Neuro-Spinal Scaffold as part of this trial has been published previously. The patient was a 25-year-old man with a T11–12 fracture-dislocation following a motocross accident. At 3 months after implantation, neurological function had improved, and no complications were seen during the follow-up [31, 59].

5. Exoskeleton

In the past decade, research in SCI rehabilitation has expanded to include robotic devices that initiate or augment movement. These robotic devices are used with two goals: to enhance recovery through functional movement and to act as a mobility aid beyond orthoses and wheelchairs [60]. In fact, exoskeleton training has been developed as a rehabilitation tool and is approved for the rehabilitation of individuals with SCI. Several studies have shown that robotic exoskeleton gait training has positive effects in terms of spasticity and pain reduction, as well as improved gait function without physical assistance [61–66].

Robotic devices may offer the greatest advantages for patients with incomplete SCI, turning measurable but functionally insignificant motor function into true mobility and independence. However, the global effects of restoring motion to the skeleton and joints in terms of cardiovascular benefits, prevention of contractures, osteoclastic activity, and psychological health have not yet been measured [67].

6. Conclusion

Significant advances over the past decades have decrease the morbidity and mortality following SCI. Unfortunately, these advances have not impacted on the majority of patients affected by SCI, decreasing long-term health and quality of life. Current treatment options for SCI are restricted to systemic delivery of MP, early surgical decompression, and rehabilitation, all of which result in minimal functional recovery. Neuroprotection as well as neuroregeneration are our current targets for both pharmacological and non-pharmacological therapies; however, further research is still needed to find the best option for SCI patients.

Author details

Diego Incontri-Abraham and José Juan Antonio Ibarra Arias*
Health Sciences Research Center (CICSA), Universidad Anáhuac México, Campus Norte Huixquilucan, Estado de México, México

*Address all correspondence to: jose.ibarra@anahuac.mx

References

[1] Van Den Berg MEL, Castellote JM, Mahillo-Fernandez I, De Pedro-Cuesta J. Incidence of spinal cord injury worldwide: A systematic review. Neuroepidemiology. 2010;34(3):184-92.

[2] McKinley WO, Seel RT, Hardman JT. Nontraumatic spinal cord injury: Incidence, epidemiology, and functional outcome. Arch Phys Med Rehabil. 1999;80(6):619-23.

[3] Alizadeh A, Dyck SM, Karimi-Abdolrezaee S. Traumatic Spinal Cord Injury: An Overview of Pathophysiology, Models and Acute Injury Mechanisms. Front Neurol. 2019;10(March):1-25.

[4] Ackery A, Tator C, Krassioukov A. A global perspective on spinal cord injury epidemiology. J Neurotrauma. 2004;21(10):1355-70.

[5] Rahimi-Movaghar V, Sayyah MK, Akbari H, Khorramirouz R, Rasouli MR, Moradi-Lakeh M, et al. Epidemiology of traumatic spinal cord injury in developing countries: A systematic review. Neuroepidemiology. 2013;41(2):65-85.

[6] Shin JC, Kim DH, Yu SJ, Yang HE, Yoon SY. Epidemiologic change of patients with spinal cord injury. Ann Rehabil Med. 2013;37(1):50-6.

[7] Mahnig S, Landmann G, Stockinger L, Opsommer E. Pain assessment according to the International Spinal Cord Injury Pain classification in patients with spinal cord injury referred to a multidisciplinary pain center. Spinal Cord [Internet]. 2016;54(10):809-15. Available from: http://dx.doi.org/10.1038/sc.2015.219

[8] Giangregorio L, McCartney N. Bone loss and muscle atrophy in spinal cord injury: epidemiology, fracture prediction, and rehabilitation strategies. J Spinal Cord Med. 2006;29(5):489-500.

[9] Krassioukov A V., Furlan JC, Fehlings MG. Medical co-morbidities, secondary complications, and mortality in elderly with acute spinal cord injury. J Neurotrauma. 2003;20(4):391-9.

[10] Hou S, Rabchevsky AG. Autonomic consequences of spinal cord injury. Compr Physiol. 2014;4(4):1419-53.

[11] Peterson MD, Kamdar N, Whitney DG, Ng S, Chiodo A, Tate DG. Psychological morbidity and chronic disease among adults with nontraumatic spinal cord injuries: a cohort study of privately insured beneficiaries. Spine J [Internet]. 2019;19(10):1680-6. Available from: https://doi.org/10.1016/j.spinee.2019.05.591

[12] Lourenco L, Blanes L, Salomé GM, Ferreira LM. Quality of life and self-esteem in patients with paraplegia and pressure ulcers: A controlled cross-sectional study. J Wound Care. 2014;23(6):331-7.

[13] Duzgun Celik H, Cagliyan Turk A, Sahin F, Yilmaz F, Kuran B. Comparison of disability and quality of life between patients with pediatric and adult onset paraplegia. J Spinal Cord Med. 2018;41(6):645-52.

[14] Kawanishi CY, Greguol M. Physical activity, quality of life, and functional autonomy of adults with spinal cord injuries. Adapt Phys Act Q. 2013;30(4):317-37.

[15] Kalyani HHN, Dassanayake S, Senarath U. Effects of paraplegia on quality of life and family economy among patients with spinal cord injuries in selected hospitals of Sri Lanka. Spinal Cord [Internet]. 2015;53(6):446-50. Available from: http://dx.doi.org/10.1038/sc.2014.183

[16] Burns AS, O'Connell C. The challenge of spinal cord injury care in the developing world. J Spinal Cord Med. 2012;35(1):3-8.

[17] Cripps RA, Lee BB, Wing P, Weerts E, MacKay J, Brown D. A global map for traumatic spinal cord injury epidemiology: Towards a living data repository for injury prevention. Spinal Cord [Internet]. 2011;49(4):493-501. Available from: http://dx.doi.org/10.1038/sc.2010.146

[18] Norenberg MD, Smith J, Marcillo A. The Pathology of Human Spinal Cord Injury: Defining the Problems. J Neurotrauma. 2004;21(4):429-40.

[19] Ahuja CS, Nori S, Tetreault L, Wilson J, Kwon B, Harrop J, et al. Traumatic Spinal Cord Injury-Repair and Regeneration. Neurosurgery. 2017;80(3):S9-22.

[20] Venkatesh K, Ghosh SK, Mullick M, Manivasagam G, Sen D. Spinal cord injury: pathophysiology, treatment strategies, associated challenges, and future implications. Cell Tissue Res. 2019;377(2):125-51.

[21] McDonald JW, Sadowsky C. Spinal-cord injury. Lancet [Internet]. 2002 Feb;359(9304):417-25. Available from: https://linkinghub.elsevier.com/retrieve/pii/S0140673602076031

[22] Batchelor PE, Wills TE, Skeers P, Battistuzzo CR, Macleod MR, Howells DW, et al. Meta-Analysis of Pre-Clinical Studies of Early Decompression in Acute Spinal Cord Injury: A Battle of Time and Pressure. PLoS One. 2013;8(8):1-12.

[23] Bracken MB. Steroids for acute spinal cord injury. Cochrane Database Syst Rev [Internet]. 2012 Jan 18;4(3):179-80. Available from: http://doi.wiley.com/10.1002/14651858.CD001046.pub2

[24] Wilson JR, Forgione N, Fehlings MG. Emerging therapies for acute traumatic spinal cord injury. Cmaj. 2013;185(6):485-92.

[25] Rouanet C, Reges D, Rocha E, Gagliardi V, Silva GS. Traumatic spinal cord injury: current concepts and treatment update. Arq Neuropsiquiatr [Internet]. 2017 Jun;75(6):387-93. Available from: http://www.scielo.br/scielo.php?script=sci_arttext&pid=S0004-282X2017000600387&lng=en&tlng=en

[26] Faden AI, Stoica B. Neuroprotection. Arch Neurol [Internet]. 2007 Jun 1;64(6):794. Available from: http://archneur.jamanetwork.com/article.aspx?doi=10.1001/archneur.64.6.794

[27] Kim YH, Ha KY, Kim S Il. Spinal cord injury and related clinical trials. CiOS Clin Orthop Surg. 2017;9(1):1-9.

[28] Kirke Rogers W, Todd M. Acute spinal cord injury. Best Pract Res Clin Anaesthesiol [Internet]. 2016;30(1):27-39. Available from: http://dx.doi.org/10.1016/j.bpa.2015.11.003

[29] Azbill RD, Mu X, Springer JE. Riluzole increases high-affinity glutamate uptake in rat spinal cord synaptosomes. Brain Res. 2000;871(2):175-80.

[30] Bhatt JM, Gordon PH. Current clinical trials in amyotrophic lateral sclerosis. Expert Opin Investig Drugs [Internet]. 2007 Aug 9;16(8):1197-207. Available from: http://www.tandfonline.com/doi/full/10.1517/13543784.16.8.1197

[31] Badhiwala JH, Ahuja CS, Fehlings MG. Time is spine: A review of translational advances in spinal cord injury. J Neurosurg Spine. 2019;30(1):1-18.

[32] Yune TY, Lee JY, Jung GY, Kim SJ, Jiang MH, Kim YC, et al. Minocycline

alleviates death of oligodendrocytes by inhibiting pro-nerve growth factor production in microglia after spinal cord injury. J Neurosci. 2007;27(29):7751-61.

[33] Casha S, Zygun D, McGowan MD, Bains I, Yong VW, John Hurlbert R. Results of a phase II placebo-controlled randomized trial of minocycline in acute spinal cord injury. Brain. 2012;135(4):1224-36.

[34] Imanaka T, Hukuda S, Maeda T. The role of GM1-ganglioside in the injured spinal cord of rats: An immunohistochemical study using GM1-antisera. J Neurotrauma. 1996;13(3):163-70.

[35] Geisler FH, Coleman WP, Grieco G, Poonian D. The Sygen® multicenter acute spinal cord injury study. Spine (Phila Pa 1976). 2001;26(24 SUPPL.):87-98.

[36] Siddiqui AM, Khazaei M, Fehlings MG. Translating mechanisms of neuroprotection, regeneration, and repair to treatment of spinal cord injury [Internet]. 1st ed. Vol. 218, Progress in Brain Research. Elsevier B.V.; 2015. 15-54 p. Available from: http://dx.doi.org/10.1016/bs.pbr.2014.12.007

[37] Nishio Y, Koda M, Kamada T, Someya Y, Kadota R, Mannoji C, et al. Granulocyte colony-stimulating factor attenuates neuronal death and promotes functional recovery after spinal cord injury in mice. J Neuropathol Exp Neurol. 2007;66(8):724-31.

[38] Takahashi H, Yamazaki M, Okawa A, Sakuma T, Kato K, Hashimoto M, et al. Neuroprotective therapy using granulocyte colony-stimulating factor for acute spinal cord injury: A phase I/IIa clinical trial. Eur Spine J. 2012;21(12):2580-7.

[39] Kamiya K, Koda M, Furuya T, Kato K, Takahashi H, Sakuma T, et al. Neuroprotective therapy with granulocyte colony-stimulating factor in acute spinal cord injury: a comparison with high-dose methylprednisolone as a historical control. Eur Spine J. 2015;24(5):963-7.

[40] Kitamura K, Fujiyoshi K, Yamane J ichi, Toyota F, Hikishima K, Nomura T, et al. Human hepatocyte growth factor promotes functional recovery in primates after spinal cord injury. PLoS One. 2011;6(11).

[41] Kitamura K, Nagoshi N, Tsuji O, Matsumoto M, Okano H, Nakamura M. Application of hepatocyte growth factor for acute spinal cord injury: The road from basic studies to human treatment. Int J Mol Sci. 2019;20(5).

[42] Dietrich WD, Levi AD, Wang M, Green BA. Hypothermic Treatment for Acute Spinal Cord Injury. Neurotherapeutics. 2011;8(2):229-39.

[43] Dehaes M, Aggarwal A, Lin PY, Rosa Fortuno C, Fenoglio A, Roche-Labarbe N, et al. Cerebral oxygen metabolism in neonatal hypoxic ischemic encephalopathy during and after therapeutic hypothermia. J Cereb Blood Flow Metab. 2014;34(1):87-94.

[44] Holzer M, Sterz F, Darby JM, Padosch SA, Kern KB, Böttiger BW, et al. Mild therapeutic hypothermia to improve the neurologic outcome after cardiac arrest. N Engl J Med. 2002;346(8):549-56.

[45] Levi AD, Green BA, Wang MY, Dietrich WD, Brindle T, Vanni S, et al. Clinical application of modest hypothermia after spinal cord injury. J Neurotrauma. 2009;26(3):407-15.

[46] Dididze M, Green BA, Dalton Dietrich W, Vanni S, Wang MY, Levi AD. Systemic hypothermia in acute cervical spinal cord injury: A case-controlled study. Spinal Cord [Internet]. 2013;51(5):395-400. Available from: http://dx.doi.org/10.1038/sc.2012.161

[47] Kwon BK, Curt AN, Belanger LM, Bernardo A, Chan D, Markez JA, et al. Intrathecal pressure monitoring and cerebrospinal fluid drainage in acute spinal cord injury: A prospective randomized trial - Clinical article. J Neurosurg Spine. 2009;10(3):181-93.

[48] Ahuja CS, Fehlings M. Concise Review: Bridging the Gap: Novel Neuroregenerative and Neuroprotective Strategies in Spinal Cord Injury. Stem Cells Transl Med [Internet]. 2016 Jul;5(7):914-24. Available from: http://doi.wiley.com/10.5966/sctm.2015-0381

[49] Dalamagkas K, Tsintou M, Seifalian A, Seifalian AM. Translational regenerative therapies for chronic spinal cord injury. Int J Mol Sci. 2018;19(6):1-17.

[50] Forgione N, Fehlings MG. Rho-ROCK inhibition in the treatment of spinal cord injury. World Neurosurg [Internet]. 2014;82(3):E535-9. Available from: http://dx.doi.org/10.1016/j.wneu.2013.01.009

[51] Fehlings MG, Theodore N, Harrop J, Maurais G, Kuntz C, Shaffrey CI, et al. A phase I/IIa clinical trial of a recombinant Rho protein antagonist in acute spinal cord injury. J Neurotrauma. 2011;28(5):787-96.

[52] Kucher K, Johns D, Maier D, Abel R, Badke A, Baron H, et al. First-in-man intrathecal application of neurite growth-promoting anti-nogo- a antibodies in acute spinal cord injury. Neurorehabil Neural Repair. 2018;32(6-7):578-89.

[53] Angeli CA, Edgerton VR, Gerasimenko YP, Harkema SJ. Altering spinal cord excitability enables voluntary movements after chronic complete paralysis in humans. Brain. 2014;137(5):1394-409.

[54] Assinck P, Duncan GJ, Hilton BJ, Plemel JR, Tetzlaff W. Cell transplantation therapy for spinal cord injury. Nat Neurosci. 2017;20(5):637-47.

[55] Incontri Abraham D, Gonzales M, Ibarra A, Borlongan C V. Stand alone or join forces? Stem cell therapy for stroke. Vol. 19, Expert Opinion on Biological Therapy. Taylor and Francis Ltd; 2019. p. 25-33.

[56] Mothe AJ, Tam RY, Zahir T, Tator CH, Shoichet MS. Repair of the injured spinal cord by transplantation of neural stem cells in a hyaluronan-based hydrogel. Biomaterials [Internet]. 2013;34(15):3775-83. Available from: http://dx.doi.org/10.1016/j.biomaterials.2013.02.002

[57] Itosaka H, Kuroda S, Shichinohe H, Yasuda H, Yano S, Kamei S, et al. Fibrin matrix provides a suitable scaffold for bone marrow stromal cells transplanted into injured spinal cord: A novel material for CNS tissue engineering. Neuropathology. 2009;29(3):248-57.

[58] Liu S, Xie YY, Wang B. Role and prospects of regenerative biomaterials in the repair of spinal cord injury. Neural Regen Res. 2019;14(8):1352-63.

[59] Theodore N, Hlubek R, Danielson J, Neff K, Vaickus L, Ulich TR, et al. First human implantation of a bioresorbable polymer scaffold for acute traumatic spinal cord injury: A clinical pilot study for safety and feasibility. Neurosurgery. 2016;79(2):E305-12.

[60] Mekki M, Delgado AD, Fry A, Putrino D, Huang V. Robotic Rehabilitation and Spinal Cord Injury: a Narrative Review. Neurotherapeutics. 2018;15(3):604-17.

[61] Baunsgaard CB, Nissen UV, Brust AK, Frotzler A, Ribeill C, Kalke YB, et al. Exoskeleton gait training after spinal cord injury: An exploratory study on secondary health conditions. J Rehabil Med. 2018;50(9):806-13.

[62] Stampacchia G, Rustici A, Bigazzi S, Gerini A, Tombini T, Mazzoleni S. Walking with a powered robotic exoskeleton: Subjective experience, spasticity and pain in spinal cord injured persons. NeuroRehabilitation. 2016;39(2):277-83.

[63] Grasmücke D, Zieriacks A, Jansen O, Fisahn C, Sczesny-Kaiser M, Wessling M, et al. Against the odds: What to expect in rehabilitation of chronic spinal cord injury with a neurologically controlled Hybrid Assistive Limb exoskeleton. A subgroup analysis of 55 patients according to age and lesion level. Neurosurg Focus. 2017;42(5).

[64] Bach Baunsgaard C, Vig Nissen U, Katrin Brust A, Frotzler A, Ribeill C, Kalke YB, et al. Gait training after spinal cord injury: Safety, feasibility and gait function following 8 weeks of training with the exoskeletons from Ekso Bionics article. Spinal Cord [Internet]. 2018;56(2):106-16. Available from: http://dx.doi.org/10.1038/s41393-017-0013-7

[65] Miller L, Zimmermann A, Herbert W. Clinical effectiveness and safety of powered exoskeleton-assisted walking in patients with spinal cord injury: systematic review with meta-analysis. Med Devices Evid Res [Internet]. 2016 Mar;455. Available from: https://www.dovepress.com/clinical-effectiveness-and-safety-of-powered-exoskeleton-assisted-walk-peer-reviewed-article-MDER

[66] Wu CH, Mao HF, Hu JS, Wang TY, Tsai YJ, Hsu WL. The effects of gait training using powered lower limb exoskeleton robot on individuals with complete spinal cord injury. J Neuroeng Rehabil. 2018;15(1):1-10.

[67] Ghobrial GM, Wang MY. The next generation of powered exoskeleton use in spinal cord injury. Neurosurg Focus. 2017;42(5):1-2.

Section 2

Therapeutic Approaches

Chapter 2

Mesenchymal Stem Cells for Clinical Use after Spinal Cord Injury

Karla Soria-Zavala, Julián García-Sánchez and Roxana Rodríguez-Barrera

Abstract

Since multipotential and immunoregulatory properties were identified in mesenchymal stem cells (MSCs) in the twentieth century, they have been proposed as an effective therapy for many degenerative and traumatic diseases such as spinal cord injury (SCI). SCI is a devastating event with a high mortality rate that evokes the loss of motor and sensory functions due to neurochemical imbalance and an exacerbated immune response as a consequence of the initial mechanical damage, which in conjunction creates a hostile microenvironment that inhibits neuronal circuitry restoration. This chapter pretends to lead the reader towards the immunomodulatory, differentiation, and tissue repairing capacities of MSCs that allow them to be a valuable candidate for clinical trials. In the first section, the physiopathology of SCI will be addressed; after that, the chapter will review the general aspects of MSCs such as origin, molecular markers, and the different mechanisms by which MSCs can heal the target tissues. Finally, we will discuss clinical trials involving autologous MSC transplantation and their limitations.

Keywords: SCI, MSCs, clinical trials

1. Introduction

Spinal cord injury (SCI) is an important clinical problem with significant socioeconomic impact worldwide.

SCI is a catastrophic event involving damage to the spinal cord (SC) that causes morphological and physiological changes leading to biomechanical and functional disorders in patients [1]. This condition induces acute and chronic inflammatory processes that can result in temporary or permanent repercussions including paraplegia, quadriplegia, or even death [2].

The pathophysiology of SCI is very complicated, and it consists of a primary and a secondary phase. The primary phase occurs immediately after the damage to the SC causing cell death at the epicenter of the injury as well as the beginning of the pro-inflammatory response [3]. The secondary phase starts 2 hours after the damage and can last up to 6 months. During this phase the extent of the injury increases in response to the augmented pro-inflammatory factors which contribute to induce local edema, ischemia, vascular alterations, ionic dysregulations, and oxidative stress [3, 4]. These prejudicial mechanisms persist during the chronic stages of the injury, and although their intensity is diminished, the neurological function continues to decline [5]. Most of the post-traumatic neuronal degeneration involves an uncontrollable cascade of destructive mechanisms that are still incompletely understood and remain a challenge for scientists [6].

The current therapy for SCI involves surgical decompression and steroid administration; however, both of them only show minimal efficiency, and the need for an effective therapy is continuously rising [7]. Therefore, the transplantation of stem cells as a novel therapeutic approach has received increasing attention due to their promising results in neurological recovery in SCI [8–10]. Among them, mesenchymal stem cells (MSCs) demonstrate to be a valuable promising therapy due to their significant autocrine and paracrine activity which help to induce the proliferation and differentiation of different cell types and to exert immunomodulatory effects in the microenvironment of the host [6, 11]. MSCs, anti-inflammatory molecules, and trophic factors are capable of supporting axonal growth to promote angiogenesis, remyelination, and protection against apoptotic cell death [12]. Furthermore, MSCs possess a varied spectrum of therapeutic properties such as neuroprotection after glutamate excitotoxicity [13, 14], reduction in protein levels associated with stress and reactive oxygen species [15] and pro-inflammatory cytokines [16], M1 macrophage polarization to the M2 pro-repair activated phenotype [17], secretion of neurotrophic factors [16, 18, 19], and their ability to produce numerous exosomes.

In addition, MSCs have minimal immunoreactivity towards the host as well as a limited chance of developing a tumor and are particularly appealing due to their wide range of advantages over other types of stem cells [20]. Finally, we will discuss clinical trials of improvement using autologous and allogeneic MSCs after acute and chronic SCI.

2. General aspects of MSCs

MSCs are adult stem cells with self-renewing and differentiation abilities. These cells can be isolated from different sources (bone marrow, adipose tissue, umbilical cord (UC), and amniotic fluid) and are easily preserved without raising any ethical issue [21]. Mammalian bone marrow is the best understood niche that harbors hematopoietic stem cells (HSCs), and MSCs are believed to provide the basis for the physical structures of the niche [22]. Moreover, MSCs are defined as multipotent cells that are thought to regulate the self-renewal, proliferation, and differentiation of the HSCs through the production of cytokines and intracellular signals that are initiated by cell-to-cell interaction. Lastly, MSCs can differentiate into cells from different lineages, such as osteoblasts, cartilage cells, fibroblasts, muscle cells, fat cells, and neurons [23, 24].

3. Markers of MSCs

Most researchers have suggested minimal criteria to define MSCs. The International Society for Cellular Therapy (ISCT) established specific criteria in order to identify unique populations of MSCs [25].

1. MSCs must be plastic adherent when maintained under standard culture conditions.

2. MSCs must be positive for CD105, CD90, CD73, CD29, CD44, CD71, and CD106 and be negative for the expression of hematopoietic markers such as CD34, CD45, HLA-DR, CD14, MHC-II, CD11b, and CD14 and express low levels of MHC-I.

3. MSCs must differentiate in vitro at least in osteoblasts, adipocytes, and chondroblasts [25, 26].

4. MSCs: biological properties

MSCs are well known for their ability to differentiate into numerous cell lineages, but, besides their cell multipotential reprogramming capacity, they promise to be an effective candidate therapy in clinical trials for different human pathologies due to their successful homing, immunomodulation, and tissue repairing [27]. Moreover, exosomes from MSCs are being considered the most important factor of the therapeutic effects of MSCs as they could be used as molecule exchangers and natural drug delivery vehicles [28].

4.1 Homing and chemotactic activity

Several studies have shown that MSCs are capable of migrating selectively and exert homing capabilities to different organs [29, 30]. Even if they are transplanted by local or systemic pathways, MSCs are principally guided to damaged tissues by the coordinate expression of specific receptors and ligands that allow them to reach their desired target and effectuate different mechanisms [31]. Additionally, MSCs possess a high chemotactic activity that increases the recruitment of different cells. Indeed, fibroblasts accelerate migration, proliferation, and integrin expression in response to MSC secretome [32, 33]. Similarly, neutrophils increase migration rate and immunological response when they are stimulated with MSCs after microbial challenge in vitro [34, 35]. In murine SCI models, the MSC-grafted SC has proven to amplify granulocytes and antigen-presenting cell recruitment in early stages by a wide variety of cytokines and chemokines such as CXCL10, CXCL12, CXCL1, and CL5 to boost SC recovery [34, 36].

4.2 Microenvironment immunomodulation

MSCs have proven to regulate the immune response through cell-to-cell contact and by the secretion of soluble mediators including cytokines, prostaglandins, enzymes, and proapoptotic and antiapoptotic molecules [27, 37–39]. Different studies involving MSC transplantation in exacerbated immune response models such as peritonitis and ulcerative colitis ameliorate inflammation by reducing the expression levels of pro-inflammatory cytokines such as interleukin-1 beta, interleukin-12, interleukin-6, and tumor necrosis factor-α (TNFα). In addition, these cells exert a decrease of the classical phenotype M1 marker and an increase of the alternative phenotype M2, as well as a marked macrophage reprogramming from M1 to M2 [17, 40–42]. Moreover, MSCs can suppress T cell activation and proliferation by downregulating the expression of costimulatory molecules on the surface of dendritic cells [43], interleukin-10, transforming growth factor-B (TGFβ), nitric oxide, and indoleamine 2,3-dioxygenase enzyme production in response to inflammation as well as interleukin-2 absorption [37, 44, 45]. Similarly, B cell activation can be disturbed, and the regulatory B cell phenotype can be promoted [46, 47].

4.3 Tissue repairing and regeneration

MSCs participate in repairing many tissues, mostly by the secretion of TGFβ and vascular endothelial growth factor (VEGF) to promote angiogenesis [48], extracellular matrix remodeling, and reduction of the scar formation in chronic wounds [49, 50]. Similarly, in pathologies where gliosis, demyelination, and neuroinflammation occur, MSCs have shown neuroprotective activities such as vascular stabilization and angiogenesis by tight junction protein expression [51], neuronal suppression apoptosis [52, 53], glia hypertrophy prevention [54], and promotion of myelinization by the activation of oligodendrocyte precursor cells [53, 55]. Additionally, MSCs promote synaptic transmission [56], neurite outgrowth, and axonal sprouting mostly by excretion of trophic factors including brain-derived neurotrophic factor (BDNF) and nerve growth factor (NGF) [12, 57]. SCI models motor skills are increased [58] inclusively; bladder and erectile dysfunction improvement have been reported [59, 60].

4.4 Multipotential capacity

Originally it was believed that MSCs could exclusively differentiate into cells from the mesodermal lineage [23, 24]; however, in the last 20 years many authors have proven that a proper microenvironment can promote greater plasticity and that MSCs from different sources can differentiate into dermal, neural, or glial cells in vitro and in vivo when they are exposed to neurotrophic factors and specific cytokines [61–63]. Smooth muscle and endothelial cells derived from MSCs can be detected and improve heart functions in ischemic myocardium models [64]. Also, skin, articular cartilage, and bone regeneration have been reported, but mostly when MSCs are combined with natural and artificial scaffolds or when genetically modified [65–67]. In order to achieve CNS regeneration, different sources of MSCs and culture methods have been tested in murine SCI models; however, transplants have demonstrated to improve functional recovery by differentiation into neurons, astrocytes, but mostly oligodendrocytes [54, 55, 58].

4.5 Exosomes as mechanisms for cell-to-cell communication and drug delivery vehicles

Exosomes are extracellular vesicles released by many cells, including MSCs. Their length is between 30 and 100nm, and they can bind to cells through receptor and ligand interaction or by fusion with the target cell membrane to deliver high amounts of cytokines, growth factors, microRNAs, and mRNAs capable of modifying peptide and protein synthesis [60]. Thus, the derived MSC exosomes could be the most attractive therapy in SCI models since neuronal differentiation from MSCs remains poor [58, 68] and several studies show that the regenerative and anti-inflammatory mechanisms are mostly mediated by paracrine factors [27, 36, 69–71]. Furthermore, MSC exosomes are natural drug delivery vehicles that can be modified and produced in high quantities [28, 72, 73]. MSCs have proven to be safe in many different preclinical studies; however, clinical trials involving exosomes in SCI therapy are not yet recruited due to the fact that optimal MSC culture conditions and protocols for exosome isolation is still to be established (www.clinicaltrials.gov).

5. MSCs in the clinic

The promising results of MSCs in preclinical studies encouraged their use in humans; however, the results obtained in the clinical trials still remain controversial and do not replicate what was previously reported in experimental animal studies. In this section we will review the results obtained from the main clinical trials involving MSC transplantation as well as their type of application, properties, limitations, and future directions.

Most of the first clinical studies describing reporting the application of MSCs were focused on describing the transplantation technique, the safety, and the evidence of any adverse reactions. Moviglia et al. conducted a preliminary report that described the intra-arterial administration of bone marrow (BM) MSCs (BM-MSCs) in two patients with chronic SCI in combination with neurorehabilitation programs. Patient 1 presented paraplegia at the eighth thoracic vertebra (T8) with a sensitive level corresponding to T6, while patient 2 presented severe quadriplegia with a lesion that extended from his third to fifth cervical vertebrae (C3–C5) and a sensitive level corresponding to C2. After 6 months, both patients improved their motor and sensory functions without having any secondary effects. The motor level of patient 1 now corresponds to his first sacral metamere (S1) and his sensitive level to the fourth sacral metamere (S4), while sensory and motor functions from patient 2 reached T1–T2 [74]. Similar results, in terms of the safety, were obtained in a pilot study conducted by Pal et al., where 30 patients with complete cervical or thoracic SCI (ASIA scale rating system class A) received intrathecal injections of MSCs via lumbar puncture and none of them presented any adverse effects in the following 1–3 years [75]. However, only the patients with less than 6 months of thoracic-level injury experienced improvement in their quality of life and degree of independence according to Barthel's Index (BI). Despite these improvements, there was no significant change in the ASIA score and in magnetic resonance imaging (MRI). Furthermore, due to the homing abilities of the MSCs, Ra et al. also tested the toxicity, tumorigenicity, and therapeutic potential of the intravenous administration of adipose tissue-derived MSCs in eight patients with more than 12 months of SCI. After 3 months the therapy demonstrated to be safe and not promoting tumor growth [76]. In addition, this study described limited motor recovery where only one patient with ASIA A demonstrated improvement to ASIA grade C. Lastly, other studies have also demonstrated the safety and lack of evidence of any severe adverse reactions with the intrathecal administration of MSCs [77, 78].

Moving forward, Sykova et al. conducted a nonrandomized phase I/phase II clinical trial comparing the functional improvement and safety of intra-arterial versus intravenous administration of BM-MSCs in 20 patients with SCI at the cervical or thoracic level. The clinical characterization described 15 patients with ASIA grade A and 5 patients with ASIA grade B (incomplete SCI). Both intra-arterial group (n=7) and the intravenous group (n=13) contained patients with acute and chronic phases of SCI. The study found significant functional improvements (motor and sensory) in five acute patients and only in one chronic patient. In the intra-arterial group, all four subacute patients exhibited a significant improvement in their ASIA score or Frankel score as well as a marked recovery of motor and somatosensory evoked potentials (MEPs and SEPs). However, in the intravenous group, only one patient demonstrated an improved ASIA score as well as electrophysiology results. Interestingly most of the patients who had functional improvements received the administration of the MSCs close to the injury site suggesting that the administration route through the vertebral artery or into the cerebrospinal fluid might lead to the best outcome. This study also describes that 3–4 weeks after the injury appears to be the best therapeutic window to administer the cells [79]. These results are also supported by another study carried out by Park et al. where they showed improved motor and sensory function in 5 out of 6 patients who received intraspinal implantation of BM-MSCs 7 days post-injury in combination with granulocyte-macrophage colony-stimulating factor (GM-CSF)

[80]. Four patients demonstrated a significant improvement in their American Spinal Injury Association Impairment Scale (AIS) grades from A to C, while one patient improved to AIS B from A. Lastly this study also describes those 3–4 weeks after the injury appears to be the best therapeutic window to administer the cells [79].

As many studies supported the safety of this therapy, more scientists focused on comparing and trying to find different types of MSC transplantation. Geffner et al. reported eight thoracic SCI cases (four acute and four chronic) with the administration of BM-MSCs through many different administration routes such as intravenous, intraspinal, and directly into the spinal canal in order to assure that the cells will reach their target. Over the course of 2 years, patients showed significant improvements in their quality of life measured by the BI score as well as certain motor recovery measured by the ASIA, Ashworth, and Frankel scores. All four patients of the acute group experienced an improvement in the ASIA score from A to C, while chronic patients had a lesser recovery improving from an ASIA score of B–C to C–D. Improvement of bladder control was the most important aspect in augmenting their quality of life; however, there were also many other important motor improvements, which cannot be correctly represented in the ASIA score [81]. In addition, other studies furtherly support the therapeutic potential of MSCs in improving the urinary functions of SCI patients which majorly contributes to increasing their self-care ability [82, 83]. This study also demonstrated the feasibility and safety of multiple administration routes. Moreover, the study conducted by Jeon et al. discussed the effectiveness of the intraspinal application of BM-MSCs in 10 patients with complete cervical SCI. After 6 months 6 patients demonstrated motor improvements in the upper limbs by measuring electrophysiological parameters (electromyography, nerve conduction velocity, SEP, MEP) as well as morphological changes described by magnetic resonance imaging (MRI) at the site of the lesion. In addition, three out of those six patients exhibited a significant increase in the performance of daily tasks. However, the ASIA/Frankel motor grade remained the same and did not reflect these motor improvements. This study also reported the absence of any major adverse effect or neoplasm growth over the course of 3 years, furtherly supporting the safety of this therapy [84].

Karamouzian et al. conducted one of the first studies to introduce a control group in the field of MSCs and SCI. This nonrandomized clinical trial discussed their therapeutic potential by comparing the outcome of 11 patients (7 males and 4 females with mean age of 33.3 ± 8.9 years) with complete subacute SCI who received BM-MSC transplantation via lumbar puncture with a control group (n=20). Five patients in the study group and 12 patients in the control group presented spinal fracture at T12 and L1 levels, while the remaining patients presented a lesion between T1 and T11. After almost 3 years of follow-up, five patients of the experimental group and three patients of the control group exhibited noticeable recovery (a two-grade improvement from baseline, i.e., from ASIA A to C); however, the results were statistically borderline, and there is no clear evidence of the therapeutic potential of these MSCs [85]. In a similar study, Dai et al. discussed the effectiveness of BM-MSCs in complete and chronic SCI. This study randomly assigned 40 patients with complete and chronic SCI into a treatment group (n=20) and a control group (n=20). After 6 months of follow-up, 50% of the treatment group demonstrated significant motor recovery as well as an improvement in ASIA score and in electrophysiological examinations. In addition, most of the patients in the treatment group exhibited a significant clinical improvement in terms of the amount of residual urinary volume, pinprick sensory, and light touch, while the control group did not exhibit any significant motor or sensorial improvements [82]. Both of these studies suggest that BM-MSCs might help improve neurological function in complete and chronic SCI, and they present no evidence of any severe complications or major adverse events in any of the patients.

Although stem cell therapy has demonstrated that they possess the therapeutic potential to be combined with neurorehabilitation, Cheng et al. analyzed the effect of UC-MSCs in comparison with neurorehabilitation and self- healing in 34 patients with thoracolumbar SCI and AIS A grading. Patients were divided into three groups: the UC-MSC treatment group, the rehabilitation group, and the control group. After 6 months around 70% of the patients in the treatment group experienced a significant motor recovery and noticeable improvement in muscle tension and self-care ability which involves an increase in the strength of the abdomen, waist, and lower limbs. Meanwhile, only 36% of the patients treated with neurorehabilitation exhibited certain improvements in these aspects, and the control group showed no significant changes in motor recovery, sensation, or self-care ability. In terms of bladder functions, the treatment group showed a decrease in residual urinary volume and maximum detrusor pressure as well as an increase in bladder capacity and urinary flow in comparison with the other two groups [86]. Later on, El-Kheir et al. decided to compare the use of BM-MSCs in combination with physical therapy with the use of physical therapy alone in 70 chronic cervical and thoracic SCI patients (25 AIS A and 45 AIS B) in a phase I/phase II controlled single-blind clinical trial. After 18 months of follow-up, 46% of the stem cell therapy group exhibited functional improvement and an increase in both motor and dermatome scores by the ASIA and AIS scoring as well as a significant improvement in motor, pinprick, and light touch sensory and functional independence scores over the treated group with physical therapy alone [87]. These studies suggest that BM-MSCs can be combined with additional therapies in order to boost their therapeutic potential.

Equally important, El-Kheir et al. described that thoracic SCI patients with smaller lesions and lower duration of the injury had a higher increase of functional improvement in comparison with patients with cervical SCI [87]. Similar results were obtained in the study carried out by Mendonca et al. which demonstrated a statistically significant correlation between the neurological recovery and both the level and size of the injury in patients with chronic (>6 months) thoracic or lumbar SCI. In addition, after the intra-lesion administration of BM-MSCs, all of the 14 patients demonstrated certain improvements in tactile sensitivity and 8 subjects showed some improvement in the motor functions of the lower limbs reflected by an improvement in their ASIA grading from A to B or C [88].

As the amount of beneficial but limited results grew, the amount of the transplanted MSCs and number of administrations started to gain attention. Vaquero et al. conducted a series of clinical trials involving different numbers of MSC administrations in SCI. The first study consisted of a clinical trial involving 12 patients with complete (ASIA A) and chronic thoracic SCI who received two separate transplantations of BM-MSCs in the subarachnoid space. All patients exhibited certain degree of sensorial improvement (pinprick sensitivity and light touch sensitivity), and 50% of the patients showed motor activity below the injury level according to clinical and neurophysiological studies (SEPs and MEPs). More than 30% of the patients improved their AIS A score from A to B or C, and 83% of the patients presented improvement in urodynamic function including possibility of voluntary micturition (5 patients), increased bladder capacity at filling in (8 patients), decreased detrusor pressure at bladder filling in (9 patients), and increased bladder compliance (10 patients). In addition, they hypothesize that the clinical improvement was dose-dependent [89]. The second study consisted of 10 patients with incomplete (ASIA B and C) cervical, thoracic, and lumbar SCI who received 4 subarachnoid administrations of MSCs. Besides the variable degree of sensorial and motor improvement, after 12 months of the first dosage almost all the patients showed noticeable improvements in bowel and bladder control as well as evidence of muscle reinnervation in electromyographic studies. Furthermore, half of them demonstrated a decrease in spasticity by the Penn and Ashworth scales, and after the third dosage of MSCs, all the patients exhibited an increase in the values of neurotrophic factors such as brain-derived neurotrophic factor (BDNF), glial-derived neurotrophic factor (GDNF), ciliary neurotrophic factor (CNF), and neurotrophin 3 (NT-3) and neurotrophin 4 (NT-4). However, the difference with the basal mean concentration was not statistically significant [90]. Lastly, their third study consisted of a phase II clinical trial with the administration of three intrathecal injections of MSCs in nine patients with chronic SCI. However, this time 44.4% of the patients demonstrated important improvements in voluntary muscle contraction, motor power, spasm, spasticity, neuropathic pain, and sexual function (IANR-SCIFRS scale) along with evidence of muscle reinnervation. In addition, more than half of the patients showed improved somatosensory and motor evoked potentials [91]. Taken all together, Vaquero and colleagues demonstrate that the subarachnoid administration of MSCs is a safe procedure and that the clinical improvement may increase in a dose-dependent manner. These results were furtherly supported by a study carried out by Oh et al. where a single intramedullary administration of MSC in 16 patients with chronic SCI ASIA B demonstrated very limited therapeutic efficacy. Only two patients demonstrated enhanced motor recovery [92].

6. Study limitations and future directions for MSCs

Overall, the use of MSCs in SCI appears to be safe and without any major evidence of severe adverse reactions. However, the results obtained in the clinical trials so far do not concrete the promising results obtained in the preclinical trials. This may be due to the fact that preclinical studies normally utilize specific animal models with standardized protocols to produce the injury as well as preestablished treatments and timing of the transplantation which cannot be replicated in a human study. In clinical trials, most of these conditions depend heavily on chance, the traumatic event, and the emergency setting which may differ a lot from the controlled atmosphere of an animal experiment. In addition, there is a great lack of phase III clinical trials due to financial and ethical reasons. As mentioned before, one of the few phase III clinical trials held by Oh et al. showed weak and limited therapeutic efficacy [92]. Further investigation is needed to determine accurate parameters for its clinical use in SCI such as optimal therapeutic protocols involving type, preparation, number of cells administered, timing of transplantation, and administration route.

On the other hand, thanks to the technological revolution, scientists have now started to investigate the use of MSCs in combination with new biomaterials in order to promote tissue repair and to improve cell survival [6]. A study conducted by Xiao et al. analyzed the therapeutic effect of MSC transplantation in combination with a collagen scaffold which is known to support cell migration and adhesion [93]. After the transplant the injury status of the patients changed from ASIA A to ASIA C accompanied by a significant improvement in motor, sensory, and urinary functions [94]. Furthermore, the possibility of combining MSCs with hydrogels is particularly appealing due to their capacity to be injected with minimal invasion and to be loaded with specific drugs that can be furtherly released in a controlled manner [95]. Moreover, MSCs' ability to induce the production of neurotrophic, immunomodulating, and neuroprotective factors needs further investigation in order to be fully understood and furtherly enhanced, aiming to improve the clinical outcomes. Lastly, the homing properties of the MSCs could be useful to transport specific target drugs to the site of the lesion and thus acting as a vector [96].

7. Conclusion

In conclusion, MSCs represent a practical therapy in the search for a new treatment for SCI; this may be due to the fact that MSC therapy presents a large spectrum of favorable assets that make it particularly appealing. First, MSCs can be isolated from non-embryonic tissues (BM, adipose tissue, UC, and amniotic fluid, among others) via noninvasive techniques and are easily preserved and expanded in vitro. Furthermore, MSCs possess migratory properties that allow them to be administered through different routes and have minimal immunoreactivity towards the host, as well as a limited chance of developing a tumor. Numerous clinical trials have demonstrated their safety for transplantation in humans as well as their lack of any major side effects. However, an enormous improvement in motor recovery and sensory function is still missing, bringing out that additional investigation and new phase III clinical trials are needed in order to fully understand the mechanism of action of MSCs as well as the pathological mechanisms which prevent the restoration of neural circuits in SCI. Lastly, the use of combinatory strategies with specific drugs, biomaterials, or neurorehabilitation may be the key factor to translate their promising results into the clinical practice.

Author details

Karla Soria-Zavala, Julián García-Sánchez and Roxana Rodríguez-Barrera*
Centro de Investigación en Ciencias de la Salud (CICSA), Universidad Anáhuac México Campus Norte, Huixquilucan, México

*Address all correspondence to: roxana.rodriguezb@anahuac.mx

References

[1] Ahuja CS, Wilson JR, Nori S, Kotter MRN, Druschel C, Curt A, et al. Traumatic spinal cord injury. Nature Reviews. Disease Primers. 2017;**3**:17018

[2] Jain NB, Ayers GD, Peterson EN, Harris MB, Morse L, O'Connor KC, et al. Traumatic spinal cord injury in the United States, 1993-2012. Journal of the American Medical Association. 2015;**313**(22):2236-2243

[3] Norenberg MD, Smith J, Marcillo A. The pathology of human spinal cord injury: Defining the problems. Journal of Neurotrauma. 2004;**21**(4):429-440

[4] Kwon BK, Tetzlaff W, Grauer JN, Beiner J, Vaccaro AR. Pathophysiology and pharmacologic treatment of acute spinal cord injury. The Spine Journal. 2004;**4**(4):451-464

[5] Bravo G, Ibarra A, Guizar-Sahagun G, Rojas G, Hong E. Indorenate improves motor function in rats with chronic spinal cord injury. Basic & Clinical Pharmacology & Toxicology. 2007;**100**(1):67-70

[6] Cofano F, Boido M, Monticelli M, Zenga F, Ducati A, Vercelli A, et al. Mesenchymal stem cells for spinal cord injury: Current options, limitations, and future of cell therapy. International Journal of Molecular Sciences. 2019;**20**(11):2698

[7] Wilson JR, Tetreault LA, Kwon BK, Arnold PM, Mroz TE, Shaffrey C, et al. Timing of decompression in patients with acute spinal cord injury: A systematic review. Global Spine Journal. 2017;**7**(3 Suppl):95S-115S

[8] Keirstead HS, Nistor G, Bernal G, Totoiu M, Cloutier F, Sharp K, et al. Human embryonic stem cell-derived oligodendrocyte progenitor cell transplants remyelinate and restore locomotion after spinal cord injury. The Journal of Neuroscience. 2005;**25**(19):4694-4705

[9] Jin MC, Medress ZA, Azad TD, Doulames VM, Veeravagu A. Stem cell therapies for acute spinal cord injury in humans: A review. Neurosurgical Focus. 2019;**46**(3):E10

[10] Oliveri RS, Bello S, Biering-Sørensen F. Mesenchymal stem cells improve locomotor recovery in traumatic spinal cord injury: Systematic review with meta-analyses of rat models. Neurobiology of Disease. 2014;**62**:338-353

[11] Baez-Jurado E, Hidalgo-Lanussa O, Barrera-Bailón B, Sahebkar A, Ashraf GM, Echeverria V, et al. Secretome of mesenchymal stem cells and its potential protective effects on brain pathologies. Molecular Neurobiology. 2019;**56**(10):6902-6927

[12] Quertainmont R, Cantinieaux D, Botman O, Sid S, Schoenen J, Franzen R. Mesenchymal stem cell graft improves recovery after spinal cord injury in adult rats through neurotrophic and pro-angiogenic actions. PLoS One. 2012;**7**(6):e39500

[13] Lu S, Lu C, Han Q, Li J, Du Z, Liao L, et al. Adipose-derived mesenchymal stem cells protect PC12 cells from glutamate excitotoxicity-induced apoptosis by upregulation of XIAP through PI3-K/Akt activation. Toxicology. 2011;**279**(1-3):189-195

[14] Voulgari-Kokota A, Fairless R, Karamita M, Kyrargyri V, Tseveleki V, Evangelidou M, et al. Mesenchymal stem cells protect CNS neurons against glutamate excitotoxicity by inhibiting glutamate receptor expression and function. Experimental Neurology. 2012;**236**(1):161-170

[15] Lanza C, Morando S, Voci A, Canesi L, Principato MC, Serpero LD, et al. Neuroprotective mesenchymal stem cells are endowed with a potent antioxidant effect in vivo. Journal of Neurochemistry. 2009;**110**(5):1674-1684

[16] Zhou C, Zhang C, Chi S, Xu Y, Teng J, Wang H, et al. Effects of human marrow stromal cells on activation of microglial cells and production of inflammatory factors induced by lipopolysaccharide. Brain Research. 2009;**1269**:23-30

[17] Nakajima H, Uchida K, Guerrero AR, Watanabe S, Sugita D, Takeura N, et al. Transplantation of mesenchymal stem cells promotes an alternative pathway of macrophage activation and functional recovery after spinal cord injury. Journal of Neurotrauma. 2012;**29**(8):1614-1625

[18] Crigler L, Robey RC, Asawachaicharn A, Gaupp D, Phinney DG. Human mesenchymal stem cell subpopulations express a variety of neuro-regulatory molecules and promote neuronal cell survival and neuritogenesis. Experimental Neurology. 2006;**198**(1):54-64

[19] Hawryluk GW, Mothe A, Wang J, Wang S, Tator C, Fehlings MG. An in vivo characterization of trophic factor production following neural precursor cell or bone marrow stromal cell transplantation for spinal cord injury. Stem Cells and Development. 2012;**21**(12):2222-2238

[20] Lu LL, Liu YJ, Yang SG, Zhao QJ, Wang X, Gong W, et al. Isolation and characterization of human umbilical cord mesenchymal stem cells with hematopoiesis-supportive function and other potentials. Haematologica. 2006;**91**(8):1017-1026

[21] Dasari VR, Veeravalli KK, Dinh DH. Mesenchymal stem cells in the treatment of spinal cord injuries: A review. World Journal of Stem Cells. 2014;**6**(2):120-133

[22] Miura Y, Gao Z, Miura M, Seo BM, Sonoyama W, Chen W, et al. Mesenchymal stem cell-organized bone marrow elements: An alternative hematopoietic progenitor resource. Stem Cells. 2006;**24**(11):2428-2436

[23] Le Blanc K, Davies LC. MSCs-cells with many sides. Cytotherapy. 2018;**20**(3):273-278

[24] Uccelli A, Moretta L, Pistoia V. Mesenchymal stem cells in health and disease. Nature Reviews. Immunology. 2008;**8**(9):726-736

[25] Chamberlain G, Fox J, Ashton B, Middleton J. Concise review: Mesenchymal stem cells: Their phenotype, differentiation capacity, immunological features, and potential for homing. Stem Cells. 2007;**25**(11):2739-2749

[26] Squillaro T, Peluso G, Galderisi U. Clinical trials with Mesenchymal stem cells: An update. Cell Transplantation. 2016;**25**(5):829-848

[27] Baberg F, Geyh S, Waldera-Lupa D, Stefanski A, Zilkens C, Haas R, et al. Secretome analysis of human bone marrow derived mesenchymal stromal cells. Biochimica et Biophysica Acta, Proteins and Proteomics. 2019;**1867**(4):434-441

[28] Chen TS, Arslan F, Yin Y, Tan SS, Lai RC, Choo AB, et al. Enabling a robust scalable manufacturing process for therapeutic exosomes through oncogenic immortalization of human ESC-derived MSCs. Journal of Translational Medicine. 2011;**9**:47

[29] Devine SM, Cobbs C, Jennings M, Bartholomew A, Hoffman R. Mesenchymal stem cells distribute to a wide range of tissues following systemic

infusion into nonhuman primates. Blood. 2003;**101**(8):2999-3001

[30] Gao J, Dennis JE, Muzic RF, Lundberg M, Caplan AI. The dynamic in vivo distribution of bone marrow-derived mesenchymal stem cells after infusion. Cells, Tissues, Organs. 2001;**169**(1):12-20

[31] Nitzsche F, Müller C, Lukomska B, Jolkkonen J, Deten A, Boltze J. Concise review: MSC adhesion cascade-insights into homing and transendothelial migration. Stem Cells. 2017;**35**(6):1446-1460

[32] Smith AN, Willis E, Chan VT, Muffley LA, Isik FF, Gibran NS, et al. Mesenchymal stem cells induce dermal fibroblast responses to injury. Experimental Cell Research. 2010;**316**(1):48-54

[33] Sarojini H, Estrada R, Lu H, Dekova S, Lee MJ, Gray RD, et al. PEDF from mouse mesenchymal stem cell secretome attracts fibroblasts. Journal of Cellular Biochemistry. 2008;**104**(5):1793-1802

[34] Brandau S, Jakob M, Bruderek K, Bootz F, Giebel B, Radtke S, et al. Mesenchymal stem cells augment the anti-bacterial activity of neutrophil granulocytes. PLoS One. 2014;**9**(9):e106903

[35] Brandau S, Jakob M, Hemeda H, Bruderek K, Janeschik S, Bootz F, et al. Tissue-resident mesenchymal stem cells attract peripheral blood neutrophils and enhance their inflammatory activity in response to microbial challenge. Journal of Leukocyte Biology. 2010;**88**(5):1005-1015

[36] Neirinckx V, Agirman G, Coste C, Marquet A, Dion V, Rogister B, et al. Adult bone marrow mesenchymal and neural crest stem cells are chemoattractive and accelerate motor recovery in a mouse model of spinal cord injury. Stem Cell Research & Therapy. 2015;**6**:211

[37] Laing AG, Fanelli G, Ramirez-Valdez A, Lechler RI, Lombardi G, Sharpe PT. Mesenchymal stem cells inhibit T-cell function through conserved induction of cellular stress. PLoS One. 2019;**14**(3):e0213170

[38] Sato K, Ozaki K, Oh I, Meguro A, Hatanaka K, Nagai T, et al. Nitric oxide plays a critical role in suppression of T-cell proliferation by mesenchymal stem cells. Blood. 2007;**109**(1):228-234

[39] Cantinieaux D, Quertainmont R, Blacher S, Rossi L, Wanet T, Noël A, et al. Conditioned medium from bone marrow-derived mesenchymal stem cells improves recovery after spinal cord injury in rats: An original strategy to avoid cell transplantation. PLoS One. 2013;**8**(8):e69515

[40] Song WJ, Li Q, Ryu MO, Ahn JO, Bhang DH, Jung YC, et al. TSG-6 released from intraperitoneally injected canine adipose tissue-derived mesenchymal stem cells ameliorate inflammatory bowel disease by inducing M2 macrophage switch in mice. Stem Cell Research & Therapy. 2018;**9**(1):91

[41] Song JY, Kang HJ, Hong JS, Kim CJ, Shim JY, Lee CW, et al. Umbilical cord-derived mesenchymal stem cell extracts reduce colitis in mice by re-polarizing intestinal macrophages. Scientific Reports. 2017;**7**(1):9412

[42] Nakajima K, Obata H, Iriuchijima N, Saito S. An increase in spinal cord noradrenaline is a major contributor to the antihyperalgesic effect of antidepressants after peripheral nerve injury in the rat. Pain. 2012;**153**(5):990-997

[43] Zhang Y, Ge XH, Guo XJ, Guan SB, Li XM, Gu W, et al. Bone marrow Mesenchymal stem cells inhibit the function of dendritic cells by

secreting Galectin-1. BioMed Research International. 2017;**2017**:3248605

[44] Rasmusson I, Ringdén O, Sundberg B, Le Blanc K. Mesenchymal stem cells inhibit lymphocyte proliferation by mitogens and alloantigens by different mechanisms. Experimental Cell Research. 2005;**305**(1):33-41

[45] Nasef A, Chapel A, Mazurier C, Bouchet S, Lopez M, Mathieu N, et al. Identification of IL-10 and TGF-beta transcripts involved in the inhibition of T-lymphocyte proliferation during cell contact with human mesenchymal stem cells. Gene Expression. 2007;**13**(4-5):217-226

[46] Cho KA, Lee JK, Kim YH, Park M, Woo SY, Ryu KH. Mesenchymal stem cells ameliorate B-cell-mediated immune responses and increase IL-10-expressing regulatory B cells in an EBI3-dependent manner. Cellular & Molecular Immunology. 2017;**14**:895-908

[47] Asari S, Itakura S, Ferreri K, Liu CP, Kuroda Y, Kandeel F, et al. Mesenchymal stem cells suppress B-cell terminal differentiation. Experimental Hematology. 2009;**37**(5):604-615

[48] Bronckaers A, Hilkens P, Fanton Y, Struys T, Gervois P, Politis C, et al. Angiogenic properties of human dental pulp stem cells. PLoS One. 2013;**8**(8):e71104

[49] Wan J, Xia L, Liang W, Liu Y, Cai Q. Transplantation of bone marrow-derived mesenchymal stem cells promotes delayed wound healing in diabetic rats. Journal Diabetes Research. 2013;**2013**:647107

[50] Berry MF, Engler AJ, Woo YJ, Pirolli TJ, Bish LT, Jayasankar V, et al. Mesenchymal stem cell injection after myocardial infarction improves myocardial compliance. American Journal of Physiology. Heart and Circulatory Physiology. 2006;**290**(6):H2196-H2203

[51] Zacharek A, Chen J, Cui X, Li A, Li Y, Roberts C, et al. Angiopoietin1/Tie2 and VEGF/Flk1 induced by MSC treatment amplifies angiogenesis and vascular stabilization after stroke. Journal of Cerebral Blood Flow and Metabolism. 2007;**27**(10):1684-1691

[52] Gu Y, Zhang Y, Bi Y, Liu J, Tan B, Gong M, et al. Mesenchymal stem cells suppress neuronal apoptosis and decrease IL-10 release via the TLR2/NFκB pathway in rats with hypoxic-ischemic brain damage. Molecular Brain. 2015;**8**(1):65

[53] Wang F, Yasuhara T, Shingo T, Kameda M, Tajiri N, Yuan WJ, et al. Intravenous administration of mesenchymal stem cells exerts therapeutic effects on parkinsonian model of rats: Focusing on neuroprotective effects of stromal cell-derived factor-1alpha. BMC Neuroscience. 2010;**11**:52

[54] Yang C, Wang G, Ma F, Yu B, Chen F, Yang J, et al. Repeated injections of human umbilical cord blood-derived mesenchymal stem cells significantly promotes functional recovery in rabbits with spinal cord injury of two noncontinuous segments. Stem Cell Research & Therapy. 2018;**9**(1):136

[55] Jaramillo-Merchán J, Jones J, Ivorra JL, Pastor D, Viso-León MC, Armengól JA, et al. Mesenchymal stromal-cell transplants induce oligodendrocyte progenitor migration and remyelination in a chronic demyelination model. Cell Death & Disease. 2013;**4**:e779

[56] Bae JS, Jin HK, Lee JK, Richardson JC, Carter JE. Bone marrow-derived mesenchymal stem cells contribute to the reduction of amyloid-β deposits and the improvement of

synaptic transmission in a mouse model of pre-dementia Alzheimer's disease. Current Alzheimer Research. 2013;**10**(5):524-531

[57] Lu P, Jones LL, Tuszynski MH. BDNF-expressing marrow stromal cells support extensive axonal growth at sites of spinal cord injury. Experimental Neurology. 2005;**191**(2):344-360

[58] Cízková D, Rosocha J, Vanický I, Jergová S, Cízek M. Transplants of human mesenchymal stem cells improve functional recovery after spinal cord injury in the rat. Cellular and Molecular Neurobiology. 2006;**26**(7-8):1167-1180

[59] Albayrak Ö, Şener TE, Erşahin M, Özbaş-Turan S, Ekentok C, Tavukçu HH, et al. Mesenchymal stem cell therapy improves erectile dysfunction in experimental spinal cord injury. International Journal of Impotence Research. 2019

[60] Valadi H, Ekström K, Bossios A, Sjöstrand M, Lee JJ, Lötvall JO. Exosome-mediated transfer of mRNAs and microRNAs is a novel mechanism of genetic exchange between cells. Nature Cell Biology. 2007;**9**(6):654-659

[61] Woodbury D, Schwarz EJ, Prockop DJ, Black IB. Adult rat and human bone marrow stromal cells differentiate into neurons. Journal of Neuroscience Research. 2000;**61**(4):364-370

[62] Takizawa S. Differentiation of adult bone marrow cells into neurons and endothelial cells in rat brain after stroke in the presence of cytokines. Rinshō Shinkeigaku. 2003;**43**(11):830-831

[63] Kopen GC, Prockop DJ, Phinney DG. Marrow stromal cells migrate throughout forebrain and cerebellum, and they differentiate into astrocytes after injection into neonatal mouse brains. Proceedings of the National Academy of Sciences of the United States of America. 1999;**96**(19):10711-10716

[64] Jiang W, Ma A, Wang T, Han K, Liu Y, Zhang Y, et al. Homing and differentiation of mesenchymal stem cells delivered intravenously to ischemic myocardium in vivo: A time-series study. Pflügers Archiv. 2006;**453**(1):43-52

[65] De Bari C, Dell'Accio F, Luyten FP. Failure of in vitro-differentiated mesenchymal stem cells from the synovial membrane to form ectopic stable cartilage in vivo. Arthritis and Rheumatism. 2004;**50**(1):142-150

[66] Chen J, Chen H, Li P, Diao H, Zhu S, Dong L, et al. Simultaneous regeneration of articular cartilage and subchondral bone in vivo using MSCs induced by a spatially controlled gene delivery system in bilayered integrated scaffolds. Biomaterials. 2011;**32**(21):4793-4805

[67] Laverdet B, Micallef L, Lebreton C, Mollard J, Lataillade JJ, Coulomb B, et al. Use of mesenchymal stem cells for cutaneous repair and skin substitute elaboration. Pathologie Biologie. 2014;**62**(2):108-117

[68] Rooney GE, McMahon SS, Ritter T, Garcia Y, Moran C, Madigan NN, et al. Neurotrophic factor-expressing mesenchymal stem cells survive transplantation into the contused spinal cord without differentiating into neural cells. Tissue Engineering. Part A. 2009;**15**(10):3049-3059

[69] Huang JH, Yin XM, Xu Y, Xu CC, Lin X, Ye FB, et al. Systemic administration of exosomes released from mesenchymal stromal cells attenuates apoptosis, inflammation, and promotes angiogenesis after spinal cord injury in rats. Journal of Neurotrauma. 2017;**34**(24):3388-3396

[70] Liu W, Wang Y, Gong F, Rong Y, Luo Y, Tang P, et al. Exosomes derived from bone Mesenchymal stem cells repair traumatic spinal cord injury by suppressing the activation of A1 neurotoxic reactive astrocytes. Journal of Neurotrauma. 2019;**36**(3):469-484

[71] Lankford KL, Arroyo EJ, Nazimek K, Bryniarski K, Askenase PW, Kocsis JD. Intravenously delivered mesenchymal stem cell-derived exosomes target M2-type macrophages in the injured spinal cord. PLoS One. 2018;**13**(1):e0190358

[72] Yang J, Zhang X, Chen X, Wang L, Yang G. Exosome mediated delivery of miR-124 promotes neurogenesis after ischemia. Molecular Therapy--Nucleic Acids. 2017;**7**:278-287

[73] Cui GH, Guo HD, Li H, Zhai Y, Gong ZB, Wu J, et al. RVG-modified exosomes derived from mesenchymal stem cells rescue memory deficits by regulating inflammatory responses in a mouse model of Alzheimer's disease. Immunity & Ageing. 2019;**16**:10

[74] Moviglia GA, Fernandez Viña R, Brizuela JA, Saslavsky J, Vrsalovic F, Varela G, et al. Combined protocol of cell therapy for chronic spinal cord injury. Report on the electrical and functional recovery of two patients. Cytotherapy. 2006;**8**(3):202-209

[75] Pal R, Venkataramana NK, Bansal A, Balaraju S, Jan M, Chandra R, et al. Ex vivo-expanded autologous bone marrow-derived mesenchymal stromal cells in human spinal cord injury/paraplegia: A pilot clinical study. Cytotherapy. 2009;**11**(7):897-911

[76] Ra JC, Shin IS, Kim SH, Kang SK, Kang BC, Lee HY, et al. Safety of intravenous infusion of human adipose tissue-derived mesenchymal stem cells in animals and humans. Stem Cells and Development. 2011;**20**(8):1297-1308

[77] Hur JW, Cho TH, Park DH, Lee JB, Park JY, Chung YG. Intrathecal transplantation of autologous adipose-derived mesenchymal stem cells for treating spinal cord injury: A human trial. The Journal of Spinal Cord Medicine. 2016;**39**(6):655-664

[78] Satti HS, Waheed A, Ahmed P, Ahmed K, Akram Z, Aziz T, et al. Autologous mesenchymal stromal cell transplantation for spinal cord injury: A phase I pilot study. Cytotherapy. 2016;**18**(4):518-522

[79] Sykova E, Homola A, Mazanec R, Lachmann H, Konradova SL, Kobylka P, et al. Autologous bone marrow transplantation in patients with subacute and chronic spinal cord injury. Cell Transplantation. 2006;**15**(8-9):675-687

[80] Park HC, Shim YS, Ha Y, Yoon SH, Park SR, Choi BH, et al. Treatment of complete spinal cord injury patients by autologous bone marrow cell transplantation and administration of granulocyte-macrophage colony stimulating factor. Tissue Engineering. 2005;**11**(5-6):913-922

[81] Geffner LF, Santacruz P, Izurieta M, Flor L, Maldonado B, Auad AH, et al. Administration of autologous bone marrow stem cells into spinal cord injury patients via multiple routes is safe and improves their quality of life: Comprehensive case studies. Cell Transplantation. 2008;**17**(12):1277-1293

[82] Dai G, Liu X, Zhang Z, Yang Z, Dai Y, Xu R. Transplantation of autologous bone marrow mesenchymal stem cells in the treatment of complete and chronic cervical spinal cord injury. Brain Research. 2013;**1533**:73-79

[83] Kishk NA, Gabr H, Hamdy S, Afifi L, Abokresha N, Mahmoud H, et al. Case control series of intrathecal autologous bone marrow mesenchymal

stem cell therapy for chronic spinal cord injury. Neurorehabilitation and Neural Repair. 2010;**24**(8):702-708

[84] Jeon SR. Et al, Treatment of spinal cord injury with bone marrow-derived, cultured autologous mesenchymal stem cells. Journal of Tissue Engineering and Regenerative Medicine. 2010;7(3): 316-322

[85] Karamouzian S, Nematollahi-Mahani SN, Nakhaee N, Eskandary H. Clinical safety and primary efficacy of bone marrow mesenchymal cell transplantation in subacute spinal cord injured patients. Clinical Neurology and Neurosurgery. 2012;**114**(7):935-939

[86] Cheng H, Liu X, Hua R, Dai G, Wang X, Gao J, et al. Clinical observation of umbilical cord mesenchymal stem cell transplantation in treatment for sequelae of thoracolumbar spinal cord injury. Journal of Translational Medicine. 2014;**12**:253

[87] El-Kheir WA, Gabr H, Awad MR, Ghannam O, Barakat Y, Farghali HA, et al. Autologous bone marrow-derived cell therapy combined with physical therapy induces functional improvement in chronic spinal cord injury patients. Cell Transplantation. 2014;**23**(6):729-745

[88] Mendonça MV, Larocca TF, de Freitas Souza BS, Villarreal CF, Silva LF, Matos AC, et al. Safety and neurological assessments after autologous transplantation of bone marrow mesenchymal stem cells in subjects with chronic spinal cord injury. Stem Cell Research & Therapy. 2014;**5**(6):126

[89] Vaquero J, Zurita M, Rico MA, Bonilla C, Aguayo C, Montilla J, et al. An approach to personalized cell therapy in chronic complete paraplegia: The Puerta de Hierro phase I/II clinical trial. Cytotherapy. 2016;**18**(8):1025-1036

[90] Vaquero J, Zurita M, Rico MA, Bonilla C, Aguayo C, Fernández C, et al. Repeated subarachnoid administrations of autologous mesenchymal stromal cells supported in autologous plasma improve quality of life in patients suffering incomplete spinal cord injury. Cytotherapy. 2017;**19**(3):349-359

[91] Vaquero J, Zurita M, Rico MA, Aguayo C, Bonilla C, Marin E, et al. Intrathecal administration of autologous mesenchymal stromal cells for spinal cord injury: Safety and efficacy of the 100/3 guideline. Cytotherapy. 2018;**20**(6):806-819

[92] Oh SK, Choi KH, Yoo JY, Kim DY, Kim SJ, Jeon SR. A phase III clinical trial showing limited efficacy of autologous mesenchymal stem cell therapy for spinal cord injury. Neurosurgery. 2016;**78**(3):436-447. Discussion 47

[93] Tetzlaff W, Okon EB, Karimi-Abdolrezaee S, Hill CE, Sparling JS, Plemel JR, et al. A systematic review of cellular transplantation therapies for spinal cord injury. Journal of Neurotrauma. 2011;**28**(8):1611-1682

[94] Xiao Z, Tang F, Zhao Y, Han G, Yin N, Li X, et al. Significant improvement of acute complete spinal cord injury patients diagnosed by a combined criteria implanted with NeuroRegen scaffolds and mesenchymal stem cells. Cell Transplantation. 2018;**27**(6):907-915

[95] Vismara I, Papa S, Rossi F, Forloni G, Veglianese P. Current options for cell therapy in spinal cord injury. Trends in Molecular Medicine. 2017;**23**(9):831-849

[96] Wang LJ, Zhang RP, Li JD. Transplantation of neurotrophin-3-expressing bone mesenchymal stem cells improves recovery in a rat model of spinal cord injury. Acta Neurochirurgica. 2014;**156**(7):1409-1418

Chapter 3

Use of Mesenchymal Stem Cells in Pre-Clinical Models of Spinal Cord Injury

Gunel Guliyeva, Ricardo A. Torres Guzman, Francisco R. Avila Verduzco, Oluwasen O. Akinduro, Hugo Guerrero-Cazares, Paola Suarez Meade, Antonio J. Forte, Alfredo Quinones-Hinojosa and Rachel Sarabia-Estrada

Abstract

Spinal Cord Injury (SCI) is a devastating disease that causes disruption of sensorimotor function below the site of injury. Current management is based on surgical decompression of the neural tissue and pharmacotherapy; however, there is no gold standard treatment readily available for patients in the clinic. This indicates that novel therapeutic strategies for the treatment are still needed in the clinical setting. There are several alternatives that are currently under investigation for the treatment of this disease, with increasing focus in regenerative medicine treatments. Mesenchymal stem cells (MSCs) are one of the most promising candidates for stem cell therapy in SCI, as they are easily obtained, have high safety profiles, and help with neural regeneration in SCI mainly via release of trophic factors, neovascularization, and immunomodulation. In this work, authors provide an insight of the available MSC for neural regeneration, their therapeutic role, and the potential MSC-based therapies for SCI.

Keywords: mesenchymal stem cells, adipose-derived stem cells, spinal cord injury, animal model, stem cell therapy

1. Introduction

Traumatic Spinal cord injury (SCI) is a devastating disease that results in severe neural disruption and severe disabilities below the site of injury. Patients are unable to regenerate neural tissue after injury, leading to a lifelong disability. The pathophysiology of SCI is complex, consisting of a primary insult to the cord followed by a secondary cascade of events characterized mainly by inflammation, ischemia, ionic imbalance, excitotoxicity, and apoptosis [1]. This disease comprises a significant portion of health care expenditure in the United States, with an estimated annual cost of 7.7 billion dollars [2]. According to the National Spinal Cord Injury Statistical Center (NSCISC) in 2019, the incidence of SCI was about 54 cases per million people in the United States. SCI is caused by motor vehicle collisions in about 50% of cases, but other common etiologies include falls (30%), violent crime (11%), and sports-related injuries (9%) [2, 3]. SCI induced paraplegia and quadriplegia causes a significant physical and emotional toll on those inflicted, thus, there is a need for optimized strategies to better treat these patients. Although there has been significant investment into development of novel therapeutic strategies to improve outcomes for these patients, there remains little with proven benefit besides aggressive supportive care.

2. Spinal cord injury: standard of care

Spinal cord injuries can be subdivided into multiple groups depending on the mechanism of injury, anatomic location of the lesion, type and severity of the injury. The basis of treatment is surgical decompression of the spinal cord to prevent secondary damage associated with hypoxia and ischemia [4]. Besides surgery, there have been numerous neuroprotective drugs that have been assessed in clinical trials, including methylprednisolone, thyrotropin-releasing hormone, nimodipine, and naloxone [5–7]. However most of these drugs were ineffective, and some were associated with wound healing complications and infections that represents a limitation in the management of this population of patients.

The current standard of care for these patients consists of aggressive medical management. This includes prevention of secondary injury with strict maintenance of mean arterial pressure (MAP) [8, 9]. SCI patients are prone to cardiovascular instability, neurogenic shock, respiratory insufficiency, particularly when cervical levels are involved, which then leads to further secondary injury [10]. Multiple studies have shown improved outcome when these patients are managed in the intensive care unit (ICU), with strict monitoring of blood pressure parameters [11, 12]. Studies have shown that augmentation of MAPs to greater than 85 for 7 days is associated with improved outcomes as assessed by American Spinal Cord injury Association (ASIA) impairment scale.

Stems cells have become a hot topic of great interest in various fields such as cancer biology, regenerative medicine, and SCI. There are multiple types of stem cells, with varying capabilities, including embryonic stem cells, (ESC), tissue-specific stem cells, mesenchymal stem cells (MSCs), and induced pluripotent stem cells. (iPSC). MSCs were first discovered in the bone marrow, but since then have been grown from other sources such as adipose tissue, amniotic fluid and umbilical cord blood, making them more easily accessible. MSCs are typically defined as plastic adhering cell populations that can be directed to differentiate *in vitro* into cells of osteogenic, chondrogenic, adipogenic, myogenic, and various other lineages. They are known to have a beneficial effect in SCI, via release of trophic factors for neuroprotection, neovascularization, and immunomodulation [13–15]. These cells naturally secrete various trophic factors, including nerve growth factor (NGF), brain-derived neurotrophic factor (BDNF), and vascular endothelial growth factors (VEGF). BDNF is of particular interest since it has been shown to induce sprouting of corticospinal tracts in animal models of SCI [16]. MSCs derived from adipose tissue present unique advantages over other mesenchymal stem cell types as bone marrow, umbilical cord, dental pulp and others. In this chapter we'll focus in how MSCs can help in promoting spinal cord recovery after traumatic injury.

3. Mesenchymal stem cell use in the central nervous system

MSCs have been suggested for the treatment of various diseases. MSCs have also been proposed as a potential treatment for diabetes, inflammatory bowel disease, Parkinson disease, Alzheimer's disease, osteoporosis, bone regeneration, wound healing, skin aging, different inflammatory skin conditions, and others [17–27].

Among neurologic diseases, the use of MSCs in hypoxic-ischemic encephalopathy, multiple sclerosis, and glioma has been considered. The majority of studies investigating MSCs' impact on the treatment of stroke reported a decrease in the size of stroke volume and improvement in behavioral outcomes [28]. In animal studies, functional improvement, along with decreased seizures and increased long term potentiation, was seen in the hypoxic-ischemic encephalopathy model. In animal models of multiple sclerosis, demyelination and infiltrates were reduced after the treatment with MSCs. In murine studies, targeting of glioma cells with MSCs while loading them with viruses, were effective in impeding the growth of the tumor [29].

Different stem cell types have been used to treat SCI (**Figure 1**). Among them, MSCs are preferred due to several reasons:

- The simplicity of the isolation process
- The simplicity of cryoprecipitation
- Preservation of regenerative capacity and viability after cryoprecipitation at very low temperatures (−80)
- Minimal chances of cellular reaction induction
- High replication speed with high-quality progenitor cells and high potential of multilineage differentiation [30]
- Hypoimmunogenicity [31]

3.1 Bone marrow mesenchymal stem cells (BM-MSCs)

The collection of bone marrow tissue for extraction of MSCs is done by aspiration, which is not only invasive and painful for the patient, but also distressing but also carries a risk of infection [32]. Nevertheless, these risks are partially negated by the intriguing properties of BM-MSCs for neuronal regeneration. One of this

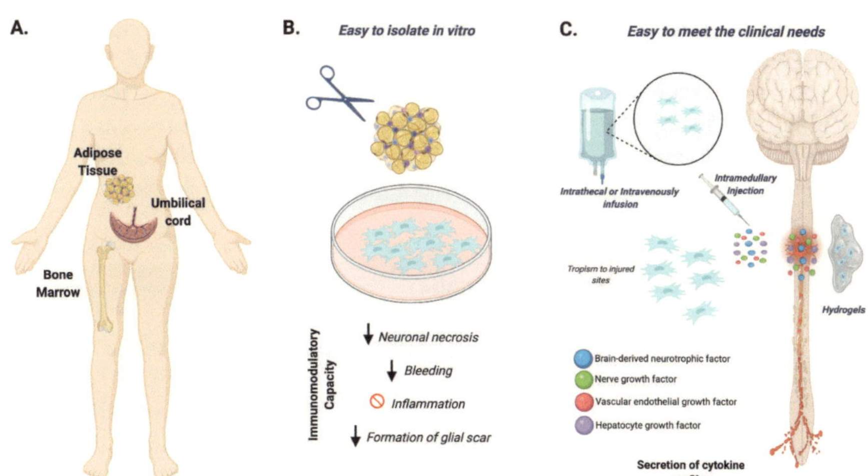

Figure 1.
Mesenchymal stem cells can be isolated from different sources (a), and can be expanded in vitro; when cultured they have a high proliferative rate (b). When applied to the SCI, they show homing properties, they are attracted by chemotactic signals and migrate towards the injured sire (c). Created with BioRender.com

properties is their plasticity potential as it allows them to differentiate into a broad spectrum other than mesodermal lineage cells as described by Wislet-Gendebien et al. [33] in which bone marrow stem cells were cultured with cerebellar granule neurons, inducing the expression the genes sox2, sox10, pax6, fzd, erbB2, and erbB4 in nestin-positive MSCs. Furthermore, with the help of electrophysiological analyses, they could establish that BM-MSCs neuron-like cells were able to fire single-action potentials and respond to the stimulation of distinct neurotransmitters such as GABA, glycine, and glutamate, concluding that nestin-positive bone marrow-derived MSCs can differentiate *in vitro* into excitable neuron-like cells.

Numerous authors have described another characteristic of this type of stem cell's source and are the capacity of MSCs to migrate to the injured tissue – a mechanism described as 'homing' - especially in BM-MSCs [34]. This characteristic makes BM-MSCs source very attractive due to the range of alternatives for applying treatment with MSCs to patients other than invasive procedures. *Andersen et al.* [35] put in practice the migration ability by injecting with BMSCs subcutaneously to an immune-deficient mouse with a bone fracture. Besides observing the homing capacity of MSCs, and is mediated by a wide range of growth factors such as PDGF and IGF-1.

BMSCs in a chimeric mice contusion SCI model was more effective in reducing the neuropathic pain and motor and thermal sensitivity if BMSCs were injected 3 days after the injury compared to injections at day 1, 7, or 14 days. This effect was mediated through the suppression of p38 MAPK and ERK1/2 activation in microglia and macrophages, CREB and PKC-c in dorsal horn neurons in the site of the injury and around it, and decreased macrophage infiltration to the epicenter. The latter reduces inflammation and restores Blood Spinal Cord Barrier [36]. Quertainmont et al. observed improved locomotor skills using open field test in the rats treated with BMSCs [37].

3.2 Adipose-derived mesenchymal stem cells (ADSC)

The abundant availability of adipose tissue, its easy accessibility under local anesthesia, a less painful procedure for the patients, and no adverse effects on animal models treated make this source desirable for the extraction, process, and administration to patients [38, 39]. A study conducted by *Ohta Y. et al.* [40] revealed that the secretion of specific growth factors, cytokines, proteases, immunomodulatory factors, and cellular matrix molecules promotes ADSCs' ability to regenerate neural tissue. However, the lack of full functional recovery results and the gap of knowledge on the description of the pro-regenerative effects are some of the limitations described on the literature on the use of MSCs that needs to be addressed in order to improve outcomes on complete functional recovery in *in vivo* models of SCI [41–43].

3.3 Umbilical cord mesenchymal stem cells

Ryu et al. [44] conducted a comparison between four sources of MSCs (Bone marrow, adipose-derived, umbilical cord blood, and Wharton's Jelly) to treat a canine model with spinal cord injury. Even though data revealed no significant differences in functional recovery among the MSCs groups, they identified essential properties such as the promotion of neuronal regeneration and anti-inflammatory activity. Umbilical cord stem cells group showed more nerve regeneration, neuroprotection, and less inflammation with reduced IL-6 and COX-2 levels than other MSCs. Moreover, researchers establish improvement in locomotion measured using the Olby and modified Tarlov scores eight weeks after the application of MSCs compared with the control group, suggesting that the use of MSCs promotes functional recovery after SCI. Additionally, preclinical studies such as the one carried by *Chua S. J. et al.* [45] have detected cytokines and growth factors known by its neuroprotective, angiogenic, and anti-inflammatory effects.

In a compression SCI rat model, both BMSCs and umbilical cord-derived stem cells caused similar results and improvement in allodynia, hyperalgesia, and functional recovery. However, UCSCs were more effective in decreasing wind-up levels [46]. 13 of 22 patients treated with UC-MSCs were better in daily living activities. They had a better motor function, better motor and tactile sensation [47].

3.4 Amniotic fetal mesenchymal stem cells

There are few preclinical studies in animal models that have to use amniotic fetal derived stem cells identified in the literature [48]. Nevertheless, the specific characteristics of this source of MSCs were observed. For instance, the multipotency, the low risk of immunogenic reaction, the ease of sample processing, and the high proliferative capacity, makes amniotic fetal derived stem cells an attractive alternative for regenerative medicine [49]. These properties are supported by data observed which showed promotion of angiogenesis and support of the surrounding tissue surplus the decreased inflammatory response and apoptosis [50–52].

In a rat model of SCI, the impact of two types of MSCs: Human umbilical cord blood-derived and Human amniotic epithelial cells were assessed for the treatment of SCI-induced thermal hyperalgesia and mechanical allodynia. None of them were effective in treating the thermal hyperalgesia. Though both improved the mechanical allodynia, human amniotic epithelial stem cells were more efficacious [53].

4. Animal models in spinal cord injury

Multiple studies described the administration of MSCs to treat spinal cord injury in a variety of animal models such as rodents, primates, sheep, dogs, cats, bovine, and even humans. Rodents are the most common animal model used [54], and the most appropriate model for spinal cord injury studies [55] since large animals and non-human primates are very expensive to care, demand additional managing requirements, and have ethical implications to consider when choosing. However, the experiments of the latter approximate more to SCIs [56].

The efficacy of MSCs were also observed in cats with SCI. Improvement in the cutaneous trunci (panniculus) reflex, pain sensation, bowel, and bladder function were noted. However, no significant change in proprioception and hyperreflexia of ataxic hind limbs were observed [57]. In dogs with SCI, treatment with BMSCs also caused the same clinical improvement with no significant recovery of low proprioceptive and hyperreflexic ataxic hind limbs [58]

4.1 Stem cell delivery methods in SCI animal models

There are currently 3 different methods to deliver mesenchymal stem cells (MSCs) in animal models of spinal cord injury (SCI). These are direct implantation, intravenous (IV) infusion, and intrathecal infusion. Direct implantation refers to the injection of MSCs directly in the injured area of the spinal cord. IV infusion refers to the injection of MSCs in a major vein of the animal model (e.g. the tail vein of a mouse or rat). Lastly, intrathecal infusion refers to the injection of MSCs directly into the subarachnoid space, in the cerebrospinal fluid. The delivery methods described in the following paragraphs concern mainly Sprague-Dawley rats. For a summary of advantages and disadvantages of delivery methods, see **Table 1**.

Direct implantation of the MSCs is done using a small syringe capable if precisely injecting cells in the damaged area [59], guaranteeing delivery to the desired site [60]. This method has been largely favored due to its high cell viability and improved survival [61], observed in higher engraftment rates in both acute and chronic SCI [59, 61, 62]. However, some authors have expressed concerns regarding the translation of this technique to clinical practice. Agglomeration of cells in the injection site, needle damage to the adjacent non-injured spinal cord, and failure of cell migration to the central parenchyma are some of the most noteworthy disadvantages of this delivery method [59–64]. Additionally, if done in humans, direct implantation of MSCs would require the patient to undergo general anesthesia and an invasive surgical procedure [61].

Since direct implantation of MSCs in humans might pose substantial risks, IV and intrathecal infusion were deemed appropriate less invasive surrogates that could potentially be clinically used. Damage to the blood-brain barrier (BBB) in SCI (particularly in traumatic SCI) allows infiltration of cells and toxic mediators that promote further neurologic damage [65]. It was initially thought that this process could improve diffusion of MSCs into the spinal cord. However, cell infusion in the first 48 hours of injury has shown conflicting evidence, with some authors reporting either the presence or absence of MSCs at the lesion site [65, 66]. Nevertheless, when present, the cell's engraftment rate with IV delivery in the spinal cord was very low in comparison to other methods [59].

Delivery method	Advantages	Disadvantages
Intralesional delivery	• Precise positioning of cells at lesion site.	• Agglomeration of cells at injection site.
	• Higher engraftment, translating into higher cell viability and increased survival.	• Needle damage to adjacent spinal cord.
	• High opportunity of differentiation	• Failure of cell migration to the central parenchyma.
		• Complicated surgical approach in animal models.
		• Would require an invasive surgical approach in humans.
Intravenous delivery	• Promotion of an anti-inflammatory environment that prevents BBB leakage and progressive damage.	• Low engraftment rates.
	• Easy administration.	• Lowest limb function recovery scores.
	• Administration of multiple doses	• Limited beneficial effects
Intrathecal delivery	• Migration of cells to different regions of the spinal cord.	• Cell attachment to other regions of the central nervous system.
	• Highest limb function recovery scores.	
		• Complicated surgical approaches in animal models.

Table 1.
Advantages and disadvantages of the three main MSC delivery methods.

The low engraftment rates in the spinal cord with IV delivery methods are considered a consequence of the cells' first pass through the systemic circulation. MSCs have been observed in the lungs and liver in the first 24-48 hours of IV infusion [66, 67], with progressive increase of cell numbers in the spleen in the following days [61, 67]. Cell engraftment in the spleen is associated with increased levels of anti-inflammatory cytokines (e.g. IL-10, TIMP-1) [67] in plasma, which is believed to decrease BBB permeability by inhibiting monocyte adhesion to the vasculature, preventing metalloproteinase release and vascular basement membrane degradation [67]. Therefore, the anti-inflammatory environment promoted by cells engrafting outside the spinal cord prevents vascular leakage at the lesion site, decreasing hemorrhage, inflammation and further damage [66, 67].

IV infusion of MSCs can be done through the femoral vein or the tail vein. In rodents, peripheral circulation is mostly accessed through the tail vein [61, 67, 68] due to its simplicity when compared to the approach required to access the femoral vein [59, 65, 66]. Additionally, inflammation around the site of injury is higher than with intrathecal administration but lower than direct injection [59]. Even though cells administered IV have low engraftment rates, animals still score better outcomes in limb function recovery scores and grip strength [67], develop less scarring [59, 68], and have higher vascularization, myelination, and axonal density than controls [68].

Intrathecal delivery of MSCs can be done via the intracisternal approach (i.e. injection into the fourth ventricle) [61, 69, 70] or by laminectomy with injection of cells through the dura [63]. When initially injected, cells occupy the whole subarachnoid space, but progressively decrease their number in this anatomical region [63]. In contrast to intralesional delivery of MSCs, intrathecally administered cells show a more extensive migration in the neural tissue, extending from the dorsal spinal cord to its center [61]. Although the number of viable cells is only second to the intralesional delivery method [61], a decrease in engrafted cells to 5% of the original cell number has been observed after 6 weeks, with some cells attaching to the pia mater [63]. Animals with intrathecally delivered MSCs obtain higher scores in limb function recovery scores when compared with intralesional and intravenous deliveries [61].

The impact of MSCs on SCI resolution can be explained by the following characteristics: immunomodulatory, anti-inflammatory, neurotrophic/neuroprotective, and angiogenetic effects. The direct impact on the regeneration of the neurons is mainly exerted by neurotrophic and neuroprotective functions. These functions are usually mediated by the secretion of neurotrophic factors.

The spinal cord injury occurs in 2 phases. The first phase occurs immediately after the trauma and is mediated by damage to the microvascular elements, cellular membrane, and the blood-spinal cord barrier. Damage to these three structures evokes series of events that give rise to axonal fragmentation, demyelination, cyst formation, and expansion and accumulation of the microglia and macrophages in and around the injury site, which leads to the secondary injury. The secondary injury is characterized by inflammation, ischemia, disruption of ion channels, free radical production, glutamatergic excitotoxicity, necrosis, axonal demyelination, and glial scar formation [30, 71].

As previously described, MSCs from different sources have been used to treat SCI. They can directly be injected to the injury site or intravenously as they have the ability to migrate to the epicenter of the injury, demonstrating their homing abilities.

Chen *et al*. reviewed 12 randomized controlled trials on rats and mice and showed that stem cell treatment improved the mechanical reflex threshold. For the mice, improvement in thermal withdrawal latency was observed. However, no improvement was seen in rat studies [72]. In a rat spinal cord hemisection model, BMSCs were noted to promote astrocyte migration to the injury epicenter. In the group treated with a combination of the BDNF with platelet-rich plasma, more astrocyte migration, and higher rates of remyelination has been documented. This group also showed remyelination and oligodendrocytes with higher activity, while only the BMSCs group showed axonal demyelination, vacuole and whirled body formation [73].

The human ADSC have been shown to be able to convert to the oligodendrocytes and to attract oligodendrocyte precursor cells, which, in turn, mediates remyelination. Unsurprisingly, the treatment caused an improvement in the motor function of the animals with focal demyelination [74]. Differentiation of neurotrophic factors secreting cells from human ADSC to oligodendrocytes was noted in a damaged spinal cord rat model. Neurotrophic factors secreting cells promoted remyelination and increased thickness of the myelin and the diameter of the axons [75].

In a rat model of spinal cord contusion, rats treated with bone marrow-derived Schwann cells experienced better functional recovery. At the same time, the size of the cystic cavity decreased, and axonal regeneration was observed [76]. Treatment with bone-derived MSCs stimulated axonal growth in the subtotal cervical hemisection rat model. An increase in the length of the axons was observed [77]. Bone marrow mesenchymal stem cells decreased the cavity volume and increased the spared white matter, the length of the neurites, the number of axons, and the neurites in a SCI rat model [78]. Rats with a moderate contusion model of spinal cord injury showed better recovery in 2 behavioral tests (Bresnahan Locomotor Rating Scale [79] and exploratory rearing [80]). All rats experienced a decrease in the size of the cyst cavity and more axons in the injury site either through an increase in spared axons or through axon regeneration [80]. In a complete spinal cord transection rat model, human umbilical mesenchymal stem cells promoted axonal regeneration, and more neurofilament-positive fibers around the epicenter of the corticospinal tract injury was observed. Additionally, proximal and dorsal to the injury site, fewer microglia and astrocytes with reactive features were found [81].

Some studies suggest that the MSCs do not have the ability to convert to neural cells. As an example, Quertainmont et al. could not detect the stem cells after grafting. The authors described tissue sparing, vascularization in the injury epicenter, but no evidence of axonal regrowth [37].

5. Use of mesenchymal stem cells in spinal cord injury in the clinical setting

The use of MSCs in the clinic has been studied thoroughly; however, results among studies are not consistent. For example, 5 patients with complete spinal cord injury were treated with autologous bone marrow cells and granulocyte macrophage-colony stimulating factor, and 4 of them showed neurologic (sensory or motor) improvement [82]. There are controversial evidences for both MSC's ability to cause and treat neuropathic pain. In one study, 9 people with SCI got treated with MSCs, and 8 of them experienced a reduction or resolution of the neuropathic pain. Improvement in peripheral nerve conduction, motor power, and sensitivity was noted. Enhancement of the voluntary muscle contraction was explained with active muscle reinnervation [83]. All 14 patients with chronic traumatic complete SCI treated with BMSCs felt an improvement in sensitivity to light touch and pinprick. The majority also experienced sacral sparing, and improvement in urologic and motor function [84].

Treatment with MSCs of 6 traumatic syringomyelia patients with paraplegia reduced the size of the syrinx. Additionally, the neuropathic pain either resolved or decreased [85]. In one case report, the patient was treated with MSCs and G-CSF, and his motor function, tactile and pain sensation were improved after the treatment. However, the patient still reported neuropathic pain, etiology of which was unknown [86].

6. Limitations in mesenchymal stem cell delivery

MSC type, dosage, delivery method, and timing of therapy are current obstacles in spinal cord injury cell therapy that limit its translation to clinical practice. Bone marrow stromal cells, bone marrow mononuclear cells, and neural stem/progenitor cells are just some examples of the cell types currently under study for this purpose, with no clear best candidate yet. Cell dosage needs further research since the appropriate therapeutic dose is still unclear. Dosage standardization is required to build a homogenized body of literature that allows for an appropriate comparison of delivery methods. The most appropriate delivery method is still debated since all poses unique benefits. Innovative methods such as subpial delivery and stem cell-derived nanovesicle are promising new alternatives that will be added to the battery of delivery techniques [87, 88].

7. Conclusions

Mesenchymal stem cell therapy has shown promising results in spinal cord injury repair. Animal studies and clinical trials performed in human patients using mesenchymal stem cells suggested that this therapy can be a promising candidate for patients suffering from spinal cord injury. MSCs derived from different sources offer potential healing in different spinal cord injury conditions.

Acknowledgements

This study was supported in part by the Mayo Clinic Center of Individualized Medicine and the Mayo Clinic Neuro-Oncology Convergence Grant.

Conflict of interest

The authors declare no conflict of interest.

Author details

Gunel Guliyeva, Ricardo A. Torres Guzman, Francisco R. Avila Verduzco, Oluwasen O. Akinduro, Hugo Guerrero-Cazares, Paola Suarez Meade, Antonio J. Forte, Alfredo Quinones-Hinojosa and Rachel Sarabia-Estrada*
Mayo Clinic, Florida, USA

*Address all correspondence to: estrada.rachel@mayo.edu

References

[1] Alizadeh A, Dyck SM, Karimi-Abdolrezaee S. Traumatic Spinal Cord Injury: An Overview of Pathophysiology, Models and Acute Injury Mechanisms. Front Neurol. 2019;10:282.

[2] DeVivo MJ. Causes and costs of spinal cord injury in the United States. Spinal Cord. 1997;35(12):809-13.

[3] Pirouzmand F. Epidemiological trends of spine and spinal cord injuries in the largest Canadian adult trauma center from 1986 to 2006. J Neurosurg Spine. 2010;12(2):131-40.

[4] Ahuja CS, Martin AR, Fehlings M. Recent advances in managing a spinal cord injury secondary to trauma. F1000Res. 2016;5.

[5] Flamm ES, Young W, Collins WF, Piepmeier J, Clifton GL, Fischer B. A phase I trial of naloxone treatment in acute spinal cord injury. J Neurosurg. 1985;63(3):390-7.

[6] Petitjean ME, Pointillart V, Dixmerias F, Wiart L, Sztark F, Lassie P, et al. [Medical treatment of spinal cord injury in the acute stage]. Ann Fr Anesth Reanim. 1998;17(2):114-22.

[7] Dumont RJ, Verma S, Okonkwo DO, Hurlbert RJ, Boulos PT, Ellegala DB, et al. Acute spinal cord injury, part II: contemporary pharmacotherapy. Clin Neuropharmacol. 2001;24(5):265-79.

[8] Ryken TC, Hurlbert RJ, Hadley MN, Aarabi B, Dhall SS, Gelb DE, et al. The acute cardiopulmonary management of patients with cervical spinal cord injuries. Neurosurgery. 2013;72 Suppl 2:84-92.

[9] Dakson A, Brandman D, Thibault-Halman G, Christie SD. Optimization of the mean arterial pressure and timing of surgical decompression in traumatic spinal cord injury: a retrospective study. Spinal Cord. 2017;55(11):1033-8.

[10] Piepmeier JM, Lehmann KB, Lane JG. Cardiovascular instability following acute cervical spinal cord trauma. Cent Nerv Syst Trauma. 1985;2(3):153-60.

[11] Levi L, Wolf A, Belzberg H. Hemodynamic parameters in patients with acute cervical cord trauma: description, intervention, and prediction of outcome. Neurosurgery. 1993;33(6):1007-16; discussion 16-7.

[12] Tator CH. Vascular effects and blood flow in acute spinal cord injuries. J Neurosurg Sci. 1984;28(3-4):115-9.

[13] Chen X, Li Y, Wang L, Katakowski M, Zhang L, Chen J, et al. Ischemic rat brain extracts induce human marrow stromal cell growth factor production. Neuropathology. 2002;22(4):275-9.

[14] Ohtaki H, Ylostalo JH, Foraker JE, Robinson AP, Reger RL, Shioda S, et al. Stem/progenitor cells from bone marrow decrease neuronal death in global ischemia by modulation of inflammatory/immune responses. Proc Natl Acad Sci U S A. 2008;105(38):14638-43.

[15] Onda T, Honmou O, Harada K, Houkin K, Hamada H, Kocsis JD. Therapeutic benefits by human mesenchymal stem cells (hMSCs) and Ang-1 gene-modified hMSCs after cerebral ischemia. J Cereb Blood Flow Metab. 2008;28(2):329-40.

[16] Zhou L, Shine HD. Neurotrophic factors expressed in both cortex and spinal cord induce axonal plasticity after spinal cord injury. J Neurosci Res. 2003;74(2):221-6.

[17] Moreira A, Kahlenberg S, Hornsby P. Therapeutic potential of mesenchymal stem cells for diabetes. J Mol Endocrinol. 2017;59(3):R109-r20.

[18] Venkatesh K, Sen D. Mesenchymal Stem Cells as a Source of Dopaminergic Neurons: A Potential Cell Based Therapy for Parkinson's Disease. Curr Stem Cell Res Ther. 2017;12(4):326-47.

[19] Aghebati-Maleki L, Dolati S, Zandi R, Fotouhi A, Ahmadi M, Aghebati A, et al. Prospect of mesenchymal stem cells in therapy of osteoporosis: A review. J Cell Physiol. 2019;234(6):8570-8.

[20] Gaur M, Dobke M, Lunyak VV. Mesenchymal Stem Cells from Adipose Tissue in Clinical Applications for Dermatological Indications and Skin Aging. Int J Mol Sci. 2017;18(1).

[21] Chakari-Khiavi F, Dolati S, Chakari-Khiavi A, Abbaszadeh H, Aghebati-Maleki L, Pourlak T, et al. Prospects for the application of mesenchymal stem cells in Alzheimer's disease treatment. Life Sci. 2019;231:116564.

[22] Mao F, Tu Q, Wang L, Chu F, Li X, Li HS, et al. Mesenchymal stem cells and their therapeutic applications in inflammatory bowel disease. Oncotarget. 2017;8(23):38008-21.

[23] Shin TH, Kim HS, Choi SW, Kang KS. Mesenchymal Stem Cell Therapy for Inflammatory Skin Diseases: Clinical Potential and Mode of Action. Int J Mol Sci. 2017;18(2).

[24] Zakirova EY, Valeeva AN, Aimaletdinov AM, Nefedovskaya LV, Akhmetshin RF, Rutland CS, et al. Potential therapeutic application of mesenchymal stem cells in ophthalmology. Experimental Eye Research. 2019;189:107863.

[25] Li H, Tian Y, Xie L, Liu X, Huang Z, Su W. Mesenchymal stem cells in allergic diseases: Current status. Allergol Int. 2020;69(1):35-45.

[26] Lazzeri E, Romagnani P, Lasagni L. Stem cell therapy for kidney disease. Expert Opin Biol Ther. 2015;15(10):1455-68.

[27] Qin Y, Guan J, Zhang C. Mesenchymal stem cells: mechanisms and role in bone regeneration. Postgrad Med J. 2014;90(1069):643-7.

[28] Zheng H, Zhang B, Chhatbar PY, Dong Y, Alawieh A, Lowe F, et al. Mesenchymal Stem Cell Therapy in Stroke: A Systematic Review of Literature in Pre-Clinical and Clinical Research. Cell transplantation. 2018;27(12):1723-30.

[29] Sherman LS, Romagano MP, Williams SF, Rameshwar P. Mesenchymal stem cell therapies in brain disease. Seminars in Cell & Developmental Biology. 2019;95:111-9.

[30] Dasari VR, Veeravalli KK, Dinh DH. Mesenchymal stem cells in the treatment of spinal cord injuries: A review. World J Stem Cells. 2014;6(2):120-33.

[31] Mundra V, Gerling IC, Mahato RI. Mesenchymal stem cell-based therapy. Mol Pharm. 2013;10(1):77-89.

[32] Hass R, Kasper C, Bohm S, Jacobs R. Different populations and sources of human mesenchymal stem cells (MSC): A comparison of adult and neonatal tissue-derived MSC. Cell Commun Signal. 2011;9:12.

[33] Wislet-Gendebien S, Hans G, Leprince P, Rigo JM, Moonen G, Rogister B. Plasticity of cultured mesenchymal stem cells: switch from nestin-positive to excitable neuron-like phenotype. Stem Cells. 2005;23(3):392-402.

[34] Zachar L, Bačenková D, Rosocha J. Activation, homing, and role of the mesenchymal stem cells in the inflammatory environment. J Inflamm Res. 2016;9:231-40.

[35] Andersen RK, Zaher W, Larsen KH, Ditzel N, Drews K, Wruck W, et al. Association between in vivo bone formation and ex vivo migratory capacity of human bone marrow stromal cells. Stem Cell Res Ther. 2015;6:196.

[36] Watanabe S, Uchida K, Nakajima H, Matsuo H, Sugita D, Yoshida A, et al. Early transplantation of mesenchymal stem cells after spinal cord injury relieves pain hypersensitivity through suppression of pain-related signaling cascades and reduced inflammatory cell recruitment. Stem Cells. 2015;33(6):1902-14.

[37] Quertainmont R, Cantinieaux D, Botman O, Sid S, Schoenen J, Franzen R. Mesenchymal stem cell graft improves recovery after spinal cord injury in adult rats through neurotrophic and pro-angiogenic actions. PloS one. 2012;7(6):e39500.

[38] De Ugarte DA, Morizono K, Elbarbary A, Alfonso Z, Zuk PA, Zhu M, et al. Comparison of multi-lineage cells from human adipose tissue and bone marrow. Cells Tissues Organs. 2003;174(3):101-9.

[39] Zuk PA, Zhu M, Mizuno H, Huang J, Futrell JW, Katz AJ, et al. Multilineage cells from human adipose tissue: implications for cell-based therapies. Tissue Eng. 2001;7(2):211-28.

[40] Ohta Y, Hamaguchi A, Ootaki M, Watanabe M, Takeba Y, Iiri T, et al. Intravenous infusion of adipose-derived stem/stromal cells improves functional recovery of rats with spinal cord injury. Cytotherapy. 2017;19(7):839-48.

[41] Kolar MK, Kingham PJ, Novikova LN, Wiberg M, Novikov LN. The therapeutic effects of human adipose-derived stem cells in a rat cervical spinal cord injury model. Stem Cells Dev. 2014;23(14):1659-74.

[42] Kim Y, Lee SH, Kim WH, Kweon OK. Transplantation of adipose derived mesenchymal stem cells for acute thoracolumbar disc disease with no deep pain perception in dogs. J Vet Sci. 2016;17(1):123-6.

[43] Menezes K, Nascimento MA, Gonçalves JP, Cruz AS, Lopes DV, Curzio B, et al. Human mesenchymal cells from adipose tissue deposit laminin and promote regeneration of injured spinal cord in rats. PLoS One. 2014;9(5):e96020.

[44] Ryu HH, Kang BJ, Park SS, Kim Y, Sung GJ, Woo HM, et al. Comparison of mesenchymal stem cells derived from fat, bone marrow, Wharton's jelly, and umbilical cord blood for treating spinal cord injuries in dogs. J Vet Med Sci. 2012;74(12):1617-30.

[45] Chua SJ, Bielecki R, Yamanaka N, Fehlings MG, Rogers IM, Casper RF. The effect of umbilical cord blood cells on outcomes after experimental traumatic spinal cord injury. Spine (Phila Pa 1976). 2010;35(16):1520-6.

[46] Yousefifard M, Nasirinezhad F, Shardi Manaheji H, Janzadeh A, Hosseini M, Keshavarz M. Human bone marrow-derived and umbilical cord-derived mesenchymal stem cells for alleviating neuropathic pain in a spinal cord injury model. Stem cell research & therapy. 2016;7:36-.

[47] Liu J, Han D, Wang Z, Xue M, Zhu L, Yan H, et al. Clinical analysis of the treatment of spinal cord injury with umbilical cord mesenchymal stem cells. Cytotherapy. 2013;15(2):185-91.

[48] Cofano F, Boido M, Monticelli M, Zenga F, Ducati A, Vercelli A, et al. Mesenchymal Stem Cells for Spinal Cord Injury: Current Options, Limitations, and Future of Cell Therapy. Int J Mol Sci. 2019;20(11).

[49] Kim EY, Lee KB, Kim MK. The potential of mesenchymal stem cells derived from amniotic membrane and amniotic fluid for neuronal regenerative therapy. BMB Rep. 2014;47(3):135-40.

[50] Bottai D, Scesa G, Cigognini D, Adami R, Nicora E, Abrignani S, et al. Third trimester NG2-positive amniotic fluid cells are effective in improving repair in spinal cord injury. Experimental neurology. 2014;254:121-33.

[51] Gao S, Ding J, Xiao HJ, Li ZQ, Chen Y, Zhou XS, et al. Anti-inflammatory and anti-apoptotic effect of combined treatment with methylprednisolone and amniotic membrane mesenchymal stem cells after spinal cord injury in rats. Neurochem Res. 2014;39(8):1544-52.

[52] Sankar V, Muthusamy R. Role of human amniotic epithelial cell transplantation in spinal cord injury repair research. Neuroscience. 2003;118(1):11-7.

[53] Roh DH, Seo MS, Choi HS, Park SB, Han HJ, Beitz AJ, et al. Transplantation of human umbilical cord blood or amniotic epithelial stem cells alleviates mechanical allodynia after spinal cord injury in rats. Cell Transplant. 2013;22(9):1577-90.

[54] Sharif-Alhoseini M, Khormali M, Rezaei M, Safdarian M, Hajighadery A, Khalatbari MM, et al. Animal models of spinal cord injury: a systematic review. Spinal Cord. 2017;55(8):714-21.

[55] Vandamme TF. Use of rodents as models of human diseases. J Pharm Bioallied Sci. 2014;6(1):2-9.

[56] Friedli L, Rosenzweig ES, Barraud Q, Schubert M, Dominici N, Awai L, et al. Pronounced species divergence in corticospinal tract reorganization and functional recovery after lateralized spinal cord injury favors primates. Sci Transl Med. 2015;7(302):302ra134.

[57] Penha EM, Aguiar PH, Barrouin-Melo SM, de Lima RS, da Silveira AC, Otelo AR, et al. Clinical neurofunctional rehabilitation of a cat with spinal cord injury after hemilaminectomy and autologous stem cell transplantation. Int J Stem Cells. 2012;5(2):146-50.

[58] Penha EM, Meira CS, Guimarães ET, Mendonça MV, Gravely FA, Pinheiro CM, et al. Use of autologous mesenchymal stem cells derived from bone marrow for the treatment of naturally injured spinal cord in dogs. Stem Cells Int. 2014;2014:437521.

[59] Paul C, Samdani AF, Betz RR, Fischer I, Neuhuber B. Grafting of human bone marrow stromal cells into spinal cord injury: a comparison of delivery methods. Spine (Phila Pa 1976). 2009;34(4):328-34.

[60] Carvalho KA, Vialle EN, Moreira GH, Cunha RC, Simeoni RB, Francisco JC, et al. Functional outcome of bone marrow stem cells (CD45(+)/CD34(−)) after cell therapy in chronic spinal cord injury in Wistar rats. Transplant Proc. 2008;40(3):845-6.

[61] Shin DA, Kim JM, Kim HI, Yi S, Ha Y, Yoon DH, et al. Comparison of functional and histological outcomes after intralesional, intracisternal, and intravenous transplantation of human bone marrow-derived mesenchymal stromal cells in a rat model of spinal cord injury. Acta Neurochir (Wien). 2013;155(10):1943-50.

[62] Kim JW, Ha KY, Molon JN, Kim YH. Bone marrow-derived mesenchymal

stem cell transplantation for chronic spinal cord injury in rats: comparative study between intralesional and intravenous transplantation. Spine (Phila Pa 1976). 2013;38(17):E1065-74.

[63] Takahashi Y, Tsuji O, Kumagai G, Hara CM, Okano HJ, Miyawaki A, et al. Comparative study of methods for administering neural stem/progenitor cells to treat spinal cord injury in mice. Cell Transplant. 2011;20(5):727-39.

[64] Ichihara K, Taguchi T, Shimada Y, Sakuramoto I, Kawano S, Kawai S. Gray matter of the bovine cervical spinal cord is mechanically more rigid and fragile than the white matter. J Neurotrauma. 2001;18(3):361-7.

[65] Osaka M, Honmou O, Murakami T, Nonaka T, Houkin K, Hamada H, et al. Intravenous administration of mesenchymal stem cells derived from bone marrow after contusive spinal cord injury improves functional outcome. Brain Res. 2010;1343:226-35.

[66] Matsushita T, Lankford KL, Arroyo EJ, Sasaki M, Neyazi M, Radtke C, et al. Diffuse and persistent blood-spinal cord barrier disruption after contusive spinal cord injury rapidly recovers following intravenous infusion of bone marrow mesenchymal stem cells. Exp Neurol. 2015;267:152-64.

[67] Badner A, Vawda R, Laliberte A, Hong J, Mikhail M, Jose A, et al. Early Intravenous Delivery of Human Brain Stromal Cells Modulates Systemic Inflammation and Leads to Vasoprotection in Traumatic Spinal Cord Injury. Stem Cells Transl Med. 2016;5(8):991-1003.

[68] Vawda R, Badner A, Hong J, Mikhail M, Lakhani A, Dragas R, et al. Early Intravenous Infusion of Mesenchymal Stromal Cells Exerts a Tissue Source Age-Dependent Beneficial Effect on Neurovascular Integrity and Neurobehavioral Recovery After Traumatic Cervical Spinal Cord Injury. Stem Cells Transl Med. 2019;8(7):639-49.

[69] Yoshihara T, Ohta M, Itokazu Y, Matsumoto N, Dezawa M, Suzuki Y, et al. Neuroprotective effect of bone marrow-derived mononuclear cells promoting functional recovery from spinal cord injury. J Neurotrauma. 2007;24(6):1026-36.

[70] Kanekiyo K, Nakano N, Homma T, Yamada Y, Tamachi M, Suzuki Y, et al. Effects of Multiple Injection of Bone Marrow Mononuclear Cells on Spinal Cord Injury of Rats. J Neurotrauma. 2017;34(21):3003-11.

[71] Witiw CD, Fehlings MG. Acute Spinal Cord Injury. Clinical Spine Surgery. 2015;28(6).

[72] Chen X, Xue B, Li Y, Song C, Jia P, Ren X, et al. Meta-analysis of stem cell transplantation for reflex hypersensitivity after spinal cord injury. Neuroscience. 2017;363:66-75.

[73] Zhao T, Yan W, Xu K, Qi Y, Dai X, Shi Z. Combined treatment with platelet-rich plasma and brain-derived neurotrophic factor-overexpressing bone marrow stromal cells supports axonal remyelination in a rat spinal cord hemi-section model. Cytotherapy. 2013;15(7):792-804.

[74] Ghasemi N, Razavi S, Mardani M, Esfandiari E, Salehi H, Zarkesh Esfahani SH. Transplantation of human adipose-derived stem cells enhances remyelination in lysolecithin-induced focal demyelination of rat spinal cord. Mol Biotechnol. 2014;56(5):470-8.

[75] Razavi S, Ghasemi N, Mardani M, Salehi H. Remyelination improvement after neurotrophic factors secreting cells transplantation in rat spinal cord injury. Iranian journal of basic medical sciences. 2017;20(4):392-8.

[76] Someya Y, Koda M, Dezawa M, Kadota T, Hashimoto M, Kamada T, et al. Reduction of cystic cavity, promotion of axonal regeneration and sparing, and functional recovery with transplanted bone marrow stromal cell-derived Schwann cells after contusion injury to the adult rat spinal cord: Laboratory investigation. Journal of neurosurgery Spine. 2009;9:600-10.

[77] Neuhuber B, Timothy Himes B, Shumsky JS, Gallo G, Fischer I. Axon growth and recovery of function supported by human bone marrow stromal cells in the injured spinal cord exhibit donor variations. Brain Research. 2005;1035(1):73-85.

[78] Gu W, Zhang F, Xue Q, Ma Z, Lu P, Yu B. Transplantation of bone marrow mesenchymal stem cells reduces lesion volume and induces axonal regrowth of injured spinal cord. Neuropathology. 2010;30(3):205-17.

[79] Basso DM, Beattie MS, Bresnahan JC. A sensitive and reliable locomotor rating scale for open field testing in rats. Journal of neurotrauma. 1995;12(1):1-21.

[80] Himes BT, Neuhuber B, Coleman C, Kushner R, Swanger SA, Kopen GC, et al. Recovery of Function Following Grafting of Human Bone Marrow-Derived Stromal Cells into the Injured Spinal Cord. Neurorehabilitation and Neural Repair. 2006;20(2):278-96.

[81] Yang CC, Shih YH, Ko MH, Hsu SY, Cheng H, Fu YS. Transplantation of human umbilical mesenchymal stem cells from Wharton's jelly after complete transection of the rat spinal cord. PloS one. 2008;3(10):e3336.

[82] Park HC, Shim YS, Ha Y, Yoon SH, Park SR, Choi BH, et al. Treatment of complete spinal cord injury patients by autologous bone marrow cell transplantation and administration of granulocyte-macrophage colony stimulating factor. Tissue Eng. 2005;11(5-6):913-22.

[83] Vaquero J, Zurita M, Rico MA, Aguayo C, Bonilla C, Marin E, et al. Intrathecal administration of autologous mesenchymal stromal cells for spinal cord injury: Safety and efficacy of the 100/3 guideline. Cytotherapy. 2018;20(6):806-19.

[84] Mendonça MVP, Larocca TF, de Freitas Souza BS, Villarreal CF, Silva LFM, Matos AC, et al. Safety and neurological assessments after autologous transplantation of bone marrow mesenchymal stem cells in subjects with chronic spinal cord injury. Stem cell research & therapy. 2014;5(6):126-.

[85] Vaquero J, Zurita M, Rico MA, Aguayo C, Fernandez C, Rodriguez-Boto G, et al. Cell therapy with autologous mesenchymal stromal cells in post-traumatic syringomyelia. Cytotherapy. 2018;20(6):796-805.

[86] Derakhshanrad N, Saberi H, Tayebi Meybodi K, Taghvaei M, Arjmand B, Aghayan HR, et al. Case Report: Combination Therapy with Mesenchymal Stem Cells and Granulocyte-Colony Stimulating Factor in a Case of Spinal Cord Injury. Basic and clinical neuroscience. 2015;6(4):299-305.

[87] Marsala M, Kamizato K, Tadokoro T, Navarro M, Juhas S, Juhasova J, et al. Spinal parenchymal occupation by neural stem cells after subpial delivery in adult immunodeficient rats. Stem Cells Transl Med. 2020;9(2):177-88.

[88] Lee JR, Kyung JW, Kumar H, Kwon SP, Song SY, Han IB, et al. Targeted Delivery of Mesenchymal Stem Cell-Derived Nanovesicles for Spinal Cord Injury Treatment. Int J Mol Sci. 2020;21(11).

Chapter 4

Strategies to Repair Spinal Cord Injuries: Single Vs. Combined Treatments

Vinnitsa Buzoianu-Anguiano and Ismael Jiménez Estrada

Abstract

Several experimental strategies have been developed in past years for the repair of damages evoked in axons, myelin, and motor functions by spinal cord injuries. This chapter briefly reviews some of such strategies. On the one hand, it examines individual procedures, such as: tissue or cell transplants (i.e. evolving cells of the olfactory glia or mesenchymal cells), implants of biomaterials (fibrine and chitosan), application of enzymes (chondroitinase and ChABC), growth factors (brain-derived neurotrophic factor, BDNF; neurotrophin-3, NT-3; or glial-derived neurotrophic factor, GDNF), and drugs (myocyclines or riluzole) among others, that induce different recovery degrees in axonal regeneration, myelination, and motor performance in experimental animals. On the other hand, it also examines the recent strategy of combining some of the previous experimental procedures to potentialize the positive effects evoked by each one in experimentally spinal cord lesioned animals and explores the possible use of this strategy in future preclinical research for the treatment of spinal cord lesions.

Keywords: spinal cord injury, cell therapy, tissue transplants, biomaterials, axonal regeneration, neuroprotection, remyelination, motor function, exogen factors

1. Introduction

It is known that the regenerative potential of the central nervous system (CNS) is limited by both extrinsic and intrinsic factors, which restrict axonal growth in adult animals. These factors include proteins associated with myelin or with the formation of a fibroglial scar, which creates a physical and chemical barrier. This barrier secretes factors from the extracellular matrix that prevents axonal growth after a traumatic spinal cord injury (TSCI) [1].

Among the myelin-associated molecules, there are NogoA, myelin-associated glycoprotein (MAG), and oligodendrocyte-associated glycoprotein (OMgp). It has been shown that, after a TSCI, these proteins favor the inhibition of axonal and neuritic growth as well as the formation of collaterals. In addition, they can form aberrant connectivity [2].

The inhibitory activity of NogoA, MAG, and Omgp after a TSCI occurs by the activation of these proteins by binding to their NGR1 receptor, which can be anchored to the GPI protein (**Figure 1**). This receptor has been reported to be specific for these proteins, promoting the inhibitory effect for axonal growth after TSCI [3]. When

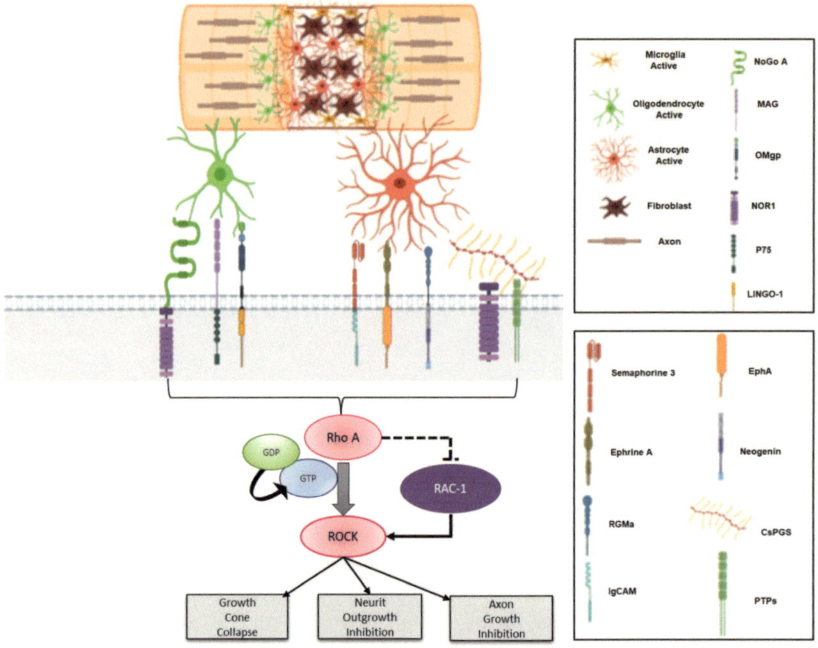

Figure 1.
Molecules that inhibit axonal growth. After a TSCI in the injury area, a fibroglial scar forms forming a physical barrier preventing axonal growth. At the same time, a chemical barrier is initiated by the activation of molecules such as MAG, NogoA, and OMgp secreted by reactive oligodendrocytes, which bind with their NGR1, P75, and Lingo receptors; or molecules secreted by reactive astrocytes such as Semaforin 3, Ephrine A, RGMa, and CsPG that also bind to their receptors such as IgCAM, EphA, Neoginine, NGR1, and PTPs; the union of these receptors with their ligands causes the activation of the RhoA pathway by GDP-GTP phosphorylation promoting the activation of ROCK kinase favoring the collapse of the axonal cone, inhibition of neuritic growth, and inhibition of axonal growth.

NgR1 is anchored to its GPI protein, in its intracellular domain, different co-receptors are activated that favor the activation of axonal inhibition signaling. In this activation, the two molecules P75 (molecule belonging to the TNF receptor) and TOY (LINGO-1) are involved. Activation of this co-receptor complex favors the activation of a RhoA kinase, which activates another ROCK kinase, in turn promoting the activation of LIM. This LIM kinase can activate the cofilin factor, thus causing the collapse of the axonal cone and depolymerization of the actin filaments [3, 4].

On the other hand, the glial reaction, which happens after the injury, promotes the recruitment of the microglia, oligodendrocyte precursors, meninges cells, and astrocytes in their reactive form at the site of the injury [5]. The result of this cell migration is the formation of a physical barrier, the fibroglial scar, which has the function of isolating the area of injury from the rest of the tissue, secreting factors that cause axonal growth to be inhibited in order to avoid aberrant connectivity. The factors that are present in the glial scar are: tenacines, semaphorins, ephrines, and chondroitin sulfate proteoglycans [1]. These molecules that are expressed from the extracellular matrix after a TSCI promote inhibition of axonal and neuritic growth as well as collapse of the axonal cone [6, 7].

The activation of all these molecules is due to an RHO-(RhoA) kinase; by activating the RhoA signaling pathway, it causes a decrease in the activity of RAC1 kinase, through binding to the PTPα receptor (transmembrane protein tyrosine phosphatase), in addition to LAR and NGR1 and 3 leukocyte-related phosphatase. This causes RhoA to be phosphorylated from Rho-GDP to Rho-GTP, activating ROCK kinase, thereby promoting inhibition of axonal growth (**Figure 1**; [6, 7]).

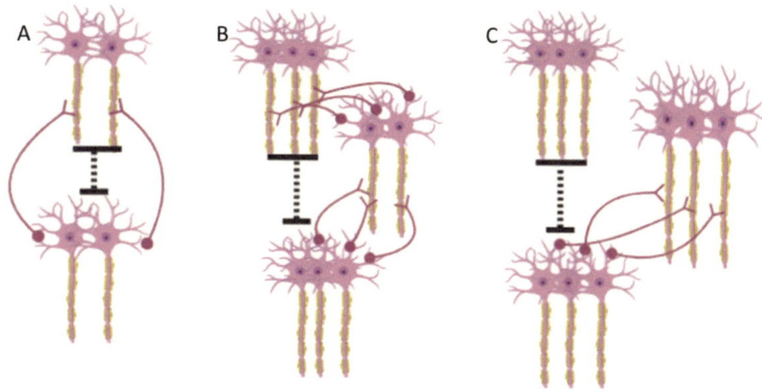

Figure 2.
Diagram of the proposed strategies for reinnervation after a spinal cord injury. (A) Long distance axonal regeneration; (B) short-distance regeneration; (C) growth of preserved axons.

Other molecules that intervene in the repulsive environment after a TSCI are the axonal repulsive guidance molecules (RGM), especially the RGMa isoform, which inhibits neuritic growth present at the site of injury (**Figure 1**). It can also cause poor axonal growth and loss of functionality [6, 8]. RGMa is activated when it binds to its neoginin receptor, causing an activation of RHO-GEF (guanine exchange factor), which in turn activates RhoA kinase. This sparks the activation of another ROCK kinase through the phosphorylation of a GTP (guanosine triphosphate). This in turn triggers the regulation of various proteins such as MCL (myosin light chain), which promotes the inhibition of neuritic growth, the LIM kinase, which causes the activation of the actin and cofilin polymerization factor, and CRMP-2 (collapsing 2 response mediator protein), which causes inhibition of neuritic growth and inhibition of axonal growth [6].

As we have seen, all these signals foster a repulsive environment for axonal growth after a spinal cord injury, which nullifies the regenerative capacity of the CNS. Some hypotheses have been proposed for reinnervation after a spinal cord injury: (1) long-distance regeneration via creating an appropriate synaptic connection by branching off new axons, which could make new connections with target cells, from originally damaged axons; (2) short-distance regeneration via enabling the formation of collateral branches that can form synaptic contacts with neighboring cells, which, in turn, can connect with the target cells of the damaged axons; and (3) growth of preserved axons which can maintain a connection with the target cells from the site of injury (**Figure 2**) [3].

2. Simple treatments that improve axonal regeneration and locomotive function

Based on the previous hypotheses, strategies have been designed with, among others, tissue transplants, biomaterials, cell therapies, and exogenous factors to favor axonal regeneration, remyelination, and improvement of locomotor function in animal models with a TSCI. We will discuss some of these strategies in this chapter.

Predegenerated peripheral nerve (PPN) transplants have been used to repair injuries to the peripheral nervous system (PNS), by being used as a bridge to promote axonal regeneration and re-functionalization [9], favoring axonal regeneration and refunctionalization after a TSCI, since they act as a neuroprotector in the medulla after transplanting it [10]. Moreover, it helps as a guide for axons to grow through the nerve and connect to both proximal and distal axons [11–14].

Axonal growth occurs due to the permissive microenvironment derived from Schwann cells and macrophages present in PPNs, which secrete growth factors such as GDNF, BDNF, NGF, NT-3, NT-4, and GM-CS [15–17]. In addition, Schwann cells form Bügner bands, which support axonal growth [18–20].

3. Use of inert bridges

The use of biomaterial bridges has been an attractive alternative for neuroregeneration. Inert bridges are temporary structures that support cell and tissue growth. These materials are biodegradable, they can foster mechanical strength, they can be fibers or porous channels, and they have the capacity of cell adhesion [21]. Hydrogels, which are biocompatible implants for repair after a TSCI, also form bridges for regeneration as well as preventing fibroglial scar formation, thus promoting a permissive environment for regeneration. Third-dimensional nanofibers have also been designed, which provide better cell adhesion and promote migration, cell proliferation, and differentiation [21].

These bridges can be made of biological materials such as collagen or fibronectin; or of natural polymers such as alignate, agarose, or chitosan; or they can also be composed of synthetic polymers such as polyhydroxy-α, poly-2-hydroxyethylmethacrylate, or polyethylene glycol [22, 23].

It has been shown that these materials in TSCI models (contusions, transection, or hemisections) can favor and direct axonal growth, since they act as bridges [24, 25]. They have also been found to be compatible when used in combination with other treatments such as cell or trophic factors, promoting a permissive environment for this axonal growth [26–28]. Furthermore, it has been observed that they help the adhesion of oligodendrocytes, or Schwann cells, thus favoring remyelination of damaged axons [29].

4. Cellular therapy

The term cellular therapy (CT) refers to any type of strategy that uses cells as a therapeutic agent. Neural transplantation has been used to repair injured SC in both acute and chronic phases. The use of cell transplants has been a positive alternative for axonal regeneration. Different cell types have been used during these transplants such as: Schwann cells, olfactory ensheathing glia (OEG) cells, embryonic stem cells, hematopoietic cells, neural stem cells and bone marrow stromal cells (BMSCs) [30].

4.1 Schwann cells

In the PNS, unlike the CNS, regeneration is efficient due to the presence of Schwann cells (Cs). Cs have been used to perform transplants in different animal models since they are capable of: engulfing cellular debris, producing trophic factors necessary for the survival of the neuron (especially brain-derived neurotrophic factor (BDNF) and neurotrophin 4/5 (NT4/5)), secreting cell matrices of inhibitory molecules that help axonal regrowth, and producing myelin layers to envelop the naked axons and increase the impulse speed of nerve cells to improve their functioning [31]. In rodent models, Cs implants have been shown to foster remyelination, thus improving motor functions in contusion and complete section injuries [32, 33]. Combination with other materials has also been shown to help guide axonal regrowth after a TSCI [34, 35].

4.2 Olfactory ensheathing glia cells

Olfactory ensheathing glia cells (OEG) are a type of glial cells that are present in the olfactory system of adult mammals. In both acute and chronic injuries, OEGs have been shown to have the ability to promote axonal regeneration and help restore axonal conduction after TSCI [36].

Ramón-Cueto et al. demonstrated that OEG aided in the regrowth of sensory axons after spinal injury [37]. Doucette et al. described the survival of the OEG after having transplanted them in brain [38]. In contusion and transection models, the ability of OEGs to help protect the tissue after transplantation has been demonstrated, since they promote axonal growth and favor the improvement of locomotor function [39, 40]. OEGs have been said to have similar properties to Schwann cells and astrocytes, which make them unique. This cell type has two important benefits: they can exist both inside and outside the central nervous system, and they can be in constant neurogenesis, producing sensitive neurons in both embryonic and adult stages in mammals [41].

4.3 Mesenchymal cells

Mesenchymal stem cells, or mesenchymal stromal cells (MSCs), are adult multipotent cells that have the capacity for self-renewal, proliferation, and differentiation. MSCs are an alternative for the experimental treatment of a spinal cord injury (contusions, transection, or ischemia). They have shown that they favor axonal regeneration and improve locomotor function [42–45]. They also have the ability to form bridging cell bundles at the TSCI epicenter [45–48] and can be differentiated both in vitro and in vivo in neurons, astrocytes, oligodendrocytes, Schwann cells, and microglia [49, 50].

Vaquero and colleagues have observed that after a TSCI, the use of MSCs and Schwann cells as therapy was beneficial not only because they observed axonal regeneration, but also because at different times (up to 9 months with transplantation), animals with severe contusions eventually recovered locomotive function (with a score of 16 on the BBB scale) [51–55]. Other studies have shown that MSCs give positive results when used in diseases or damage the nervous system by secreting growth factors such as neural growth factor (NGF), brain-derived neurotrophic factor (BDNF), neurotrophin 3 (NT-3), basic fibroblast growth factor (bFGF), vascular endothelial growth factor (VEGF), and hepatocyte growth factor (HGF). They can also secrete cytokines such as interleukin-6 (IL-6), colony stimulating factor 1 (CSF-1), monocyte chemoattractant protein (MCP), colony stimulating factor (CSF), and stromal cell derived factor (SDF-1) [42, 56]. In addition, they promote angiogenesis, proliferate after transplantation, aid neuronal survival, and decrease apoptosis [56]. Moreover, another important factor of MSCs is the immunomodulatory effect, since they are capable of secreting soluble inflammatory-mediating factors such as indolamine 2–3 dioxygenase (IDO), inducible nitric oxide synthase (iNOS), and homo-oxygenase 1. They can also secrete the human leukocyte G antigen, transforming factor β (TGF-β), interleukin 6 (IL-6), and prostaglandin E2. These soluble factors promote the inhibition of CD4+CD8+ T cells [57]. It has been shown in contusions and compressions that using MSCs helps decrease proinflammatory cytokines such as TNF-α and IL-6, and promotes the secretion of anti-inflammatory cytokines such as IL-4, IL-10, and IL-13, which promotes the activation of M2 macrophages by fostering a neuroprotective environment [58, 59].

5. Exogenous factors

Neurotrophins are structural proteins consisting of four families, which are involved in events in the development of the CNS such as survival, differentiation, and axonal growth. Among these, we find neuronal growth factor NGF, neurotrophin 3 (NT-3), neurotrophin 4/5 (NT-4/5), and brain-derived growth factor (BDNF). These neurotrophins bind directly to Trk receptors (tropomycin kinase receptors): NGF binds to its TrkA receptor, BDNF and NT4/5 bind to the same TrkB receptor, and NT-3 binds to its TrkC receptor. They also have a high affinity for the p75 receptor, NTR [60].

Studies on contusions, transections, and hemisections have shown that the most studied neurotrophins are BDNF and NT-3. The use of BDNF has been seen to promote neuroprotection, form collateral branches, and promote plasticity [61]. It also favors axonal growth, thus improving locomotor function [62, 63]. Moreover, in different models of contusion, transection, and hemisections, it was demonstrated that the exogenous use of NT-3 favors axonal regrowth and improvement of locomotor function [64, 65].

As for NGF and NT4/5, they are the least studied within TSCI models. NGF has been shown to promote the growth of sensory axons [66, 67], and in a contusion study, it reduced neuronal death, thus promoting an improvement in locomotive function [68]. NT4/5, like BDNF, can promote neuroprotection and axonal growth in a full-section model [69].

Another factor used chondroitinase ABC (ChABC), an enzyme from the bacteria *Proteus Vulgaris*. ChABC can bind to the chains of the GAG glycosaminoglycans, within the disaccharides, which favors the digestion of chondroitin sulfates (CSPGs) [70]. It has been seen that both in hemisection and transection models, this enzyme favors axonal growth [71, 72]. Moreover, in the presence of growth factors such as NT-3 and BDNF, it promotes the proliferation of oligodendrocytes, increasing remyelination and favoring improvement in locomotor function [71, 73, 74].

6. Pharmacological use

Successful drug trials on animals have been carried out and have advanced to human clinical trials; however, none of them has shown a clear improvement on patients. Some of the drugs used in TSCIs will be mentioned.

Methylprednisolone (MPP) is a synthetic steroid from the glucocorticoid group, which is used for its immunosuppressive and anti-inflammatory properties. Its mechanism of action is to inhibit the formation of arachidonic acid and decrease inflammation. In studies of animals with a TSCI, it has been observed that the administration of MPP favors the reduction of apoptosis. It also induces the interaction with the glucocorticoid receptor HIF-1α, which decreases the damage of oligodendrocytes [75]. In clinical studies with acute injuries, the use of MPP has been shown to improve functionality and sensitivity when compared to patients who only took the placebo [76–78].

Another drug used is riluzole, a benzothiasilic anticonvulsant, which acts as a blocker of sodium channels. Fehlings and colleagues compared the effect of riluzole with phenytoin in an acute contusion injury model, where they observed promoted functional recovery [79]. In studies with patients with acute injury, riluzole has been observed to prompt sensory and locomotor improvement [80].

Minocycline, a second-generation synthetic tetracycline, has also been used as an antibacterial agent. This medication can stay in the CNS longer than the usual tetracycline since it can cross the blood-brain barrier. It can act as a neuroprotector by reducing inflammation and preventing cell death [81]. In studies with patients with acute cervical and thoracic injuries, it was observed that the administration of minocycline did not cause side effects in patients. Additionally, in patients with cervical injuries, it improved locomotor function when compared to patients who took only the placebo. However, in patients with thoracic lesions, no changes were observed. In this study, it was concluded that the effect of minocycline with more patients should be evaluated to verify its efficacy [82].

7. Combined treatments

As described in previous paragraphs, the use of different strategies as simple treatments in TSCI models promotes neuroprotection, axonal growth, and remyelination of damaged axons, and facilitates the improvement of locomotor function. Therefore, it has been determined that the combination of different strategies should be able to more effectively facilitate axonal growth and remyelination, helping to increase locomotor function.

The effect of using PPN transplantation in combination with ChABC or growth factors has been evaluated. It was shown that the animals with combined treatment had a greater number of regenerated axons and an increase in the improvement of locomotor function, unlike those animals with simple treatment [83, 84]. It was also demonstrated that by, in comparison with single treatments, combining PPN with FGFα, and PPN with ChABC, a favorable microenvironment was formed, increasing axonal growth [11, 85].

The effect of MSCs combined with chitosan bridges or with growth factors such as the granulocyte colony-stimulating factor (G-CSF) has also been studied, and it was observed that animals on combined treatments, compared to simple treatments, had greater axonal growth, thus improving locomotor function [46, 86]. In a chronic phase compression model, the combination of MSCs with ChABC increased axonal growth in comparison to single treatments [87].

It was also observed that animals, after 2 months of PPN and MSC transplants in a full-section model, had a greater number of growing axons by detecting GAP43 as well as an improvement in remyelination by detection of PBM and by electron microscopy, unlike animals treated with simple transplantation [88]. When making a triple combination of PPN with MSCs and ChABC, an increase in axonal regeneration was observed after 3 months, improving locomotor function [89].

On the other hand, the combination of ChABC with growth factors such as BDNF and NT-3 can promote greater axonal growth and favor the proliferation of oligodendrocytes, thus increasing remyelination compared to animals that only had separate treatments [71, 73, 74]. Also, in a full section model in the acute phase, the combination of ChABC with NT-3 increased axonal growth and improved locomotor function, unlike groups with single treatments [73]. It was also demonstrated in a chronic transection model that a ChABC injection with rehabilitation inhibited the formation of chondroitin sulfates, promoting increased axonal growth, unlike single treatment groups [72].

8. Clinical trials

Independent of the type of traumatic spinal lesión (contusion, compression, or sectioning), the treatment of a spinal cord injury patient often begins at the site of the accident. Emergency personnel must gently and quickly immobilize and check the vital signs (urine retention, respiratory, and cardiovascular difficulty and formation

Treatment	Function	Advantages	Disadvantages	References
Neuroprotective				
Methylprednisolone	Corticosteroid drug that reduces inflammation	It has been shown in patients with complete SCI that improves locomotor function	Adverse events, infections, pneumonia, sepsis	[90–92]
Minocycline	Tetracycline, second generation antibiotics, with anti-inflammatory, antioxidant and anti-apoptotic effects	In patients with incomplete acute lesions, only very few present improvements in motor functions	No side effects are present	[90–92]
Riluzole	Anti-epileptic drug that blocks excitotoxic, blocking sodium channels	Increased motor function of patients with incomplete acute injuries	Increments of liver enzymes	[90–92]
Gacycline	NMDA receptor agonist	Patients with incomplete acute injuries showed no motor or sensory improvement	No adverse effects	[90–92]
Neuroregenerative				
FGF	Growth factor that binds to heparin protein and stimulates axonal regeneration, survival of neurons and decreases the fibroglial scar	No changes in motor and sensory function were observed in patients with complete spinal cord lesions	No side effects	[91, 93–95]
Cethrine	Transferase C3, toxin produced by Clostridium botulinum that blocks Rho kinase	Promotes axonal regeneration and improves the motor function of patients with complete acute phase injuries	No adverse effects	[91, 93–95]
Anti-Nogo A	Nogo A is a myelin protein that inhibits neuronal growth. Anti-NogoA antibody that inhibits Nogo A and promotes axonal regeneration	In patients with complete acute phase injuries, they showed no differences in motor and sensory function	No adverse effects	[91, 93–95]
Ganglioside GM1	Gangliosides— acidic glycoproteins present in cell membranes, which favor axonal regeneration	In patients with incomplete acute injuries improves motor function	No adverse effects	[91, 93–95]
Schwann cells	Myelinizing cells that function as an axonal support. They favor the myelinization of axons in the PNS	In patients with chronic complete injury it has been shown to promote motor and sensory recovery	Produce few adverse effects, muscle spasms and non-permanent paresthesia	[91, 93–95]

Treatment	Function	Advantages	Disadvantages	References
Olfactory ensheathing cells	Glial cells, with astrocyte properties. Promote axonal regeneration and improves locomotor function	In patients with chronic complete injuries showed scarce improvement in motor function	No adverse effects	[91, 93–95]
Mesenchymal cells	Induce the secretion of growth factors and promotes axonal regeneration, myelination and improvement of function	In patients with chronic complete injuries, it has been shown to promote motor improvement	No adverse effects	[91, 93–95]
Neural precursor cells	Multipotent CNS cells that reduce inflammation, promote cell replacement, and promote axonal regeneration	Patients with complete chronic injuries shows few improvements in motor function	No adverse effects	[91, 93–95]
Oligodendrocyte progenitor cells	They are able to secrete growth factors, promote axonal myelination and improved locomotor function	In patients with chronic complete injuries improves their motor function	No adverse effects	[91, 93–95]

Table 1.
Clinical trials of treatments for spinal cord injuries.

of coagules in extremities) and prepare the patient for transport. In the clinic, doctors may apply anti-inflammatory drugs or lower the body temperature—a condition known as hypothermia—for 24–48 h to help prevent damaging inflammation. The patient is subjected to a careful medical inspection and examination, testing for sensory function and movement, and by asking some questions about the accident. In addition, X-rays, computerized tomography (CT) scanning, and/or magnetic resonance imaging (MRI) tests may be needed to reveal vertebral (spinal column) problems such as: tumors, fractures or degenerative changes in the spine, herniated disks, blood clots, or other masses that may be compressing the spinal cord. Often, a surgery intervention is necessary to remove fragments of bones, foreign objects, herniated disks, or fractured vertebrae that appear to be compressing the spine. Subsequently to these tests, doctors begin to analyze which treatment will be applied to the SCI patient.

Over the past few decades, several therapeutic strategies have been developed to target TSCI pathology in clinic, including single and combined treatments with the main objective to cover two important aspects: neuroprotection and neuroregeneration. **Table 1** summarizes several clinic trials used for the treatment of TSCI, which have advantages and disadvantages in their application. However, it needs to be mentioned that until now there are no effective treatments for TSCI, which promote complete regeneration and restoration of motor and systemic functions in humans. Since spinal cord injury research has relied on animal models to understand the mechanisms of disease and develop pre-clinical models of treatment, there is no successful translation from pre-clinical to patient interventions that could be attributed to the limited understanding of biological differences between human and animal model systems.

9. Conclusions

As it can be seen, in this chapter, some of the strategies used in models of spinal cord injury were discussed, showing that they favor axonal regeneration, remyelination, and improvement of locomotor function. However, they have been insufficient as single treatments for preclinical and clinical therapies, which leads us to propose that the best option when dealing with TSCIs is to use combined treatments to increase the beneficial effects of each of the strategies, which could yield optimal results in clinical practice.

Author details

Vinnitsa Buzoianu-Anguiano[1] and Ismael Jiménez Estrada[2*]

1 Neuro-Regenerative Chemical Group, Paraplegic National Hospital, Healthcare Service of Castilla-la-Mancha (SESCAM), Toledo, Spain

2 Department of Physiology, Biophysics and Neurosciences, CINVESTAV, Instituto Politécnico Nacional (IPN), México, Mexico

*Address all correspondence to: ijimenez@fisio.cinvestav.mx

References

[1] Silver J, Miller JH. Regeneration beyond the glial scar. Nature Reviews. Neuroscience. 2004;**5**:146-156. DOI: 10.1038/nrn1326

[2] Schwab ME, Strittmatter SM. Nogo limits neural plasticity and recovery from injury. Current Opinion in Neurobiology. 2014;**1**:233-245. DOI: 10.1016/j.dcn.2011.01.002.The

[3] Giger RJ, Hollis ER, Tuszynski MH. Guidance molecules in axon regeneration. Cold Spring Harbor Perspectives in Biology. 2010;**2**:a001867. DOI: 10.1101/cshperspect.a001867

[4] Filbin MT. Myelin-associated inhibitors of axonal regeneration in the adult mammalian CNS. Nature Reviews. Neuroscience. 2003;**4**:703-713. DOI: 10.1038/nrn1195

[5] Chacón SC, Nieto-sampedro M. Pathophysiology of spinal cord injury. A review. MedVet. 2005;**36**:75-86

[6] Fujita Y, Yamashita T. Axon growth inhibition by rho A/ROCK in the central nervous system. Frontiers in Neuroscience. 2014;**8**:1-12. DOI: 10.3389/fnins.2014.00338

[7] Ohtake Y, Li S. Molecular mechanisms of scar-sourced axon growth inhibitors. Brain Research. 2015:1-14. DOI: 10.1016/j.brainres.2014.08.064

[8] Kubo T, Yamashita T. Rho-ROCK inhibitors for the treatment of CNS injury. Recent Patents on CNS Drug Discovery. 2007;**2**:173-179. DOI: 10.2174/157488907782411738

[9] Côté M-P, Amin AA, Tom VJ, Houle JD. Peripheral nerve grafts support regeneration after spinal cord injury. Neurotherapeutics. 2011a;**8**:294-303. DOI: 10.1007/s13311-011-0024-6

[10] Guizar-Sahagun G, Grijalva I, Madrazo I, Franco-Bourland R, Salgado-Ceballos H, Ibarra A, et al. Neuroprotection of completely lacerated spinal cord of adult rats by homotopic and heterotopic transplantation. Restorative Neurology and Neuroscience. 1994;**7**:61-70. DOI: 10.3233/RNN-1994-7201

[11] Côté M, Ph D, Hanna A, Lemay MA, Ollivier- K, Santi L, et al. Peripheral nerve grafts after cervical spinal cord injury in adult cats. Experimental Neurology. 2011;**225**:173-182. DOI: 10.1016/j.expneurol.2010.06.011. Peripheral

[12] Evans GRD. Peripheral nerve injury: A review and approach to tissue engineered constructs. The Anatomical Record. 2001;**404**:396-404. DOI: 10.1002/ar.1120

[13] Houle JD, Tom VJ, Mayes D, Wagoner G, Phillips N, Silver J. Combining an autologous peripheral nervous system "bridge" and matrix modification by chondroitinase allows robust, functional regeneration beyond a hemisection lesion of the adult rat spinal cord. The Journal of Neuroscience. 2006;**26**:7405-7415. DOI: 10.1523/JNEUROSCI.1166-06.2006

[14] Tom VJ, Sandrow-feinberg HR, Miller K, Santi L, Lemay MA, Houlé JD. Combining peripheral nerve grafts and chondroitinase promotes functional axonal regeneration in the chronically injured spinal cord. The Journal of Neuroscience. 2010;**29**:14881-14890. DOI: 10.1523/JNEUROSCI.3641-09.2009.Combining

[15] Bozkurt A, Deumens R, Beckmann C, Olde Damink L, Schügner F, Heschel I, et al. In vitro cell alignment obtained with a Schwann cell enriched microstructured nerve guide with longitudinal guidance channels.

Biomaterials. 2009;**30**:169-179. DOI: 10.1016/j.biomaterials.2008.09.017

[16] Höke A, Gordon T, Zochodne DW, Sulaiman OAR. A decline in glial cell-line-derived neurotrophic factor expression is associated with impaired regeneration after long-term Schwann cell denervation. Experimental Neurology. 2002;**173**:77-85. DOI: 10.1006/exnr.2001.7826

[17] Michalski B, Bain JR, Fahnestock M. Long-term changes in neurotrophic factor expression in distal nerve stump following denervation and reinnervation with motor or sensory nerve. Journal of Neurochemistry. 2008;**105**:1244-1252. DOI: 10.1111/j.1471-4159.2008.05224.x

[18] Ribeiro-Resende VT, Koenig B, Nichterwitz S, Oberhoffner S, Schlosshauer B. Strategies for inducing the formation of bands of Büngner in peripheral nerve regeneration. Biomaterials. 2009;**30**:5251-5259. DOI: 10.1016/j.biomaterials.2009.07.007

[19] Tom VJ, Houle JD. Peripheral nerve graft-mediated axonal regeneration. In: Neural Regeneration. Elsevier Inc.; 2015. DOI: 10.1016/B978-0-12-801732-6.00019-7

[20] Zhang Y, Campbell G, Anderson PN, Martini R, Schachner M, Lieberman AR. Molecular basis of interactions between regenerating adult rat thalamic axons and Schwann cells in peripheral nerve grafts. I. Neural cell adhesion molecules. The Journal of Comparative Neurology. 1995;**361**:193-209. DOI: 10.1002/cne.903610202

[21] Tsintou M, Dalamagkas K, Seifalian AM. Advances in regenerative therapies for spinal cord injury: A biomaterials approach. Neural Regeneration Research. 2015;**10**:726-742. DOI: 10.4103/1673-5374.156966

[22] Raspa A, Pugliese R, Maleki M, Gelain F. Recent therapeutic approaches for spinal cord injury. Biotechnology and Bioengineering. 2015;**113**:253-259. DOI: 10.1002/bit.25689

[23] Sakiyama-Elbert S, Johnson PJ, Hodgetts SI, Plant GW, Harvey AR. Scaffolds to promote spinal cord regeneration. In: Handbook of Clinical Neurology. 1st ed. Elsevier B.V; 2012. DOI: 10.1016/B978-0-444-52137-8.00036-X

[24] GÜnther MI, Weidner N, MÜller R, Blesch A. Cell-seeded alginate hydrogel scaffolds promote directed linear axonal regeneration in the injured rat spinal cord. Acta Biomaterialia. 2015;**27**:140-150. DOI: 10.1016/j.actbio.2015.09.001

[25] Tsai EC, Dalton PD, Shoichet MS, Tator CH. Matrix inclusion within synthetic hydrogel guidance channels improves specific supraspinal and local axonal regeneration after complete spinal cord transection. Biomaterials. 2006;**27**:519-533. DOI: 10.1016/j.biomaterials.2005.07.025

[26] Taylor L, Jones L, Tuszynski MH, Blesch A. Neurotrophin-3 gradients established by lentiviral gene delivery promote short-distance axonal bridging beyond cellular grafts in the injured spinal cord. The Journal of Neuroscience. 2006;**26**:9713-9721. DOI: 10.1523/JNEUROSCI.0734-06.2006

[27] Tobias CA, Han SSW, Shumsky JS, Kim D, Tumolo M, Dhoot NO, et al. Alginate encapsulated BDNF-producing fibroblast grafts permit recovery of function after spinal cord injury in the absence of immune suppression. Journal of Neurotrauma. 2005;**22**:138-156. DOI: 10.1089/neu.2005.22.138

[28] Zhang J, Lu X, Feng G, Gu Z, Sun Y, Bao G, et al. Chitosan scaffolds induce human dental pulp stem cells to neural

differentiation: Potential roles for spinal cord injury therapy. Cell and Tissue Research. 2016;**12**:1-14. DOI: 10.1007/s00441-016-2402-1

[29] King VR, Phillips JB, Hunt-Grubbe H, Brown R, Priestley JV. Characterization of non-neuronal elements within fibronectin mats implanted into the damaged adult rat spinal cord. Biomaterials. 2006;**27**:485-496. DOI: 10.1016/j.biomaterials.2005.06.033

[30] Watt FM, Driskell RR. The therapeutic potential of stem cells. Philosophical Transactions of the Royal Society of London. Series B, Biological Sciences. 2010;**365**:155-163. DOI: 10.1098/rstb.2009.0149

[31] Garza-Castro OD, Martínez-Rodríguez HG, Gabriela S. Schwann cell precursor transplant in a rat spinal cord injury model. Revista de Investigacion Clinica. 2018;**70**:88-95. DOI: 10.24875/RIC.18002466

[32] Guest JD, Rao A, Olson L, Bunge MB, Bunge RP. The ability of human Schwann cell grafts to promote regeneration in the transected nude rat spinal cord. Experimental Neurology. 1997;**148**:502-522. DOI: 10.1006/exnr.1997.6693

[33] Zurita M, Aguayo C, Bonilla C, Vaquero J. Co-cultivo de células madre adultas mesenquimales y células de Schwann en presencia de membranas de policarbonato. Neuroscience Letters. 2007;**5**:103-109

[34] Liu S, Sandner B, Schackel T, Nicholson L, Chtarto A, Tenenbaum L, et al. Regulated viral BDNF delivery in combination with Schwann cells promotes axonal regeneration through capillary alginate hydrogels after spinal cord injury. Acta Biomaterialia. 2017;**1**:1-14. DOI: 10.1016/j.actbio.2017.07.024

[35] Oudega M, Xu X-M. Schwann cell transplantation for repair of the adult spinal cord. Journal of Neurotrauma. 2006;**23**:453-467. DOI: 10.1089/neu.2006.23.453

[36] Lim PAC, Tow AM. Recovery and regeneration after spinal cord injury: A review and summary of recent literature. Annals of the Academy of Medicine, Singapore. 2007;**36**:49-57

[37] Ramón-Cueto A, Plant GW, Avila J, Bunge MB. Long-distance axonal regeneration in the transected adult rat spinal cord is promoted by olfactory ensheathing glia transplants. The Journal of Neuroscience. 1998;**18**:3803-3815

[38] Smale KA, Doucette R, Kawaja MD. Implantation of olfactory ensheathing cells in the adult rat brain following fimbria-fornix transection. Experimental Neurology. 1996;**137**:225-233

[39] López-Vales R, Forés J, Navarro X, Verdú E. Chronic transplantation of olfactory ensheathing cells promotes partial recovery after complete spinal cord transection in the rat. Glia. 2007;**55**:303-311. DOI: 10.1002/glia.20457

[40] Torres-Espín A, Redondo-Castro E, Hernández J, Navarro X. Bone marrow mesenchymal stromal cells and olfactory ensheathing cells transplantation after spinal cord injury—A morphological and functional comparison in rats. The European Journal of Neuroscience. 2014;**39**:1704-1717. DOI: 10.1111/ejn.12542

[41] Mackay-sim A. Olfactory ensheathing cells and spinal cord repair. Glia. 2005;**54**:8-14

[42] Lu P, Jones LL, Tuszynski MH. BDNF-expressing marrow stromal cells

support extensive axonal growth at sites of spinal cord injury. Experimental Neurology. 2005;**191**:344-360

[43] Neuhuber B, Timothy Himes B, Shumsky JS, Gallo G, Fischer I. Axon growth and recovery of function supported by human bone marrow stromal cells in the injured spinal cord exhibit donor variations. Brain Research. 2005;**1035**:73-85

[44] Ohta M, Suzuki Y, Noda T, Ejiri Y, Dezawa M, Kataoka K, et al. Bone marrow stromal cells infused into the cerebrospinal fluid promote functional recovery of the injured rat spinal cord with reduced cavity formation. Experimental Neurology. 2004;**187**:266-278

[45] Wu S, Suzuki Y, Ejiri Y, Noda T, Bai H, Kitada M, et al. Bone marrow stromal cells enhance differentiation of cocultured neurosphere cells and promote regeneration of injured spinal cord. Journal of Neuroscience Research. 2003;**72**:343-351

[46] Chen X, Yang Y, Yao J, Lin W, Li Y, Chen Y, et al. Bone marrow stromal cells-loaded chitosan conduits promote repair of complete transection injury in rat spinal cord. Journal of Materials Science. Materials in Medicine. 2011;**22**:2347-2356. DOI: 10.1007/s10856-011-4401-9

[47] Gu W, Zhang F, Xue Q, Ma Z, Lu P, Yu B. Transplantation of bone marrow mesenchymal stem cells reduces lesion volume and induces axonal regrowth of injured spinal cord. Neuropathology. 2010;**30**:205-217

[48] Hofstetter CP, Schwarz EJ, Hess D, Widenfalk J, El Manira A, Prockop DJ, et al. Marrow stromal cells form guiding strands in the injured spinal cord and promote recovery. Proceedings of the National Academy of Sciences of the United States of America. 2002;**99**:2199-2204. DOI: 10.1073/pnas.042678299

[49] Chopp M, Zhang XH, Li Y, Wang L, Chen J, Lu D, et al. Spinal cord injury in rat: Treatment with bone marrow stromal cell transplantation. Neuroreport. 2000;**11**:3001-3005

[50] Woodbury D, Reynolds K, Black IB. Adult bone marrow stromal stem cells express germline, ectodermal, endodermal, and mesodermal genes prior to neurogenesis. Journal of Neuroscience Research. 2002;**69**:908-917. DOI: 10.1002/jnr.10365

[51] Chiba Y, Kuroda S, Maruichi K, Osanai T, Hokari M, Yano S, et al. Transplanted bone marrow stromal cells promote axonal regeneration and improve motor function in a rat spinal cord injury model. Neurosurgery. 2009;**64**:991-999. discussion 999-1000

[52] Vaquero J, Zurita M. Functional recovery after severe CNS trauma: Current perspectives for cell therapy with bone marrow stromal cells. Progress in Neurobiology. 2011;**93**:341-349

[53] Vaquero J, Zurita M. Bone marrow stromal cells for spinal cord repair: A challenge for contemporary neurobiology. Histology and Histopathology. 2009;**24**:107-116

[54] Zurita M, Vaquero J. Functional recovery in chronic paraplegia after bone marrow stromal cells transplantation. Neuroreport. 2004;**15**:1105-1108

[55] Zurita M, Vaquero J, Bonilla C, Santos M, De Haro J, Oya S, et al. Functional recovery of chronic paraplegic pigs after autologous transplantation of bone marrow stromal cells. Transplantation. 2008;**86**:845-853

[56] Chen J-R, Cheng G-Y, Sheu C-C, Tseng G-F, Wang T-J, Huang Y-S. Transplanted bone marrow stromal cells migrate, differentiate

and improve motor function in rats with experimentally induced cerebral stroke. Journal of Anatomy. 2008;**213**:249-258. DOI: 10.1111/j.1469-7580.2008.00948.x

[57] Jorgensen C. Mesenchymal stem cells immunosuppressive properties: Is it specific to bone marrow-derived cells? Stem cell res. Stem Cell Research & Therapy. 2010;**1**:15. DOI: 10.1186/scrt15

[58] Nakajima H, Uchida K, Guerrero AR, Watanabe S, Sugita D, Takeura N, et al. Transplantation of mesenchymal stem cells promotes an alternative pathway of macrophage activation and functional recovery after spinal cord injury. Journal of Neurotrauma. 2012;**29**:1614-1625. DOI: 10.1089/neu.2011.2109

[59] Urdzíková L, Růžička J, LaBagnara M, Kárová K, Kubinová Š, Jiráková K, et al. Human mesenchymal stem cells modulate inflammatory cytokines after spinal cord injury in rat. International Journal of Molecular Sciences. 2014;**15**:11275-11293. DOI: 10.3390/ijms150711275

[60] Harvey AR, Lovett SJ, Majda BT, Yoon JH, Wheeler LPG, Hodgetts SI. Neurotrophic factors for spinal cord repair: Which, where, how and when to apply, and for what period of time? Brain Research. 2015;**1619**:36-71. DOI: 10.1016/j.brainres.2014.10.049

[61] Kovalchuk Y, Holthoff K, Konnerth A. Neurotrophin action on a rapid timescale. Current Opinion in Neurobiology. 2004;**14**:558-563. DOI: 10.1016/j.conb.2004.08.014

[62] Ollivier-Lanvin K, Fischer I, Tom V, Houle JD, Lemay MA. Either brain-derived neurotrophic factor or neurotrophin-3 only neurotrophin-producing grafts promote locomotor recovery in untrained spinalized cats. Neurorehabilitation and Neural Repair. 2015;**29**:90-100. DOI: 10.1177/1545968314532834

[63] Ziemlińska E, Kügler S, Schachner M, Wewiór I, Czarkowska-Bauch J, Skup M. Overexpression of BDNF increases excitability of the lumbar spinal network and leads to robust early locomotor recovery in completely spinalized rats. PLoS One. 2014;**9**. DOI: 10.1371/journal.pone.0088833

[64] Johnson PJ, Tatara A, Shiu A, Sakiyama-Elbert SE. Controlled release of neurotrophin-3 and platelet-derived growth factor from fibrin scaffolds containing neural progenitor cells enhances survival and differentiation into neurons in a subacute model of SCI. Cell Transplantation. 2010;**19**:89-101. DOI: 10.3727/096368909X477273

[65] Wang L-J, Zhang R-P, Li J-D. Transplantation of neurotrophin-3-expressing bone mesenchymal stem cells improves recovery in a rat model of spinal cord injury. Acta Neurochirurgica. 2014;**156**:1409-1418. DOI: 10.1007/s00701-014-2089-6

[66] Feng S, Kong X, Liu Y, Ban D, Ning G, Chen J, et al. Regeneration of spinal cord with cell and gene therapy. Orthopaedic Surgery. 2009;**1**:153-163. DOI: 10.1111/j.1757-7861.2009.00018.x

[67] Huang EJA, Reichardt LF. Neurotrophins: Roles in neuronal development and function. Annual Review of Neuroscience. 2001;**24**:677-736. DOI: 10.1016/j.biotechadv.2011.08.021.Secreted

[68] Zhang H, Wu F, Kong X, Yang J, Chen H, Deng L, et al. Nerve growth factor improves functional recovery by inhibiting endoplasmic reticulum stress-induced neuronal apoptosis in rats with spinal cord injury. Journal of Translational Medicine. 2014;**12**:130. DOI: 10.1186/1479-5876-12-130

[69] Blesch A, Yang H, Weidner N, Hoang A, Otero D. Axonal responses to cellularly delivered NT-4/5 after spinal cord injury. Molecular and Cellular Neurosciences. 2004;**27**:190-201. DOI: 10.1016/j.mcn.2004.06.007

[70] Zhao RR, Fawcett JW. Combination treatment with chondroitinase ABC in spinal cord injury—Breaking the barrier. Neuroscience Bulletin. 2013;**29**:477-483. DOI: 10.1007/s12264-013-1359-2

[71] Jefferson SC, Tester NJ, Howland DR. Chondroitinase ABC promotes recovery of adaptive limb movements and enhances axonal growth caudal to a spinal hemisection. The Journal of Neuroscience. 2011;**31**:5710-5720. DOI: 10.1523/JNEUROSCI.4459-10.2011. Chondroitinase

[72] Wang D, Ichiyama RM, Zhao R, Andrews MR, Fawcett JW. Chondroitinase combined with rehabilitation promotes recovery of forelimb function in rats with chronic spinal cord injury. The Journal of Neuroscience. 2011;**31**:9332-9344. DOI: 10.1523/JNEUROSCI.0983-11.2011

[73] García-Alías G, Petrosyan HA, Schnell L, Horner PJ, Bowers WJ, Mendell LM, et al. Chondroitinase ABC combined with neurotrophin NT-3 secretion and NR2D expression promotes axonal plasticity and functional recovery in rats with lateral hemisection of the spinal cord. The Journal of Neuroscience. 2011;**31**:17788-17799. DOI: 10.1523/JNEUROSCI.4308-11.2011

[74] Karimi-Abdolrezaee S, Schut D, Wang J, Fehlings MG. Chondroitinase and growth factors enhance activation and oligodendrocyte differentiation of endogenous neural precursor cells after spinal cord injury. PLoS One. 2012;**7**:1-16. DOI: 10.1371/journal.pone.0037589

[75] do Vale Ramos RC, Alegrete N. The role of pharmacotherapy in modifying the neurological status of patients with spinal and spinal cord injuries. Revista Brasileira de Ortopedia. 2015;**50**:617-624. DOI: 10.1016/j.rboe.2015.09.001

[76] Bowers CA, Kundu B, Rosenbluth J, Hawryluk GWJ. Patients with spinal cord injuries favor administration of methylprednisolone. PLoS One. 2016;**11**:e0145991. DOI: 10.1371/journal.pone.0145991

[77] Evaniew N, Belley-Cote EP, Fallah N, Noonan V, Rivers CS, Dvorak MF. Methylprednisolone for the treatment of patients with acute spinal cord injuries: A systematic review and meta-analysis 1. Journal of Neurotrauma. 2015;**481**:468-481. DOI: 10.1089/neu.2015.4192

[78] Fehlings MG, Wilson JR, Cho N. Methylprednisolone for the treatment of acute spinal cord injury: Counterpoint. Neurosurgery. 2014;**61**:36-42. DOI: 10.1227/NEU.0000000000000412

[79] Fehlings MG, Nakashima H, Nagoshi N, Chow DSL, Grossman RG, Kopjar B. Rationale, design and critical end points for the riluzole in acute spinal cord injury study (RISCIS): A randomized, double-blinded, placebo-controlled parallel multi-center trial. Spinal Cord. 2015:1-8. DOI: 10.1038/sc.2015.95

[80] Nagoshi N, Nakashima H, Fehlings MG. Riluzole as a neuroprotective drug for spinal cord injury: From bench to bedside. Molecules. 2015;**20**:7775-77789. DOI: 10.3390/molecules20057775

[81] Stirling DP, Koochesfahani KM, Steeves JD, Tetzlaff W. Minocycline as a neuroprotective agent.

Neuroscience. 2005;**11**:308-322. DOI: 10.1177/1073858405275175

[82] Casha S, Zygun D, McGowan MD, Bains I, Yong VW, John Hurlbert R. Results of a phase II placebo-controlled randomized trial of minocycline in acute spinal cord injury. Brain. 2012;**135**:1224-1236. DOI: 10.1093/brain/aws072

[83] Feng S-Q, Zhou X-F, Rush RA, Ferguson IA. Graft of pre-injured sural nerve promotes regeneration of corticospinal tract and functional recovery in rats with chronic spinal cord injury. Brain Research. 2008;**1209**:40-48. DOI: 10.1016/j.brainres.2008.02.075

[84] Fausto PG, Soares JG, de Freitas LM, de Paiva Cavalcanti JRL, Oliveira FG, Araujo JF, et al. Sciatic nerve grafting and inoculation of FGF-2 promotes improvement of motor behavior and fiber regrowth in rats with spinal cord transection. Restorative Neurology and Neuroscience. 2012;**30**:265-275. DOI: 10.3233/RNN-2012-110184

[85] Kuo H-S, Tsai M-J, Huang M-C, Chiu C-W, Tsai C-Y, Lee M-J, et al. Acid fibroblast growth factor and peripheral nerve grafts regulate Th2 cytokine expression, macrophage activation, polyamine synthesis, and neurotrophin expression in transected rat spinal cords. The Journal of Neuroscience. 2011;**31**:4137-4147. DOI: 10.1523/JNEUROSCI.2592-10.2011

[86] Luo J, Zhang H, Jiang X, Xue S, Ke Y. Combination of bone marrow stromal cell transplantation with mobilization by granulocyte-colony stimulating factor promotes functional recovery after spinal cord transection. Acta Neurochirurgica. 2009;**151**:1483-1492. DOI: 10.1007/s00701-009-0402-6

[87] Lee SH, Kim Y, Rhew D, Kuk M, Kim M, Kim WH, et al. Effect of the combination of mesenchymal stromal cells and chondroitinase ABC on chronic spinal cord injury. Cytotherapy. 2015;**17**:1374-1383. DOI: 10.1016/j.jcyt.2015.05.012

[88] Buzoianu-AnguianoV,Orozco-SuárezS, García-Vences E, Caballero-Chacón S, Guizar-Sahagún G, Chavez-Sanchez L, et al. The morphofunctional effect of the transplantation of bone marrow stromal cells and predegenerated peripheral nerve in chronic paraplegic rat model via spinal cord transection. Neural Plasticity. 2015:2015. DOI: 10.1155/2015/389520

[89] Buzoianu-Anguiano V, Rivera-Osorio J, Orozco-Suárez S, Angélica V-G, Elisa G-V, Stephanie S-T, et al. Single vs. combined therapeutic approaches in rats with chronic spinal cord injury. Frontiers in Neurology. 2020;**11**:1-11. DOI: 10.3389/fneur.2020.00136

[90] Badhiwala JH, Wilson JR, Kwon BK, Casha S, Fehlings MG. A review of clinical trials in spinal cord injury including biomarkers. Journal of Neurotrauma. 2018;**35**:1906-1917. DOI: 10.1089/neu.2018.5935

[91] Donovan J, Kirshblum S. Clinical trials in traumatic spinal cord injury. Neurotherapeutics. 2018;**15**:654-668. DOI: 10.1007/s13311-018-0632-5

[92] Kim YH, Ha KY, Kim SI. Spinal cord injury and related clinical trials. Clinics in Orthopedic Surgery. 2017;**9**:1-9. DOI: 10.4055/cios.2017.9.1.1

[93] Ahuja CSFM. Concise review: Bridging the gap: Novel neuroregenerative and neuroprotective strategies in spinal cord injury. Stem Cells Translational Medicine. 2015:1131-1143. DOI: 10.5966/sctm.2013-0207

[94] Badhiwala JH, Ahuja CS, Fehlings MG. Time is spine: A review of translational advances in spinal

cord injury. Journal of Neurosurgery. Spine. 2019;**30**:1-18. DOI: 10.3171/2018.9.SPINE18682

[95] Tetzlaff W, Okon EB, Karimi-Abdolrezaee S, Hill CE, Sparling JS, Plemel JR, et al. A systematic review of cellular transplantation therapies for spinal cord injury. Journal of Neurotrauma. 2011;**28**:1611-1682. DOI: 10.1089/neu.2009.1177

Chapter 5

Mesenchymal Stem Cell Therapies for Paraplegia: Preclinical and Clinical Studies

Fereshteh Azedi, Kazem Mousavizadeh and Mohammad Taghi Joghataei

Abstract

Paraplegia is the damage or loss of function in motor and/or sensory abilities. This insult can be observed in the thoracic, lumbar, or sacral parts of spinal column. Besides, paraplegia may be occurring because of any injuries or diseases of the lower segments or peripheral nerves or by cerebral palsy (CP). This damage can be seen as a result of a tumor or blood clot on the spinal cord. By now, there is not any curative treatment for paraplegia. Using mesenchymal stem cells (MSCs) in the treatment of spinal cord injury is a promising tested strategy because of their simplicity of isolation/preservation and their properties. Several preclinical studies in this field can be found; however, MSCs showed weak and conflicting outcomes in trials. In this chapter book, we will discuss about the therapeutic role of these cells in the treatment of paraplegia, with emphasis on their characterization, relevance, boundaries, and prospect views.

Keywords: paraplegia, stem cell therapy, mesenchymal stem cell, preclinical study, clinical study

1. Introduction

Paralysis of the lower parts of the body (paraplegia) can be caused by any damage to the spinal cord [1, 2]. Traumatic and nontraumatic injuries are classifications of this disease [3]. Paraplegia causes severe and in most cases lasting changes in the patient's lifetime and lifestyle [4, 5].

Attempts to find a complete cure for paraplegia and several discoveries show that in adult mammalian, by the preparation of appropriate microenvironment, regeneration of spinal cord axons can be obtained [6]. But then, why can we see the huge delay in the processing of bench to bedside in spite of these findings? Unfortunately, spinal cord scientists find a new barrier in the regeneration field. In fact, axons do regenerate up and down through a graft or transplant placed at the damage site; however, when they reach healthy cord tissue beyond the injury zone, they fail to regenerate more at once [7]. The most important cause for this provision is that the axons of neural networks need to cross through during sufficient stabilized conditions which are unreceptive and intractable to new restoration. Successful elongated distance regeneration is probable only within destabilized neural tissues [8].

Recently, rapid progresses in multipotent stem cell (routinely called mesenchymal stromal/stem cells) investigations increase the interest of scientists to study about the cell therapy and regenerative medicine [9–11].

Mesenchymal stem cell transplantation in patients suffering paraplegia is considered as a strategy for increasing neuroregeneration [12–14]. Notably, because of the disproportion in the technique and method of MSC preparation for paraplegia treatment like how they administrate and which criteria are chosen for selecting patients, MSC transplantation is in the initial stages, and there is confusion about the consequences at present [15].

MSCs have various sources in the body including the bone marrow [16, 17], adipose [18], muscle [19], peripheral blood [20], umbilical cord [21–23], placenta [24], endometrial [25, 26] and menstrual blood [27–29], fetal tissue [30], and amniotic fluid [31]. Previous finding indicated that these clonal cells can adhere to plastic; express cluster of differentiation (CD) markers like CD73, CD90, and CD105 markers [32]; and can differentiate into adipogenic [33], chondrogenic [34], osteogenic [35, 36], and neurogenic [37–39] lineages in the experimental condition (in vitro). However, it can be observed many different reports in their strength and self-renewal potential [40]. Accordingly, when we compare previous surveys, variable or even conflicting results can be seen. The lack of uniform methods in MSC characterization, both in preclinical and clinical studies, contributes to this confusion. It is interesting that even the name "MSCs" has still been gradually questioned. Actually, an urgent demand is required to understand the novel sources and potencies of MSCs especially for applying in SCI treatment.

Previous findings showed that the optimistic effect of MSC in treatment of spinal cord and peripheral nerve injury ascribed to their differentiation ability. They can differentiate into various cell lineages and modulate the inflammation process and immunomodulatory responses. [41] MSCs can diminish cell apoptosis and secrete various neurotrophic factors [42, 43].

According to previous studies, transplanting enough cells is important to obtain the best outcome after MSC transplantation and also applying especial techniques for achieving the highest possible survival of MSCs. Likewise, it seems that repeated doses of MSC therapy might be helpful [44].

Findings obtained about clinical trials for SCI treatment demonstrated that the efficacy of MSCs in human studies is not beneficial like in preclinical studies [45]. For these reasons protocol standardization of basic and preclinical studies using MSCs should emphasize to translate to the clinical setting. This chapter book is based on preclinical studies and clinical trials dealing with MSC therapy for paraplegia with emphasis on the challenges in this field.

2. Paraplegia: mechanisms of degeneration

SCI is included in two mechanisms: primary and secondary damage. When the direct physical injury to the spinal cord happened like any contusion, compression, contraction, and laceration, it can be called primary injury [46]. In this condition, axons separate from each other, mechanical injury to cells occurs directly, and blood vessels rupture. The progress of the injury site can occur in secondary phase, and it can be led to the restorative process [47]. This phase is including alterations in concentration of local ionic, blood pressure dysregulation (local and systemic), decrease of blood flow in the spine, disruption in the blood-brain barrier (BBB), diffusion of proteins from serum into the spinal cord, alterations in inflammatory chemokines and cytokines, cell apoptosis, excitotoxicity, activation of calpain proteases, accumulation of neurotransmitter, production of free radicals, lipid peroxidation, and activation of matrix metalloproteinases (MMPs). All of these changes can lead to demyelination of axons and also ischemia, necrosis, and apoptosis of spinal cord tissue [48]. As a result of these alterations, the inhibitory prospect overcomes, and axonal regrowth constrains. By this reason, injured axons cannot regenerate for a second time [49].

3. Mesenchymal stem cells: a historical outline

The pathologist Cohnheim in 1867 could show the first evidence of nonhematopoietic stem cells in the bone marrow (BM) and their potency to be the source of fibroblasts involved in wound healing [50]. However, only a century later (50 years ago), the isolation and culture of these cells in an experimental condition successfully could be done. Friedenstein and his colleagues found that, when isolated cells from the rat bone marrow are cultured, a population of fibroblastic-shape nonhematopoietic cells that adhered to the plastic of the cell culture dish could be seen. Then these cells were called as a colony-forming unit fibroblast (CFU-F). These cells were capable of self-maintenance and multi-lineage differentiation like adipocytes, chondrocytes, and osteocytes in vitro and also could support hematopoietic stroma when a single cell was transplanted into animal models [51]. In 1988, Owen showed that a stromal system existed, with a stromal stem cell (CFU-F) at the base of the hierarchy, popularizing the stromal cell terminology [52]. Altogether, this information was generated from in vivo studies.

Only in 1992, Haynesworth and his colleagues enriched and expanded cells in culture with the osteochondrogenic potential of the human bone marrow [53]. In the early 1990s, the proliferation and differentiation potency of these cells in an experimental condition and also multipotency and self-renewal properties after transplantation lead to characteristics of the "stemness" [54]. Thus, the term mesenchymal stem cell (MSC) was proposed by Caplan for progenitor cells, which were isolated from the human adult bone marrow (BM) instead of the term "stromal" or "osteogenic" stem cell and acquired a broad recognition [55]. **Figure 1** shows the representation of the most imperative results related to MSC discovery, characterization, and clinical relevance.

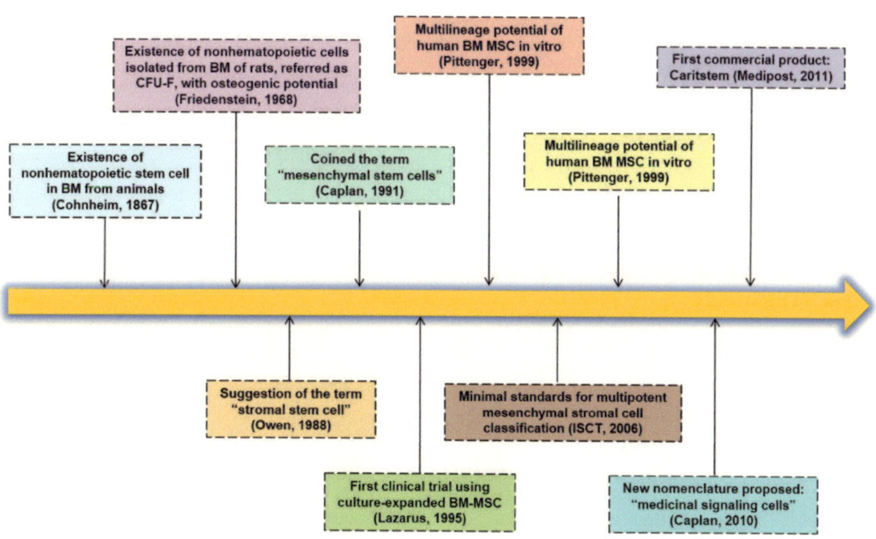

Figure 1.
Representation of the most significant findings associated with MSC discovery, description, and clinical purpose.

4. Preclinical researches using mesenchymal stem cells for paraplegia treatment

Transplantation of MSCs has been well established by several researchers. MSCs have significant effects on the several cellular and molecular cascades. Therefore,

Animal	Type of lesion	Cell source	Route of administration	Effects on neural regeneration	Ref.
Rat	Contusion	Human mesenchymal precursor cells	Lesion site	Functional recovery enhancement and tissue sparing and cyst volume decrease	[69]
Rat	Contusion	Human bone marrow MSCs	Lesion site, intracisternal, intravenous	Improvement in functional recovery	[70]
Rat	Hemisection	Bone marrow MSCs induced in Schwann cells	Lesion site	Progress in locomotor and sensory scores, axonal regeneration and remyelination	[71]
Rat	Contusion	Bone marrow MSCs	Lesion site, intravenous	Enhancement in locomotor scores and nerve growth factor (NGF) expression	[72]
Rat	Transection to the dorsal columns and tracts	Bone marrow MSCs, adipose derived-MSCs	Lesion site	Progress in locomotor scores, increased angiogenesis, preserved axons, reduced numbers of ED1-positive	[73]
Rat	Hemisection	Human umbilical cord-derived MSCs	Lesion site	Suppression of mechanical allodynia modulation of microglia in the spinal cord	[74]
Rat	Hemisection	Human bone marrow MSCs	Lesion site	Improvement of locomotor aspect, shorter latency of somatosensory-evoked potentials and different cell types	[75]
Rat	Hemisection	Bone marrow-MSCs	Lesion site	Enhancement in locomotor aspect and reduction of lesion cavity formation	[76]

Animal	Type of lesion	Cell source	Route of administration	Effects on neural regeneration	Ref.
Rat	Contusion	Human bone marrow MSCs	Lesion site	Improvement in functional recovery, tissue sparing and decrease in the volume of lesion cavity and in the white matter loss	[77]
Mouse	Compression	Bone marrow MSCs	Lesion site	Improvement in locomotor and sensory scores and reduced lesion volume	[78]
Mouse	Transection	Bone marrow MSCs	Lesion site	Improvement in functional recovery and neuronal survival, reduction of cavity volume and decrease of inflammation, progress in angiogenesis, and reduction of cavity formation	[79]
Dog	Compression	Bone marrow, adipose, Wharton's jelly, umbilical cord derived MSCs	Lesion site	Improvement in functional recovery scores, elevated numbers of surviving neurons, lesser lesion sizes and fewer microglia, and reactive astrocytes in the epicenter of the lesion	[80]
Dog	Compression	Neural-induced adipose derived-MSCs	Lesion site	Improvement in functional recovery and neuronal regeneration and decline of fibrosis	[81]
Dog	Compression	Umbilical cord MSCs	Lesion site	Improvement in functional recovery, promotion of neuronal regeneration, and diminishing of fibrosis	[82]
Dog	Compression	Human umbilical cord MSCs	Lesion site	Amelioration in functional recovery and remyelination	[83]

Animal	Type of lesion	Cell source	Route of administration	Effects on neural regeneration	Ref.
Dog	Chronic paraplegia (≥6 months)	Adipose tissue derived MSCs	Lesion site, intraparenchymal	Improved locomotion, no adverse effects or complexity, no changes in deep pain perception	[84]
Monkey	Dorsal SCI	Differentiated BM-MSCs into neural lineage cells	Lesion site	Motor-evoked potential (MEP), somatosensory-evoked potential in cortex (CSEP), and functional recovery and de novo neurogenesis	[85]

Table 1.
Summary of preclinical surveys using MSCs for treatment of paraplegia.

they can be regarded as a possible candidate for treating of CNS diseases [56]. MSCs have anti-inflammatory representation [57], immunomodulatory regulation [58, 59], and neuroprotective [60] effects. Moreover, previous findings showed that these cells could secrete trophic factors; thus they could motivate axon regeneration finally leading to functional recovery improvement [61, 62].

Regarding to the paracrine effect, MSCs can produce trophic and neurotropic factors such as insulin-like growth factor (IGF), brain-derived neurotrophic factor (BDNF) [63], vascular endothelial growth factor (VEGF) [64], granulocyte-macrophage colony-stimulating factor (GMCSF), fibroblast growth factor-2 (FGF2) [65], and transforming growth factor beta (TGF-β) [66]. In addition, gene therapy is another field that MSC therapy can be combined with, for example, introducing special genes into MSCs to generate molecules that have great curative ability and can increase neural survival and regeneration [67, 68]. **Table 1** presents a summary of preclinical studies by applying MSCs for paraplegia.

5. Clinical trials using mesenchymal stem cell for paraplegia

The clinical trials conducted for the treatment of paraplegia include three different phases. Phase 1 trials begin with the cell transplantation to a human participant, and the aim of these trials is to study any events such as adverse or toxic effects and also the safety of this intervention. During these trials, subjects may be exposed to some risks and obtain low benefits at the end. In phase 2, the goal of the trial is to determine the potential and variety of an intervention compared to a control group. Typically, the participants are recruited and arbitrarily assigned to the groups as experimental or control, and both participants and investigators are in blind condition, which means they do not have any insight about which of them have been assigned [86]. In phase 3, the conclusive clinical trial and the objective normally affirm the preliminary results obtained at the phase 2, with a significant clinical profit of the therapeutic intervention which has been proved by statistic methods. The number of participants is also larger, and manifold centers are elaborated in the trial [87]. By now, the majority of the studies using MSCs for paraplegia treatment are in phase 1 or 2 (**Table 2**).

Title	Lesion type	Cell source	Phase of the study	Effects on neural regeneration	ClinicalTrials.gov identifier
Safety study of local administration of autologous bone marrow stromal cells in chronic paraplegia (CME-LEM1)	Chronic paraplegia	Autologous bone marrow stromal cells	Phase I, completed	Motor enhancement, alteration in the chronic pain, improvement of neurophysiological parameters, and morphology changes in the spinal cord on neuroimaging follow-up	NCT01909154
Autologous mesenchymal stem cells transplantation in thoracolumbar chronic and complete spinal cord injury spinal cord injury	Thoracolumbar chronic and complete SCI	Autologous bone marrow mesenchymal stem cells	Phase II, not yet recruiting	Not informed	NCT02574585
Autologous mesenchymal stem cells transplantation for spinal cord injury—a phase I clinical study	Traumatic spinal cord injury at the thoracic level	Autologous BM MSCs	Completed	Intrathecal administration of BMMSCs is safe with no adverse events	NCT02482194
The effect of intrathecal transplantation of autologous adipose tissue derived MSCs in the patients with SCI, phase I clinical study	Clinical diagnosis of SCI	Autologous adipose-derived MSCs	Phase I, completed	Mild improvements in neurological function, free of serious adverse events	NCT01624779
Phase I, single center, trial to assess safety and tolerability of the intrathecal infusion of ex-vivo expanded bone-marrow derived MSCs for the treatment of SCI	SCI clinical diagnosis (ASIA A)	Autologous bone marrow MSCs	Active, not recruiting	Not informed	NCT01162915
Study the safety and efficacy of bone marrow derived autologous cells for the treatment of SCI	SCI clinical diagnosis	Autologous bone marrow MSCs	Recruiting	Not informed	NCT01730183
Phase I study of autologous bone marrow stem cell transplantation in patients with spinal cord injury	Traumatic thoracic or lumbar SCI	Autologous bone marrow MSCs	Phase I	Transplantation of autologous BMSCs is a feasible and safe technique	NCT01325103
Surgical transplantation of autologous bone marrow stem cells with glial scar resection for patients of chronic SCI and intra-thecal injection for acute and subacute injury—a preliminary study	Complete transection of spinal cord	Autologous bone marrow MSCs	Completed	Not informed	NCT01186679

Title	Lesion type	Cell source	Phase of the study	Effects on neural regeneration	ClinicalTrials.gov identifier
Autologous adipose derived MSCs transplantation in patient with spinal cord injury	Clinical diagnosis of spinal cord injury	Autologous AD MSCs	Phase I, completed	Intravenous administration of AD-MSCs is safe with no adverse events	NCT01274975
Difference between rehabilitation therapy and stem cells transplantation in patients with spinal cord injury in China	Traumatic injury, spinal cord injury	U-MSCs	Phase II, completed	Patients receiving U-MSCs demonstrate improved urinary control, muscle tension, motion, and self-care ability	NCT01393977

Table 2.
Summary of trials using mesenchymal stem cell for treatment of paraplegia.

Currently, clinical trials with applying mesenchymal stem cells for treatment of paraplegia are growing, suggesting that despite the existence of numerous questions at primary and preclinical levels, the MSC is considered supposedly valuable for translational researches [46].

6. Why mesenchymal stem cell functions do not soundly shift these cells toward clinic yet?

It is well established that, despite promising preclinical findings about mesenchymal stem cells, clinical trials failed to be impressive in SCI treatment and are still away from obtaining behavioral and functional improvement and repairing neural circuits totally [88].

Regarding the previous researches, studies using animal models are usually performed by applying standardized protocols of lesions, treatments, and specific timings of transplantation in each group of investigation [89]. However, these conditions are often incomparable with human subjects because timing and therapies are dependent on emergency setting and many variables such as lesion site damage at the cord [90]. Most of animal studies are necessarily done with rodents such as mice and rat, and, despite many anatomical or behavioral similarities, clinical trials with human participants should be the main goal of stem cell research. Therefore, making a strong bridge between preclinical and clinical studies is mandatory for finding the best trail in cell therapy [91].

As well, it is necessary to run more rigorous clinical trials such as RCTs and also animal researches in providing MSC therapy as a safe, effective, and beneficial approach for various diseases. Already, completed human trials displayed only limited outcome. However, applying MSCs in SCIs seems to cause no harm. Different trials [92, 93] indicated the safety of MSC therapy showing no side effects [94]. Regardless of these findings about safety of stem cell therapy, clinical outcomes showed poor results compared to expectations. Among the others, it seems that not many studies particularly encourage cell therapy [95].

Consequently, ongoing trials will almost certainly help and develop comprehension about the outcomes of stem cell therapy [96]. Unfortunately, translation of encouraging data from preclinical studies into clinical administration seems intricate. This probably reflects the multivariable and sophisticated paraplegia physiopathology, requiring a multi-aspect curative approach. To tell the truth, many points require further illuminating and depicting, such as:

1. The best therapeutic protocols with respect to the preparation method, type, and amount of stem cells transplanted.

2. The paracrine effects and their impact on behavioral and functional improvement.

3. The rout of stem cell delivery and timing of transplantation.

4. The substance of cellular matrix and microenvironment.

5. The ability of neuroplasticity and production of new connections from injured neuronal cells.

6. The ethical aspects and financial challenges associated with stem cell research [97].

As a result, prospect preclinical and clinical studies based on MSCs should put emphasis on multivariable factors [98]. For instance, considering donor-related properties like sex, age, and comorbidities that may have an effect on the capacity and excellence of cells is important. Moreover, a better appreciation of the accurate and beneficial methods of action calling for ad hoc investigations will also able to scrutinize MSC complexity, for instance, stem versus stromal. MSC interactions with host tissues have to be considered too. The development of precious in vitro and in vivo models is to be applied in a number of medical conditions; and choosing reagents and techniques that may be administrated from experimental studies to clinical developments for preserving cell consistency and eventually reducing manufacturing expenses is imperative markedly [99].

7. Conclusion

Nowadays, the advancements in cell marketing with the progress in cell isolation, description, and quality control will positively encourage scientists to apply MSCs for treating several diseases and disorders, even with all remaining challenges.

Preclinical studies revealed the importance of MSC therapy in the SCI and paraplegia field. Unluckily, the effect of MSC therapy is not typically seen in the human studies, and the results need a long time from being similar to preclinical studies. Consequently, among other concerns, the protocol standardization in source of cells, culture conditions, time of cell delivery after paraplegia, number and administration rout of cells, plasticity, and potential of MSCs after isolation and expansion in vitro is of urgency. Confidently, preliminary studies with emphasis on these key points will be helpful in terms of their winning implementation of human studies.

Conflict of interest

The authors declare no conflict of interest.

Author details

Fereshteh Azedi[1,2], Kazem Mousavizadeh[1,3] and Mohammad Taghi Joghataei[1,2]*

1 Cellular and Molecular Research Center, Iran University of Medical Sciences, Tehran, Iran

2 Department of Neuroscience, Faculty of Advanced Technologies in Medicine, Iran University of Medical Sciences, Tehran, Iran

3 Department of Molecular Medicine, Faculty of Advanced Technologies in Medicine, Iran University of Medical Sciences, Tehran, Iran

*Address all correspondence to: mt.joghataei@yahoo.com

References

[1] Besalti O, Aktas Z, Can P, Akpinar E, Elcin AE, Elcin YM. The use of autologous neurogenically-induced bone marrow-derived mesenchymal stem cells for the treatment of paraplegic dogs without nociception due to spinal trauma. The Journal of Veterinary Medical Science. 2016;**78**(9):1465-1473

[2] McDonald JW, Sadowsky C. Spinal-cord injury. Lancet. 2002;**359**(9304):417-425

[3] Dubey A, Tomar S, Gupta A, Khandelwal D. Delayed paraplegia in an adult patient with spinal cord injury without radiographic abnormality of dorsal spine: A lesson learned. Asian Journal of Neurosurgery. 2018;**13**(3):867-869

[4] Ke X, Wang Y, Zhang A, Jiang Y, Dong C, Wang Q, et al. Neurological protection effects of "paraplegia-triple-needling method" on rats with incomplete spinal cord injury. Zhongguo Zhen Jiu. 2015;**35**(6):585-589

[5] Courtine G, van den Brand R, Musienko P. Spinal cord injury: Time to move. Lancet. 2011;**377**(9781):1896-1898

[6] Fitch MT, Silver J. CNS injury, glial scars, and inflammation: Inhibitory extracellular matrices and regeneration failure. Experimental Neurology. 2008;**209**(2):294-301

[7] Nash M, Pribiag H, Fournier AE, Jacobson C. Central nervous system regeneration inhibitors and their intracellular substrates. Molecular Neurobiology. 2009;**40**(3):224-235

[8] Busch S, Silver J. The role of extracellular matrix in CNS regeneration. Current Opinion in Neurobiology. 2007;**17**:120-127

[9] Oh SK, Jeon SR. Current concept of stem cell therapy for spinal cord injury: A review. Korean Journal of Neurotrauma. 2016;**12**(2):40-46

[10] Jeong SK, Choi I, Jeon SR. Current status and future strategies to treat spinal cord injury with adult stem cells. Journal of Korean Neurosurgical Association. 2020;**63**(2):153-162

[11] Yong KW, Choi JR, Dolbashid AS, Wan Safwani WKZ. Biosafety and bioefficacy assessment of human mesenchymal stem cells: What do we know so far? Regenerative Medicine. 2018;**13**(2):219-232

[12] Zhang D, He X. A meta-analysis of the motion function through the therapy of spinal cord injury with intravenous transplantation of bone marrow mesenchymal stem cells in rats. PLoS One. 2014;**9**(4):e93487

[13] Alessandrini M, Preynat-Seauve O, De Bruin K, Pepper MS. Stem cell therapy for neurological disorders. South African Medical Journal. 2019 10;**109**(8b):70-77

[14] Mukhamedshina Y, Shulman I, Ogurcov S, Kostennikov A, Zakirova E, Akhmetzyanova E, et al. Mesenchymal stem cell therapy for spinal cord contusion: A comparative study on small and large animal models. Biomolecules. 2019;**9**(12):811

[15] Goel A. Stem cell therapy in spinal cord injury: Hollow promise or promising science? Journal of Craniovertebral Junction and Spine. 2016;**7**(2):121-126

[16] Vaquero J, Zurita M. Bone marrow stromal cells for spinal cord repair: A challenge for contemporary neurobiology. Histology and Histopathology. 2009;**24**(1):107-116

[17] An H, Li Q, Wen J. Bone marrow mesenchymal stem cells encapsulated thermal-responsive hydrogel network bridges combined photo-plasmonic nanoparticulate system for the treatment of urinary bladder dysfunction after spinal cord injury. Journal of Photochemistry and Photobiology. B. 2020;**203**:111741

[18] Radtke C, Schmitz B, Spies M, Kocsis J, Vogt P. Peripheral glial cell differentiation from neurospheres derived from adipose mesenchymal stem cells. International Journal of Developmental Neuroscience. 2009;**27**:817-823

[19] Latil M, Rocheteau P, Châtre L, Sanulli S, Mémet S, Ricchetti M, et al. Skeletal muscle stem cells adopt a dormant cell state post mortem and retain regenerative capacity. Nature Communications. 2012;**3**:903. DOI: 101038/ncomms1890

[20] Dunac A, Frelin C, Popolo-Blondeau M, Chatel M, Mahagne M, Philip P. Neurological and functional recovery in human stroke are associated with peripheral blood CD34+ cell mobilization. Journal of Neurology. 2007;**254**:327-332

[21] Shahbazi A, Safa M, Alikarami F, Kargozar S, Asadi MH, Joghataei MT, et al. Rapid induction of neural differentiation in human umbilical cord matrix mesenchymal stem cells by cAMP-elevating agents. International Journal of Molecular and Cellular Medicine. 2016;**5**(3):167-177

[22] Tian DZ, Deng D, Qiang JL, Zhu Q, Li QC, Yi ZG. Repair of spinal cord injury in rats by umbilical cord mesenchymal stem cells through P38MAPK signaling pathway. European Review for Medical and Pharmacological Sciences. 2019;**23** (3 Suppl):47-53

[23] Bagher Z, Azami M, Ebrahimi-Barough S, Mirzadeh H, Solouk A, Soleimani M, et al. Differentiation of Wharton's jelly-derived mesenchymal stem cells into motor neuron-like cells on three-dimensional collagen-grafted nanofibers. Molecular Neurobiology. 2015;**53**(4):2397-2408

[24] Long C, Lankford L, Kumar P, Grahn R, Borjesson DL, Farmer D, et al. Isolation and characterization of canine placenta-derived mesenchymal stromal cells for the treatment of neurological disorders in dogs. Cytometry. Part A. 2017;**93**(1):82-92

[25] Sahoo AK, Das JK, Nayak S. Isolation, culture, characterization, and osteogenic differentiation of canine endometrial mesenchymal stem cell. Veterinary World. 2018;**10**(12):1533-1541

[26] Gargett CE, Masuda H. Adult stem cells in the endometrium. Molecular Human Reproduction. 2010;**16**(11):818-834

[27] Azedi F,Kazemnejad S, Zarnani A, Behzadi G, Vasei M, Khanmohammadi M, et al. Differentiation potential of menstrual blood- versus bone marrow stem cells into glial-like cells. Cell Biology International. 2014;**38**(2014):615-624

[28] Azedi F, Kazemnejad S, Zarnani A, Soleimani M, Shojaei A, Arasteh S. Comparative capability of menstrual blood versus bone marrow derived stem cells in neural differentiation. Molecular Biology Reports. 2017;**44**(1):169-182

[29] Allickson JG, Sanchez A, Yefimenko N, Borlongan CV, Sanberg PR. Recent studies assessing the proliferative capability of a novel adult stem cell identified in menstrual blood. Open Stem Cell Journal. 2011;**3**(2011):4-10

[30] Bachoud-Levi A, Gaura V, Brugieres P, et al. Effect of fetal neural transplants in patients with

Huntington's disease 6 years after surgery: A long-term follow-up study. Lancet Neurology. 2006;**5**:303-309

[31] Harrell CR, Gazdic M, Fellabaum C, Jovicic N, Djonov V, Arsenijevic N, et al. Therapeutic potential of amniotic fluid derived mesenchymal stem cells based on their differentiation capacity and immunomodulatory properties. Current Stem Cell Research & Therapy. 2019;**14**(4):327-336

[32] Ding DC, Shyu WC, Lin SZ. Mesenchymal stem cells. Cell Transplantation. 2011;**20**(1):5-14

[33] Baer PC, Koch B, Hickmann E, Schubert R, Cinatl J Jr, Hauser IA, et al. Isolation, characterization, differentiation and immunomodulatory capacity of mesenchymal stromal/stem cells from human perirenal adipose tissue. Cell. 2019;**8**(11):0. DOI: 10.3390/cells8111346

[34] Khanmohammadi M, Khanjani S, Bakhtyari MS, Zarnani AH, Edalatkhah H, Akhondi MM, et al. Proliferation and chondrogenic differentiation potential of menstrual blood- and bone marrow-derived stem cells in two-dimensional culture. International Journal of Hematology. 2012;**95**(5):484-493

[35] Atmani H, Chappard D, Basle M. Proliferation and differentiation of osteoblasts and adipocytes in rat bone marrow stromal cell cultures: Effects of dexamethasone and calcitriol. Journal of Cellular Biochemistry. 2003;**2**:364-372

[36] Darzi S, Zarnani AH, Jeddi-Tehrani M, Entezami K, Mirzadegan E, Akhondi MM, et al. Osteogenic differentiation of stem cells derived from menstrual blood versus bone marrow in the presence of human platelet releasate. Tissue Engineering. Part A. 2012;**18**(15-16):1720-1728

[37] Hernandez R, Jimenez-Luna C, Perales-Adan J, Perazzoli G, Melguizo C, Prados J. Differentiation of human mesenchymal stem cells towards neuronal lineage: Clinical trials in nervous system disorders. Biomolecules & Therapeutics (Seoul). 2019;**28**(1):34-44

[38] Zemelko V, Kozhukharova I, Alekseenko L, Reshetnikova G, Puzanov M, Grinchuk T, et al. Neurogenic potential of human mesenchymal stem cells isolated from bone marrow, adipose tissue and endometrium: A comparative study. Cell and Tissue Biology. 2013;**7**(3):235-244

[39] Woodbury D, Schwarz EJ, Prockop DJ, Black IB. Adult rat and human bone marrow stromal cells differentiate into neurons. Journal of Neuroscience Research. 2000;**61**:364-370

[40] Bhat IA, Sivanarayanan TB, Somal A, Pandey S, Bharti MK, Panda BSK, et al. An allogenic therapeutic strategy for canine spinal cord injury using mesenchymal stem cells. Journal of Cellular Physiology;**234**(3):2705-2718

[41] Chaudhary D, Trivedi RN, Kathuria A, Goswami TK, Khandia R, Munjal A. In vitro and in vivo Immunomodulating properties of mesenchymal stem cells. Recent Patents on Inflammation & Allergy Drug Discovery. 2018;**12**(1):59-68

[42] Leyendecker A Jr, Pinheiro CCG, Amano MT, Bueno DF. The use of human mesenchymal stem cells as therapeutic agents for the in vivo treatment of immune-related diseases: A systematic review. Frontiers in Immunology. 2018;**9**:2056

[43] Liu X, Xu W, Zhang Z, Liu H, Lv L, Han D, et al. VEGF-transfected BMSC improve the recovery of motor and sensory functions of rats with spinal cord injury. Spine (Phila Pa 1976). 2020;**45**(7):E364-E372

[44] Gong Z, Xia K, Xu A, Yu C, Wang C, Zhu J, et al. Stem cell transplantation: A promising therapy for spinal cord injury. Current Stem Cell Research & Therapy. 2020;**15**(4):321-331

[45] Huang H, Chen L, Sanberg P. Cell therapy from bench to bedside translation in CNS neurorestoratology era. Cell Medicine. 2010;**1**(1):15-46

[46] Blanco Martinez AM, Goulart C, Ramalho BS, Oliveira J, Almeida F. Neurotrauma and mesenchymal stem cells treatment: From experimental studies to clinical trials. World Journal of Stem Cells. 2014;**6**(2):179-194

[47] Granger N, Carwardine D. Acute spinal cord injury: Tetraplegia and paraplegia in small animals. The Veterinary Clinics of North America. Small Animal Practice. 2014;**44**(6):1131-1156

[48] Dumont R, Okonkwo D, Verma S, Hurlbert R, Boulos P, Ellegala D, et al. Acute spinal cord injury, part I: Pathophysiologic mechanisms. Clinical Neuropharmacology. 2001;**24**:254-264

[49] McKerracher L, David S, Jackson D, Kottis V, Dunn R, Braun P. Identification of myelin-associated glycoprotein as a major myelin-derived inhibitor of neurite growth. Neuron. 1994;**13**:805-811

[50] Chamberlain G, Fox J, Ashton B, Middleton J. Concise review: Mesenchymal stem cells: Their phenotype, differentiation capacity, immunological features, and potential for homing. Stem Cells. 2007;**25**(11):2739-2749

[51] Friedenstein A, Chailakhjan R, Lalykina K. The development of fibroblast colonies in monolayer cultures of Guinea-pig bone marrow and spleen cells. Cell and Tissue Kinetics. 1970;**3**(4):393-403

[52] Meirelles L, Fontes A, Covas D, Caplan A. Mechanisms involved in the therapeutic properties of mesenchymal stem cells. Cytokine & Growth Factor Reviews. 2009;**20**(5):419-427

[53] Haynesworth S, Goshima J, Goldberg V, Caplan A. Characterization of cells with osteogenic potential from human marrow. Bone. 1992;**13**(1):81-88

[54] Nombela-Arrieta C, Ritz J, Silberstein L. The elusive nature and function of mesenchymal stem cells. Nature Reviews. Molecular Cell Biology. 2011;**12**(2):126-131

[55] Torre M, Lucarelli E, Guidi S. Ex vivo expanded mesenchymal stromal cell minimal quality requirements for clinical application. Stem Cells and Development. 2015;**24**(6):677-685

[56] Matthay M, Pati S, Lee J. Concise review: Mesenchymal stem (stromal) cells: Biology and preclinical evidence for therapeutic potential for organ dysfunction following trauma or sepsis. Stem Cells. 2017;**35**:316-324

[57] Najar M, Krayem M, Merimi M, Burny A, Meuleman N, Bron D, et al. Insights into inflammatory priming of mesenchymal stromal cells: Functional biological impacts. Inflammation Research. 2018;**67**(6):467-477

[58] Bai L, Lennon D, Eaton V, Maier K, Caplan A, Miller S, et al. Human bone marrow-derived mesenchymal stem cells induce Th2-polarized immune response and promote endogenous repair in animal models of multiple sclerosis. Glia. 2009;**57**:1192-1203

[59] Salami F, Tavassoli A, Mehrzad J, Parham A. Immunomodulatory effects of mesenchymal stem cells on leukocytes with emphasis on neutrophils. Immunobiology;**223**(12):786-791

[60] Chen X, Wu J, Sun R, Zhao Y, Li Y, Pan J, et al. Tubular scaffold with

microchannels and an H-shaped lumen loaded with BMSCs promotes neuroregeneration and inhibits apoptosis after spinal cord injury. Journal of Tissue Engineering and Regenerative Medicine. 2020;**14**(3):397-411

[61] Chudickova M, Vackova I, Machova Urdzikova L, Jancova P, Kekulova K, Rehorova M, et al. The effect of Wharton jelly-derived mesenchymal stromal cells and their conditioned media in the treatment of a rat spinal cord injury. International Journal of Molecular Sciences. 2019;**20**(18):4516

[62] Li C, Jiao G, Wu W, Wang H, Ren S, Zhang L, et al. Exosomes from bone marrow mesenchymal stem cells inhibit neuronal apoptosis and promote motor function recovery via the Wnt/beta-catenin signaling pathway. Cell Transplantation. 2019;**28**(11):1373-1383

[63] Zhang T, Liu C, Chi L. Suppression of miR-10a-5p in bone marrow mesenchymal stem cells enhances the therapeutic effect on spinal cord injury via BDNF. Neuroscience Letters. 2019;**714**:134562

[64] Xu ZX, Zhang LQ, Zhou YN, Chen XM, Xu WH. Histological and functional outcomes in a rat model of hemisected spinal cord with sustained VEGF/NT-3 release from tissue-engineered grafts. Artificial Cells, Nanomedicine and Biotechnology. 2020;**48**(1):362-376

[65] Huang XR, Xu H, Zhang Y, Jiang YB, Xia CL, Fang SC. Repair effect of bFGF combined with bone marrow mesenchymal stem cells on spinal cord injury in rats. Zhongguo Gu Shang. 2019;**32**(7):653-657

[66] Sohrabi Akhkand S, Amirizadeh N, Nikougoftar M, Alizadeh J, Zaker F, Sarveazad A, et al. Evaluation of umbilical cord blood CD34+ hematopoietic stem cells expansion with inhibition of TGF-beta receptorII in co-culture with bone marrow mesenchymal stromal cells. Tissue & Cell. 2016;**48**(4):305-311

[67] Huang JH, Xu Y, Yin XM, Lin FY. Exosomes derived from miR-126-modified MSCs promote angiogenesis and neurogenesis and attenuate apoptosis after spinal cord injury in rats. Neuroscience. 2019;**424**:133-145

[68] Wang X, Ye L, Zhang K, Gao L, Xiao J, Zhang Y. Upregulation of microRNA-200a in bone marrow mesenchymal stem cells enhances the repair of spinal cord injury in rats by reducing oxidative stress and regulating Keap1/Nrf2 pathway. Artificial Organs. 2020;**44**(7):744-752

[69] Hodgetts S, Simmons P, Plant G. A comparison of the behavioral and anatomical outcomes in sub-acute and chronic spinal cord injury models following treatment with human mesenchymal precursor cell transplantation and recombinant decorin. Experimental Neurology. 2013;**248**:343-359

[70] Shin D, Kim J, Kim H, Yi S, Ha Y, Yoon DH, et al. Comparison of functional and histological outcomes after intralesional, intracisternal, and intravenous transplantation of human bone marrow-derived mesenchymal stromal cells in a rat model of spinal cord injury. Acta Neurochirurgica. 2013;**155**:1943-1950

[71] Zaminy A, Shokrgozar M, Sadeghi Y, Noroozian M, Heidari M, Piryaei A. Mesenchymal stem cells as an alternative for Schwann cells in rat spinal cord injury. Iranian Biomedical Journal. 2013;**17**:113-122

[72] Kang E, Ha K, Kim Y. Fate of transplanted bone marrow derived mesenchymal stem cells following spinal cord injury in rats by transplantation

routes. Journal of Korean Medical Science. 2012;**27**:586-593

[73] Zhou Z, Chen Y, Zhang H, Min S, Yu B, He B, et al. Comparison of mesenchymal stromal cells from human bone marrow and adipose tissue for the treatment of spinal cord injury. Cytotherapy. 2013;**15**:434-448

[74] Roh D, Seo M, Choi H, Park S, Han H, Beitz A, et al. Transplantation of human umbilical cord blood or amniotic epithelial stem cells alleviates mechanical allodynia after spinal cord injury in rats. Cell Transplantation. 2013;**22**:1577-1590

[75] Choi J, Leem J, Lee K, Kim S, Suh-Kim H, Jung S, et al. Effects of human mesenchymal stem cell transplantation combined with polymer on functional recovery following spinal cord hemisection in rats. The Korean Journal of Physiology & Pharmacology. 2012;**16**:405-411

[76] Wei X, Wen Y, Zhang T, Li H. Effects of bone marrow mesenchymal stem cells with acellular muscle bioscaffolds on repair of acute hemi-transection spinal cord injury in rats. Zhongguo Xiu Fu Chong Jian Wai Ke Za Zhi. 2012;**26**:1362-1368

[77] Alexanian A, Fehlings M, Zhang Z, Maiman D. Transplanted neurally modified bone marrow-derived mesenchymal stem cells promote tissue protection and locomotor recovery in spinal cord injured rats. Neurorehabilitation and Neural Repair. 2011;**25**:873-880

[78] Boido M, Garbossa D, Fontanella M, Ducati A, Vercelli A. Mesenchymal stem cell transplantation reduces glial cyst and improves functional outcome after spinal cord compression. World Neurosurgery. 2014;**81**:183-190

[79] Zhang W, Yan Q, Zeng Y, Zhang X, Xiong Y, Wang J, et al. Implantation of adult bone marrow-derived mesenchymal stem cells transfected with the neurotrophin-3 gene and pretreated with retinoic acid in completely transected spinal cord. Brain Research. 2010;**1359**:256-271

[80] Ryu H, Lim J, Byeon Y, Park J, Seo M, Lee Y, et al. Functional recovery and neural differentiation after transplantation of allogenic adiposederived stem cells in a canine model of acute spinal cord injury. Journal of Veterinary Science. 2009;**10**:273-284

[81] Gu W, Zhang F, Xue Q, Ma Z, Lu P, Yu B. Transplantation of bone marrow mesenchymal stem cells reduces lesion volume and induces axonal regrowth of injured spinal cord. Neuropathology. 2010;**30**:205-217

[82] Park S, Byeon Y, Ryu H, Kang B, Kim Y, Kim W, et al. Comparison of canine umbilical cord blood-derived mesenchymal stem cell transplantation times: Involvement of astrogliosis, inflammation, intracellular actin cytoskeleton pathways, and neurotrophin-3. Cell Transplantation. 2011;**20**:1867-1880

[83] Lee J, Chung W, Kang E, Chung D, Choi C, Chang H, et al. Schwann cell-like remyelination following transplantation of human umbilical cord blood (hUCB)-derived mesenchymal stem cells in dogs with acute spinal cord injury. Journal of the Neurological Sciences. 2011;**300**:86-96

[84] Escalhão C, Ramos I, Hochman-Mendez C. Safety of allogeneic canine adipose tissue-derived mesenchymal stem cell intraspinal transplantation in dogs with chronic spinal cord injury. Stem Cells International. 2017;**2017**:3053759

[85] Deng Y, Liu X, Liu Z, Liu X, Liu Y, Zhou G. Implantation of BM mesenchymal stem cells into injured

spinal cord elicits de novo neurogenesis and functional recovery. Cytotherapy. 2006;**8**:210-214

[86] Steeves J, Lammertse D, Curt A, Fawcett J, Tuszynski M, Ditunno J, et al. Guidelines for the conduct of clinical trials for spinal cord injury (SCI) as developed by the ICCP panel: Clinical trial outcome measures. Spinal Cord. 2007;**45**:206-202

[87] Lammertse D, Tuszynski M, Steeves J, Curt A, Fawcett J, Rask C, et al. Guidelines for the conduct of clinical trials for spinal cord injury as developed by the ICCP panel: Clinical trial design. Spinal Cord. 2007;**45**:232-242

[88] Mastrolia I, Foppiani E, Murgia A, Candini O, Samarelli A, Grisendi G, et al. Challenges in clinical development of mesenchymal stromal/stem cells: Concise review. Stem Cells Translational Medicine. 2019;**8**:1135-1148

[89] Wyatt L, Keirstead H. Stem cell-based treatments for spinal cord injury. Progress in Brain Research. 2012;**201**:233-252

[90] Cho S, Kim Y, Kang H, Yim S, Park C, Min YH, et al. Functional recovery after the transplantation of neurally differentiated mesenchymal stem cells derived from bone marrow in a rat model of spinal cord injury. Cell Transplantation. 2016;**25**(7):1423

[91] Kabat M, Bobkov I, Kumar S, Grumet M. Trends in mesenchymal stem cell clinical trials 2004-2018: Is efficacy optimal in a narrow dose range? Stem Cells Translational Medicine. 2020;**9**:17-27

[92] Lalu M, McIntyre L, Pugliese C. Safety of cell therapy with mesenchymal stromal cells (SafeCell): A systematic review and meta-analysis of clinical trials. PLoS One. 2012:e47559

[93] Tsuji W, Schnider J, McLaughlin M. Effects of immunosuppressive drugs on viability and susceptibility of adipose- and bone marrow-derived mesenchymal stem cells. Frontiers in Immunology. 2015;**6**:131

[94] Ra J, Shin I, Kim S, Kang S, Kang B, Lee H. Safety of intravenous infusion of human adipose tissue-derived mesenchymal stem cells in animals and humans. Stem Cells and Development. 2011;**20**:1297-1308

[95] Jin M, Medress Z, Azad T, Doulames V, Veeravagu A. Stem cell therapies for acute spinal cord injury in humans: A review. Neurosurgical Focus. 2019;**46**(3):E10

[96] Osaka M, Honmou O, Murakami T. Intravenous administration of mesenchymal stem cells derived from bone marrow after contusive spinal cord injury improves functional outcome. Brain Research. 2010;**1343**:226-235

[97] Jossen V, van den Bos C, Eibl R. Manufacturing human mesenchymal stem cells at clinical scale: Process and regulatory challenges. Applied Microbiology and Biotechnology. 2018;**102**:3981-3994

[98] Reger R, Prockop D. Should publications on mesenchymal stem/progenitor cells include in-process data on the preparation of the cells? Stem Cells Translational Medicine. 2014;**3**:632-635

[99] Martin I, Galipeau J, Kessler C. Challenges for mesenchymal stromal cell therapies. Science Translational Medicine. 2019;**11**:1-3

Section 3

Rehabilitation Approaches

Chapter 6

Rehabilitation Therapies in Spinal Cord Injury Patients

Brenda Rodríguez-Mendoza, Paola A. Santiago-Tovar, Marco A. Guerrero-Godinez and Elisa García-Vences

Abstract

Spinal cord injury (SCI) represents a neurological life-changing condition that causes devastating physical, social, psychological, and economic consequences in the injured patient. It is due to traumatic causes that affect the motor and sensory functions, limiting daily life activities. Since rehabilitation is a fundamental process of recovery, this chapter will review diverse approaches in rehabilitation to restore or improve patients' capability. In the first section, functionality and quality of life tools will be discussed. Subsequently, rehabilitation strategies and their adoption will be explained. Ultimately, rehabilitation goals, according to the level of injury, will be reviewed.

Keywords: spinal cord injury, rehabilitation, exoskeleton, functional electrical stimulation, rehabilitation goals

1. Introduction

Spinal cord injury (SCI) is attributable to trauma caused by accidents like car crashes, falls or sports such as diving or gymnastics, and violent causes like gunshots or injuries by cold weapon [1] and also caused by nontraumatic causes like primary or metastatic tumors, compressive myelopathy such as cervical spondylotic myelopathy, neurodegenerative diseases such as motor neuron disease, autoimmune diseases like multiple sclerosis, infections such as epidural abscess, and vascular diseases such as medullary infarction, as well as genetic causes, for example, spinal muscular atrophy [2] that affect spinal cord motor and sensory function, also causing neurogenic bladder or bowel.

The global prevalence rate, including both traumatic and nontraumatic causes, is 40–80 cases per million people; however 90% of cases are due to traumatic causes, with a male-to-female ratio of 2:1, respectively [3], presenting with a bimodal age peak of young people and 60-year-old people [4]. To estimate the economic burden, the first year after injury treatment cost is estimated to be $334,170 USD rising to $1,023,924 USD [5]. The main causes of SCI are vehicle accidents, falls, violence [6], compressive myelopathy, tumors, and multiple sclerosis [2]. Most damaged anatomical regions are the lower cervical spine, cervicothoracic union, and thoracic-lumbar union [6]. Prognosis depends on the level of injury [4].

To the present day, there are no medical or surgical procedures to reverse neurological damage in SCI patients; therefore new rehabilitation strategies have been designed to avoid deterioration in many patient scopes. This process has to be coordinated by a multidisciplinary SCI expert team so that biopsychosocial impact on patients is reduced.

2. Evaluation and assessment tools in rehabilitation

There are several tools to assess the patient with SCI; some of them are the following, ASIA scale, Spinal Cord Independence Measure (SCIM) scale, Walking Index for Spinal Cord Injury II (WISCI II) scale, and Short-Form Health Survey (SF-36) quality of life test, which will be discussed in detail below. These are very useful instruments that ease decision-making on treatment and rehabilitation, taking into consideration patient capacity and expectations to integrate into society.

2.1 ASIA scale

This scale developed by the American Spinal Injury Association is considered the gold standard for SCI clinical evaluation. The scale significance relies on its capacity to determine the level of injury, whether it is a complete or incomplete injury, predict prognosis, and serve as guidance for treatment.

It consists of the examination of dermatomes and myotomes. For evaluation of sensory function, 28 key dermatomes are explored using a piece of cotton and a monofilament. For motor examination, five upper and five lower key muscle groups are evaluated. S4 and S5 dermatome evaluation is useful to determine if the injury is complete or incomplete by looking for external anal sphincter contraction and anal pressure sense.

Patients are classified from A, which means an injury is complete, to E, where patients have normal functionality (**Table 1**). This tool provides a long-term reliable prognosis, but it does not take into account pain and spasticity [7, 8].

According to this scale, an accurate prognosis can be established if a 72-h post-injury evaluation is made. 80% of patients with an A-type injury will remain in this classification; meanwhile, 10% will convert into a B-type injury and the 10% remaining will convert into a C-type injury; from the conversion percentage, only 14% of the patients will gain some aided gait capacity. Patients with B-type injury are considered to gain 33% of gait capacity, C-type injury patients will gain approximately 75% of gait capacity, and D-type injury patients will have a very good prognosis since most of them will be able to walk in 1-year post-injury [9, 10].

2.2 SCIM scale

The Spinal Cord Independence Measure is a tool that assesses an SCI patient capacity to perform daily life activities. This instrument evaluates 19 areas and contains 4 subscales: self-caring (0–20 points), breathing and sphincter control (0–40 points), room and bathroom mobility (0–10 points), and interior and exterior mobility (0–30 points). Besides these subscales, feeding, bed mobility, pressure ulcer prevention, and transfer from wheelchair to the car and floor are included [11].

The maximum score to obtain is 100 points; a high score means that the patient is independent for daily life activities. This is a self-assessment tool, so there is no need for qualified personnel to evaluate it [12].

A	Complete	No motor and sensory function
B	Incomplete	Sensory function preserved. No motor function below the level of injury, including S4-S5 level
C	Incomplete	Motor function preserved below the level of injury and more than half of the key muscles below the level of injury with less than 3/5 strength
D	Incomplete	Motor function preserved below the level of injury and at least half of key muscles with strength more than 3/5
E	Normal	Normal sensory and motor function

Table 1.
ASIA scale.

2.3 WISCI II

The Walking Index for Spinal Cord Injury II is a reliable and trustworthy tool to measure walking improvement in SCI patients [13]. It comprises 21 levels that evaluate gait, considering the use of walking aids. It goes from 0 (the patient is not able to walk) to 20 (the patient walks at least 10 m without crutches or assistance) [14].

2.4 SF-36

The Short-Form Health Survey questionnaire is a nonspecific generic test broadly used to evaluate the quality of life, considering both positive and negative subjects, in patients with chronic conditions and mobility diseases [15]. It is easy to answer and takes approximately 5 to 10 min.

The test comprises 36 items, divided into 8 subscales that evaluate the following areas: physical function (10 items), role limitations due to physical issues (4 items), pain (2 items), general health appreciation (5 items), vitality (4 items), social function (2 items), role limitations due to emotional issues (3 items), mental health (5 items), and an additional item that compares actual health with previous year perception of health [16]. Many studies have found with this instrument that SCI has a negative influence on the quality of life of patients [17].

3. Rehabilitation strategies

SCI is a neurological condition that demands a long rehabilitation period, coordinated by a multidisciplinary team because of the damage that it entails. To avoid complications as much as possible, to improve function, and to achieve the most independence, numerous rehabilitation strategies have been shown in many studies to have an impact in patient recovery; some of them are the following: strength, range of movement and stretching exercises, functional electrical stimulation (FES), epidural electrical stimulation (EES) of the spinal cord, occupational therapy, dry needling, and exoskeleton.

3.1 Range of movement, strength, and stretching exercises

Range of movement refers to the normal movement of a joint; hence range of movement exercises are those that promote joint mobility and flexibility.

Studies have observed that these exercises improve function for daily life activities [18], prevent contractures, protect tenodesis effect [19], strengthen paralyzed muscles, promote nerve and cerebral remodeling, and improve spinal microenvironment and functional prognosis [20]. For protection of the joint structure and preservation of muscle tone, sandbags, pillows, or orthotics are usually used. Exercise is important for strengthening the muscles of the upper limbs, emphasizing on rotation of the shoulders for the use of crutches or wheelchair. These exercises will help in the mobilization and independence in daily life activities. In patients with incomplete SCI, walking potential is high, so sitting, parallel bars, and balance exercises should be done [19].

3.2 Functional electrical stimulation

Functional electrical stimulation is a technique that artificially activates sensory-motor systems through electrical current pulses, producing action potentials in afferent and efferent neural pathways to stimulate muscles and generate movement [21]. This procedure is added to other therapies to increase mobility, sensory feedback, and muscle activity to decrease atrophy. It also provides cardiorespiratory fitness; improves posture and trunk stability [22]; prevents contractures, pressure ulcers, and orthostatic hypotension [23]; promotes nerve restoration; and prevents peripheral nerve deterioration [24].

Functional electrical stimulation is a technique that artificially activates sensory-motor systems through electrical current pulses, producing action potentials in afferent and efferent neural pathways to stimulate muscles and generate movement [21]. The main elements of a FES system are the battery, an electronic stimulator, control unit, wiring, and electrodes. The controller can work through a switch, joystick, or voice. There are different types of electrodes, superficial, intramuscular percutaneous, implantable, and epimysial; however the commercially available are the superficial ones, which should be placed over the skin above the nerves to be stimulated; the rest of the electrodes are for research purpose only. The electrodes must be of low-impedance, flexible, and easy to don and doff [22]. The electrical parameters of these systems are waveforms, amplitude, pulse width, reciprocity, ramp, and duration; all of these are combined to generate an electrical current and must be adjusted to achieve the desired response [22, 23].

It is important to evaluate the patient to determine if he or she is a candidate for this therapy. Some exclusion criteria for FES are the following: if the patient has an electrical implantable device, history of cancer, osteomyelitis, epilepsy, and thrombosis [23].

FES systems can be applied to different sites. In patients with cervical SCI, hand function recovery is the main priority, so there are FES systems developed for the upper limb that work through neuroprosthetics with a stimulator for forearm and hand muscles; patients with injuries at C5-C6 level can benefit with this therapy. The only commercially available systems for the upper limb are NESSH200 and Compex. NESSH200 consists of an adjustable wrist prosthetic with five electrodes for finger flexors and extensors, allowing handgrip [24, 25]. There are FES systems for lower limbs that allow sitting and mobility. The best candidates for this therapy are patients with injuries at T4-T12 level, which have more impact in patients with incomplete injuries. The FES neuroprosthetics for the lower limbs stimulate the knees and hips [24]. A commercially available FES system in the USA is the Parastep, which works through 4–6 channels to stimulate the quadriceps and gluteal muscles. Battery is placed on the waist and controls are over a walker [25]. FES cycling systems are also commercially available; one of them is developed by Restorative Therapies, Inc. [24] and the other one, ERGYS, developed by

Therapeutic Technologies, Inc. which has six electrodes to stimulate the quadriceps, hamstrings, and gluteal muscles [22].

This procedure is added to other therapies to increase mobility, sensory feedback, and muscle activity to decrease atrophy. It also provides cardiorespiratory fitness; improves posture and trunk stability [26]; prevents contractures, pressure ulcers, and orthostatic hypotension [27]; promotes nerve restoration; and prevents peripheral nerve deterioration [28].

3.3 Epidural electrical stimulation of the spinal cord

This strategy requires a device to be implanted through a laminectomy over the dura mater of the spinal cord [25]. The device delivers a rhythmical afferent electrical current to posterior nerve roots to activate central circuits that regulate movement, pain, and the cardiorespiratory system [22].

It is believed that EES activates two pathways: The first one stimulates afferent dorsal pathways that synapse with motor neurons; the second pathway directly stimulates motor neurons through stimulation of efferent motor nerves [26].

Studies in SCI patients have shown that this strategy decreases fatigue [25], improves cardiovascular and respiratory fitness, increases lean body mass, and improves bladder voiding [26]. The main disadvantage of EES is that it requires surgery for device insertion, which implicates the risk of infection, hematoma, or injury because of the device [25].

This experimental strategy requires a device to be implanted through a laminectomy over the dura mater of the spinal cord [29]. The device delivers a rhythmical afferent electrical current to posterior nerve roots to activate central circuits that regulate movement, pain, and the cardiorespiratory system [26].

It is believed that EES activates two pathways: The first one stimulates afferent dorsal pathways that synapse with motor neurons; the second pathway directly stimulates motor neurons through stimulation of efferent motor nerves [30].

Studies in SCI patients have shown that this strategy decreases fatigue [29], improves cardiovascular and respiratory fitness, increases lean body mass, and improves bladder voiding [30]. The main disadvantages of EES are that it requires surgery for device insertion, which implicates the risk of infection, hematoma, or injury because of the device [29], it is expensive, and it does not yet establish a standard number of sessions and parameter configurations since multiple studies have shown that outcomes vary in each patient due to SCI heterogeneity [30].

It is worth mentioning that this technique is used merely for research purpose only and it is not approved by health authorities. The evidence that exists to date is not enough to justify its use, since it has been studied only in specific small cohorts of patients or single patients with SCI and there are no clinical trials with this method [29, 30].

3.4 Transcutaneous electrical nerve stimulation (TENS)

TENS is a high- and low-frequency electrical current therapy. It is used for pain management, but many other benefits have been observed, such as balance and proprioception improvement and spasticity decrease [31]. To date, its mechanism of action is unknown; however, different theories assume it works by modulating inhibitory spinal circuits, by activating afferent neurons, or by inducing central nervous system plasticity [32]. When applying it, it is necessary to consider electrode positioning, frequency, and pulse intensity; though, there is not a consensus on how long sessions should last and how much frequency has to be applied. The main advantages of this therapy are that it is low cost, it is easy to apply since the patient can do it by himself/herself, and there are no side effects reported yet [31, 33].

3.5 Occupational therapy

Occupational therapy is a crucial process in rehabilitation since it eases societal role finding [19]. It focuses on enhancing daily life activity execution and fine movement, by searching for total independence or performing compensatory strategies to adapt [34–36] as well as patient's environment adaption (home, transportation, or workplace) to achieve total inclusion with its remaining abilities.

It demands equipment and techniques for transferring from one surface to another, dressing, bathing, grooming, feeding, cooking, respiratory exercises, and vesical and intestinal control. Besides, it also trains on wheelchair use and provides counseling for house modification like ramp addition, bath chair incorporation, and current insulation [34, 37].

3.6 Dry needling

Dry needling is an invasive procedure that consists of reaching muscle myofascial trigger points (MTPs) with a needle [38]. MTPs are small, tense muscle nodules that cause pain, cause weakness, and limit range of motion [39].

It is considered that dry needling stimulation inhibits spontaneous electrical activity in MTPs by diminishing the availability of acetylcholine in the motor end plate (it is believed that MTP originates here); consequently, muscle fiber relaxes, promoting pain and spasticity reduction and improving gait speed and stability in patients with incomplete injury [39, 40]. It is worth mentioning that more studies have to be made to set the frequency, duration, and intensity of sessions to obtain desirable outcomes [41].

3.7 Exoskeletons

Exoskeletons are battery-powered robotic devices that adjust to the patients' limbs; it can be operated with manual or oral control or micromovement detector to ease mobility and gait [26, 34].

Two main objectives of exoskeletons are promoting recovery through repeated movements to increase neural plasticity and assist mobility [42]. ReWalk™ and Indego™ are two community use exoskeletons [43] that enable walking, sitting, and climbing stairs up and down [44, 45]. Their use has shown improvements in quality of life, body composition, bone density, neuropathic pain, and spasticity [42] and an increase in gait speed [43], number of steps, and distance test before and after 90 days of training [34]. Restraints for certain users are height, weight, articular rigidity, and high cost ($80,000 USD) [43].

4. Electrical stimulation outcome measurement

Electrical stimulation outcome measurement can be performed through different methods, depending on the evaluated function. After FES, cycling outcomes can be measured by tridimensional analysis of the gait, estimation of oxygen consumption by indirect calorimetry, and muscle tone evaluation with Modified Ashworth Scale [46]. To evaluate outcomes after EES, the following methods can be applied: Motor activity can be evaluated by electromyography and motor tasks, the cardiovascular status might be evaluated by blood pressure measurement after tilt table testing; sexual performance can be assessed by the achievement of orgasm, and for bladder control evaluation, the Neurogenic Bladder Symptom Score (NBSS) can be applied, or post-void residual volume and voluntary urination capacity can be evaluated [47]. In other studies, the outcomes have been measured through motor task performance such as sitting and balance, body fat mass measurement, and respiratory function or inspiratory function by coughing; all cases are compared before and after therapy application [30].

5. Cardiovascular rehabilitation

Cardiovascular rehabilitation is critical because daily life activities are not enough to preserve cardiovascular health. It is estimated that the prevalence of cardiovascular diseases in patients with SCI is 60–70% and these represent, just as in able population, the main cause of death [48]. Besides, if the level of injury is higher, so will be the sedentarism and risk [49]. Another detail to consider is that SCI patients have a higher risk of complications such as thromboembolism, autonomic dysreflexia (AD), orthostatic hypotension, pain, and cardiac atrophy [34].

5.1 Cardiovascular health

For cardiovascular status enhancement in the SCI patient, it is suggested to: (1) do body weight-supported training for it has advantageous effects on cardiac rhythm and blood pressure; (2) do upper limb exercise with moderate to strenuous intensity 3 days a week for at least 6 weeks; and (3) train with functional electrical stimulation 3 days a week for at least 2 months. This kind of training improves the patient lipid profile because it reduces triglycerides and LDL cholesterol [48].

5.2 Orthostatic hypotension

After a long resting period, patients may suffer orthostatic hypotension. Training with a tilt table can be useful to get patients used to a vertical position, with a gradual beginning until tolerance of position is achieved. Afterward, patients should sit on the border of the bed by their own 3 or 4 times a day to keep balance. This is important because the position is needed for wheelchair use [19].

5.3 Glycemic control

For optimal glycemic control, aerobic exercise and EES 30 min a day for at least 3 times a week for 8 weeks is recommended [48].

5.4 Autonomic dysreflexia

Autonomic dysreflexia consists of a sudden blood pressure elevation caused by stimuli such as bladder overdistension or lack of bowel voiding, tight clothes, or pressure ulcers.

AD is considered when systolic blood pressure increases to 20–40 mmHg over the baseline. This usually occurs in patients with injuries in or over T6 level. AD happens because the previously mentioned stimuli start an uncontrolled adrenergic response due to an abnormal supraspinal regulatory signal, causing blood pressure elevation and bradycardia as a compensatory response.

AD is an emergency since it can cause serious complications such as hypertensive encephalopathy, seizures, cardiac arrest, or even death. To prevent patients from

AD, stimuli should be avoided. Some pharmacological treatments used are nitrates, nifedipine, prazosin, capsaicin, and botulinum toxin for refractory cases [50, 51].

6. Pulmonary rehabilitation

Pulmonary rehabilitation is critical in the acute and chronic phases of SCI, particularly in patients with high-level injuries because there are respiratory muscle paralysis limiting thoracic expansion, low pulmonary volumes, and weak cough [52]. Previously mentioned issues cause hypoventilation, mucus plugs, surfactant decrease, pneumonia, atelectasis, or respiratory failure that may result in death if not properly cared [53].

Additionally, due to respiratory mechanics compromise, certain voice characteristics are affected such as less syllable production per breathing, less volume, and more roughness [54].

The next section discusses the strategies to improve pulmonary function: (1) postural changes and early mobilization; (2) breathing techniques, spontaneous cough, and cough aid; (3) secretion management and respiratory muscle training [19, 34, 53]; and (4) pulmonary percussion and vibration therapy [26].

7. Neurofacilitation techniques

Neurofacilitation techniques are frequently used in patients who suffered a stroke but these can also be applied to patients with SCI. It consists of a group of techniques whose main objectives are functionality recovering through noninvasive neuropsychological stimulation, promoting nerve regeneration, and neural systems reorganization [55]. Some of these techniques are mentioned below.

7.1 Constraint-induced movement therapy

It is useful for upper limb rehabilitation. It consists of repeatedly training the limb mobility; meanwhile the contralateral limb is immobilized. However, there has to be some mobility remaining to be applied [55].

7.2 Body weight-supported treadmill training

This is a functional movement training in which the patient stands over a treadmill with a harness, aided by therapists to move the legs and keep balance. It can be beneficial since it is an aerobic exercise [55].

7.3 Bobath method

Bobath method consists of a group of complex, specific, and individualized techniques based on postural control and task execution, taking advantage of neuromuscular plasticity to achieve problem-solving in people with movement disorders. It is possible to control posture, reduce spasticity, increase muscle tone, and improve standing ability through this method [56, 57].

8. Neurogenic bladder

Up to 80% of patients with SCI suffer neurogenic bladder as a result of detrusor hyperactivity disorder, sphincter dyssynergia, or detrusor areflexia; they have an increased risk of urinary incontinence, recurrent infections, vesicoureteral reflux, and renal and bladder lithiasis [58].

Most of the patients will need management for dry, incomplete voiding, to ensure the low-pressure reservoir function of the bladder. This management begins with anticholinergic medication and intermittent catheterization; patients who failed these treatments need more invasive treatments such as sphincterotomy, botulinum toxin applications, and stent insertion [59].

Imaging and urodynamic studies should be performed for the initial evaluation of the patient [60]. Catheterization techniques are detailed below.

8.1 Clean intermittent catheterization

This is the most used method for bladder drainage without the need for a permanent catheter. A catheter is inserted in an interval of 4–6 h. It prevents complications such as hydronephrosis and kidney and bladder stones. It must be done by patients who have enough manual ability (writing and feeding) or a caregiver willing to do it [60].

8.2 Permanent catheterizations

It consists of the insertion of a suprapubic or urethral catheter. This catheterization is suggested for patients with poor manual ability, cognitive deficits, and limited assistance [60].

8.3 Credé method

It is the application of suprapubic pressure for drainage of the bladder. It is used when the bladder is flaccid or when it is necessary to increase the contraction; the Valsalva method is also used to drain the bladder [60].

8.4 Surgery

Transurethral sphincterotomy, stent colocation, or ileocystoplasty can be done.

9. Neurogenic bowel

Neurogenic bowel dysfunction occurs 95% of the time as constipation and 75% as fecal incontinence. Hemorrhoids, abdominal pain, prolapse, rectal bleeding, and anal fissures also occur and can trigger episodes of autonomic dysreflexia.

The management of this dysfunction requires a history of bowel habits in addition to a complete physical examination [61]. It is recommended to establish a schedule to defecate in a comfortable position, implementing changes in diet and lifestyle before using laxatives or suppositories. The caregiver must perform an examination or digital stimulation; manual removal of feces is also preferable [60, 61]. Enemas are another treatment [62].

10. Sexual rehabilitation

After SCI, sexual function is affected since it alters the motor, sensory, and autonomous functionality, and its importance relies in the fact that the number of patients with SCI is young in a childbearing age. There is damage to male fertility, vaginal lubrication, erection, and ejaculation [63].

The causes of sexual dysfunction are multifactorial: altered sensitivity, erectile dysfunction, and side effects of medical therapy.

In men with SCI, some dysfunctions can present as a delayed orgasm, erectile or ejaculatory disorder, seminal abnormalities such as hypomotility, or low sperm viability [64].

10.1 Male sexual quotient (MSQ)

It is a questionnaire designed to assess the sexual function and satisfaction in men. This instrument includes 10 questions where physical and emotional aspects are considered; scores go from 0 to 100 points [65].

10.2 Medical management for erectile dysfunction

Administration of phosphodiesterase-5 inhibitors is helpful in inhibition of guanosine monophosphate degradation causing smooth muscle relaxation. Other methods are intracavernous application of phentolamine, papaverine, and alprostadil or intraurethral application of alprostadil [64].

10.3 Management for ejaculatory dysfunction

Vibratory stimulation can be done until antegrade ejaculation is achieved. Another method is electroejaculation, which electrically stimulates prostatic nerves and muscles and seminal vesicles; if retrograde ejaculation occurs, a catheter is needed to collect residual semen from the bladder [64].

In women, sexual function after SCI has not been sufficiently studied as in male dysfunction. Sexual rehabilitation in women focuses on psychological matters and sphincter control during sexual activities. In addition, vaginal lubrication depends on neurological factors and vascular factors [66, 67].

11. Skin care

SCI causes an alteration in the microenvironment of the skin, causing excessive sweating, thinning, onychogryphosis, paronychia, tinea, seborrheic dermatitis, and cellulitis [68, 69]; besides, keeping the same position for a long time damages the integrity causing pressure ulcers [70].

Pressure ulcers are the result of applying pressure to tissue over a bone prominence, exceeding the 12–32 mmHg capillary pressure collapsing the capillaries and causing ischemia. Pressure ulcers represent a major problem for patients with SCI in the acute and chronic stages, also considering the cost involved in treatment [71]. For correct management, pressure must be decreased, and special mattresses, heel protectors, and turns and transfers are recommended. Regarding turns, these must be done in intervals of 2–4 h. Lateral positioning should be limited to minimize pressure on bony prominences. When the patient is in supine position, the bed must incline less than 30° or the limbs must be elevated. Patients using a wheelchair should be trained to distribute pressure by tilting at intervals of 15–30 min [62].

12. Nutritional support

Since life expectancy in patients with SCI has been prolonged, the incidence of metabolic syndrome, diabetes, cardiovascular diseases, but also malnutrition has increased substantially; therefore, it is important to make a nutritional plan.

There are no nutritional guidelines for patients with SCI; however, the following general measures are suggested:

1. Abundant consumption of fruits and vegetables to obtain fiber and avoid constipation; it is recommended to adjust the amount of it to avoid bloating and diarrhea.

2. Plenty intake of water (minimum 1.5 l).

3. Protein consumption of 0.8 g/kg per day is recommended, and if a pressure ulcer is present, this amount can be 1.2 g/kg, rising up to 2 g/kg if the ulcers are grade III or IV. The purpose of increasing protein consumption is to decrease the negative nitrogen balance, which is greater in acute stages of the disease; it is also helpful in preserving muscle mass and avoiding glucose intolerance. Liquid protein supplements that contain leucine may be recommended.

4. High-fat diets should be avoided since the patient lipid profile is altered and predisposes to metabolic syndrome.

5. Omega-3 is recommended because of its neuro- and cardioprotective effects; however more studies are required.

6. Micronutrients such as vitamins A, B5, D, E, and C and biotin and minerals such as calcium, chlorine, magnesium, and potassium are usually low consumed, so their intake should increase to improve glucose metabolism.

Nutritional plans must be individualized according to the objectives, the age of the patient, and the level of the injury [72, 73].

13. Psychological management of the patient with SCI

Psychological management after SCI is essential for the patient in order to return to activities of daily living. After an injury, there are many psychological stages in the readjustment process: shock and denial, depression, anxiety, anger, negotiation, and adaptation.

Psychological rehabilitation should start in the intensive care unit because the patient can experience disorientation, depression, anxiety, and sensory and sleep deprivation.

Psychotherapy groups are helpful to provide emotional support, educate in the development of new skills, and minimize social aversion. Similarly, family psychotherapy groups make it easier for the family to adjust to the new situation since similar emotional reactions also occur in them [74].

14. SCI patient rehabilitation stages through time

14.1 Acute phase

This rehabilitation begins since the patient is admitted to the hospital until the stabilization. It can be a period of 6–12 weeks, depending on the existence of complications. Rehabilitation in the acute phase is important to increase the patient strength and stability for postural adaptation and orthostatic hypotension [19, 28].

Passive exercises have been observed to decrease the risk of spasticity [43]. Other early interventions in rehabilitation are bed mobility with rotation at 2–3-h intervals to prevent pressure ulcers [19, 34].

14.2 Chronic phase

This rehabilitation is focused on the patient capacity to reintegrate into society. The goals are aimed to develop motor skills such as walking, transferring using the upper limbs, and wheelchair use [28], restore psychological status as much as possible, and perform occupational therapy [19].

15. Goals in rehabilitation

Despite the fact that most of the patients with SCI want to be able to walk again, the goals of rehabilitation are mainly focused on restoring quality of life [75], and these should be individualized according to the ASIA classification.

The following functional goals can be considered in the first 5 months according to the level of injury (time may vary depending on the patient ASIA classification he/she has):

- C4: independence with a motorized wheelchair, partial or assisted ventilation, and dependence on activities of daily living.

- C5: independence with a motorized wheelchair with hand control; may require extra respiratory care, performance of some activities of daily living, adapted driving is possible.

- C6: independence with a manual wheelchair, assistance in transfer with a sliding table, control of supporting points, can do certain activities of daily life; extension of the wrist is possible; adapted driving is possible.

- C7: this is a key level for wheelchair mobility, independent transfers without sliding board support.

- C8-L2: advanced wheelchair skills, independent daily life activities, driving with adaptations.

- L3 and lower: home and community ambulation with aid devices, independence in daily life activities [19, 34].

16. Conclusion

SCI is a relevant health issue because of the impact it has on the patient, his/her family, and health system. Even though there is active research for treatment development, being surgical or medical, in order to achieve motor recovery, in the present time, there are only treatments to reduce the damage after SCI and prevent future damage so none of this therapies are curative; one of this treatments is rehabilitation, which must be coordinated by a multidisciplinary team to reduce possible complications that may arise.

To achieve better outcomes at clinical level, it is recommended to perform an integral rehabilitation therapy that combines different strategies, for example, functional, transcutaneous, or epidural electrical stimulation in addition to musculoskeletal rehabilitation exercises to decrease complications associated with this pathology. It is important to emphasize that some rehabilitation strategies have not yet been approved by health authorities for commercial use and to date have only shown results in very small populations with very particular characteristics, which impede their general application in patients with SCI, in addition to the heterogeneity of spinal cord injuries due to the level of injury, age, treatments used before, or time since injury.

The ultimate goal of these interventions is to achieve patient's societal reintegration and become independent in most of the activities according to the severity of their condition; therefore improving and updating these strategies create opportunities for novel innovative research, as well as implementing rehabilitation strategies as a complement for regenerative pharmacological and non-pharmacological strategies for the SCI patient.

Author details

Brenda Rodríguez-Mendoza[1†], Paola A. Santiago-Tovar[1†], Marco A. Guerrero-Godinez[2] and Elisa García-Vences[1*]

1 Facultad de Ciencias de la Salud, Centro de Investigación en Ciencias de la Salud (CICSA), Universidad Anáhuac México Campus Norte, Mexico

2 Instituto Nacional de Rehabilitación Luis Guillermo Ibarra Ibarra, Mexico

*Address all correspondence to: edna.garcia@anahuac.mx

† These authors contributed equally.

References

[1] Chen Y, Tang Y, Vogel LC, Devivo MJ. Causes of spinal cord injury. Topics in Spinal Cord Injury Rehabilitation. 2013;**19**(1):1-8

[2] Grassner L, Marschallinger J, Dünser MW, Novak HF, Zerbs A, Aigner L, et al. Nontraumatic spinal cord injury at the neurological intensive care unit: Spectrum, causes of admission and predictors of mortality. Therapeutic Advances in Neurological Disorders. 2016;**9**(2):85-94

[3] Salud OMdl. Lesiones Medulares. 2013. Available from: http://www.who.int/es/news-room/fact-sheets/detail/spinal-cord-injury

[4] Alizadeh A, Dyck SM, Karimi-Abdolrezaee S. Traumatic spinal cord injury: An overview of pathophysiology, models and acute injury mechanisms. Frontiers in Neurology. 2019;**10**:282

[5] Ma VY, Chan L, Carruthers KJ. Incidence, prevalence, costs, and impact on disability of common conditions requiring rehabilitation in the United States: Stroke, spinal cord injury, traumatic brain injury, multiple sclerosis, osteoarthritis, rheumatoid arthritis, limb loss, and back pain. Archives of Physical Medicine and Rehabilitation. 2014;**95**(5):986-995.e1

[6] Sekhon L, Fehlings M. Epidemiology, demographics, and pathophysiology of acute spinal cord injury. Spine. 2001;**26**(24S):S2-S12

[7] Roberts TT, Leonard GR, Cepela DJ. Classifications in brief: American spinal injury association (ASIA) impairment scale. Clinical Orthopaedics and Related Research. 2017;**475**(5):1499-1504

[8] Van Middendorp JJ, Goss B, Urquhart S, Atresh S, Williams RP, Schuetz M. Diagnosis and prognosis of traumatic spinal cord injury. Global Spine Journal. 2011;**1**(1):1-8

[9] Scivoletto G, Tamburella F, Laurenza L, Torre M, Molinari M. Who is going to walk? A review of the factors influencing walking recovery after spinal cord injury. Frontiers in Human Neuroscience. 2014;**8**:141

[10] Vazquez XM, Rodriguez MS, Peñaranda JMS, Concheiro L, Barus JIM. Determining prognosis after spinal cord injury. Journal of Forensic and Legal Medicine. 2008;**15**(1):20-23

[11] Catz A, Itzkovich M. Spinal cord independence measure: Comprehensive ability rating scales for the spinal cord lesion patient. JRRD. 2007;**44**(1):65-68

[12] Harvey L, Anderson K. The spinal cord independence measure. Journal of Physiotherapy. 2015;**61**(2):99

[13] Burns AS, Delparte JJ, Patrick M, Marino RJ, Ditunno JF. The reproducibility and convergent validity of the walking index for spinal cord injury (WISCI) in chronic spinal cord injury. Neurorehabilitation and Neural Repair. 2011;**25**(2):149-157

[14] Morganti B, Scivoletto G, Ditunno P, Ditunno JF, Molinari M. Walking index for spinal cord injury (WISCI): Criterion validation. Spinal Cord. 2005;**43**(1):27-33

[15] Tate DG, Kalpakjian CZ, Forchheimer MB. Quality of life issues in individuals with spinal cord injury. Archives of Physical Medicine and Rehabilitation. 2002;**83**:S18-S25

[16] Aquarone RL, e Faro ACM. Scales on quality of life in patients with spinal cord injury: Integrative review. Einstein (São Paulo). 2014;**12**(2):245-250

[17] Gurcay E, Bal A, Eksioglu E, Cakci A. Quality of life in patients with spinal cord injury. International Journal of Rehabilitation Research. 2010;**33**(4):356-358

[18] Tseng C-N, Chen CC-H, Wu S-C, Lin L-C. Effects of a range-of-motion exercise programme. Journal of Advanced Nursing. 2007;**57**(2):181-191

[19] Nas K, Yazmalar L, Şah V, Aydın A, Öneş K. Rehabilitation of spinal cord injuries. World Journal of Orthopedics. 2015;**6**(1):8-16

[20] Fu J, Wang H, Deng L, Li J. Exercise training promotes functional recovery after spinal cord injury. Neural Plasticity. 2016;**2016**:4039580

[21] Popović DB. Advances in functional electrical stimulation (FES). Journal of Electromyography and Kinesiology. 2014;**24**(6):795-802

[22] Gorman PH. An update on functional electrical stimulation after spinal cord injury. Neurorehabilitation and Neural Repair. 2000;**14**(4):251-263

[23] Martin R, Sadowsky C, Obst K, Meyer B, McDonald J. Functional electrical stimulation in spinal cord injury:: From theory to practice. Topics in Spinal Cord Injury Rehabilitation. 2012;**18**(1):28-33

[24] Ho CH, Triolo RJ, Elias AL, Kilgore KL, DiMarco AF, Bogie K, et al. Functional electrical stimulation and spinal cord injury. Physical Medicine and Rehabilitation Clinics of North America. 2014;**25**(3):631-654

[25] Ragnarsson KT. Functional electrical stimulation after spinal cord injury: Current use, therapeutic effects and future directions. Spinal Cord. 2008;**46**(4):255-274

[26] Hachem LD, Ahuja CS, Fehlings MG. Assessment and management of acute spinal cord injury: From point of injury to rehabilitation. The Journal of Spinal Cord Medicine. 2017;**40**(6):665-675

[27] Bersch I, Tesini S, Bersch U, Frotzler A. Functional electrical stimulation in spinal cord injury: Clinical evidence versus daily practice. Artificial Organs. 2015;**39**(10):849-854

[28] Harvey LA. Physiotherapy rehabilitation for people with spinal cord injuries. Journal of Physiotherapy. 2016;**62**(1):4-11

[29] Mayr W, Krenn M, Dimitrijevic MR. Epidural and transcutaneous spinal electrical stimulation for restoration of movement after incomplete and complete spinal cord injury. Current Opinion in Neurology. 2016;**29**(6):721-726

[30] Calvert JS, Grahn PJ, Zhao KD, Lee KH. Emergence of epidural electrical stimulation to facilitate sensorimotor network functionality after spinal cord injury. Neuromodulation: Technology at the Neural Interface. 2019;**22**(3):244-252

[31] Fernández-Tenorio E, Serrano-Muñoz D, Avendaño-Coy J, Gómez-Soriano J. Transcutaneous Electrical Nerve Stimulation for Spasticity: A Systematic Review | Neurología (English Edition) [Internet]. Spain: Elsevier; 2019

[32] Sivaramakrishnan A, Solomon J, Manikandan N. Comparison of transcutaneous electrical nerve stimulation (TENS) and functional electrical stimulation (FES) for spasticity in spinal cord injury—A pilot randomized cross-over trial. The Journal of Spinal Cord Medicine. 2017;**41**(4):397-406

[33] Barroso F, Pascual-Valdunciel A, Torricelli D, Moreno JC, Del Ama-Espinosa A, Laczko J, et al. Noninvasive modalities used in spinal cord injury rehabilitation. In: Spinal Cord Injury Therapy. London: IntechOpen, 2019

[34] Mazwi NL, Adeletti K, Hirschberg RE. Traumatic spinal cord injury: Recovery, rehabilitation, and prognosis. Current Trauma Reports. 2015;**1**(3):182-192

[35] Bolt M, Ikking T, Baaijen R, Saenger S. Occupational therapy and primary care. Primary Health Care Research & Development. 2019;**20**:e27

[36] Arsh A, Anwar Z, Zeb A, Ilyas SM. Effectiveness of occupational therapy in improving activities of daily living performance in complete cervical tetraplegic patients; A quasi-experimental study. Pakistan Journal of Medical Sciences. 2020;**36**(2):96-99

[37] Foy T, Perritt G, Thimmaiah D, Heisler L, Offutt JL, Cantoni K, et al. The SCIRehab project: Treatment time spent in SCI rehabilitation. Occupational therapy treatment time during inpatient spinal cord injury rehabilitation. The Journal of Spinal Cord Medicine. 2011;**34**(2):162-175

[38] Cruz-Montecinos C, Núñez-Cortés R, Bruna-Melo T, Tapia C, Becerra P, Pavez N, et al. Dry needling technique decreases spasticity and improves general functioning in incomplete spinal cord injury: A case report. The Journal of Spinal Cord Medicine. 2018:1-5

[39] Shah JP, Thaker N, Heimur J, Aredo JV, Sikdar S, Gerber L. Myofascial trigger points then and now: A historical and scientific perspective. PM & R : The Journal of Injury, Function, and Rehabilitation. 2015;7(7):746-761

[40] Abbaszadeh-Amirdehi M, Ansari NN, Naghdi S, Olyaei G, Nourbakhsh MR. The neurophysiological effects of dry needling in patients with upper trapezius myofascial trigger points: Study protocol of a controlled clinical trial. BMJ Open. 2013;**3**(5):e002825

[41] Dunning J, Butts R, Mourad F, Young I, Flannagan S, Perreault T. Dry needling: A literature review with implications for clinical practice guidelines. The Physical Therapy Review. 2014;**19**(4):252-265

[42] Mekki M, Delgado AD, Fry A, Putrino D, Huang V. Robotic rehabilitation and spinal cord injury: A narrative review. Neurotherapeutics: The journal of the American Society for Experimental NeuroTherapeutics. 2018;**15**(3):604-617

[43] Kandilakis C, Sasso-Lance E. Exoskeletons for personal use after spinal cord injury. Archives of Physical Medicine and Rehabilitation. 2019;S0003-9993(19)30396-X

[44] Guanziroli E, Cazzaniga M, Colombo L, Basilico S, Legnani G, Molteni F. Assistive powered exoskeleton for complete spinal cord injury: Correlations between walking ability and exoskeleton control. European Journal of Physical and Rehabilitation Medicine. 2019;**55**(2):209-216

[45] Hartigan C, Kandilakis C, Dalley S, Clausen M, Wilson E, Morrison S, et al. Mobility outcomes following five training sessions with a powered exoskeleton. Topics in Spinal Cord Injury Rehabilitation. 2015;**21**(2):93-99

[46] Yaşar E, Yılmaz B, Göktepe S, Kesikburun S. The effect of functional electrical stimulation cycling on late functional improvement in patients with chronic incomplete spinal cord injury. Spinal Cord. 2015;**53**(12):866-869

[47] Darrow D, Balser D, Netoff TI, Krassioukov A, Phillips A, Parr A, et al. Epidural spinal cord stimulation facilitates immediate restoration of dormant motor and autonomic supraspinal pathways after chronic neurologically complete spinal cord injury. Journal of Neurotrauma. 2019;**36**(15):2325-2336

[48] Warburton DER, Eng JJ, Krassioukov A, Sproule S. Cardiovascular health and exercise rehabilitation in spinal cord injury. Topics in Spinal Cord Injury Rehabilitation. 2007;**13**(1):98-122

[49] Krassioukov AV, Currie KD, Hubli M, Nightingale TE, Alrashidi AA, Ramer L, et al. Effects of exercise interventions on cardiovascular health in individuals with chronic, motor complete spinal cord injury: Protocol for a randomized controlled trial [cardiovascular health/outcomes: Improvements created by exercise and education in SCI (CHOICES) study]. BMJ Open. 2019;**9**(1):e023540

[50] Eldahan KC, Rabchevsky AG. Autonomic dysreflexia after spinal cord injury: Systemic pathophysiology and methods of management. Autonomic Neuroscience. 2018;**209**:59-70

[51] Sharif H, Hou S. Autonomic dysreflexia: A cardiovascular disorder following spinal cord injury. Neural Regeneration Research. 2017;**12**(9):1390-1400

[52] Berlowitz DJ, Wadsworth B, Ross J. Respiratory problems and management in people with spinal cord injury. Breathe (Sheffield, England). 2016;**12**(4):328-340

[53] Galeiras Vázquez R, Rascado Sedes P, Mourelo Fariña M, Montoto Marqués A, Ferreiro Velasco ME. Respiratory management in the patient with spinal cord injury. BioMed Research International. 2013;**2013**:168757

[54] Ward EC, Jarman L, Cornwell PL, Amsters DI. Impact of voice and communication deficits for individuals with cervical spinal cord injury living in the community. International Journal of Language & Communication Disorders. 2016;**51**(5):568-580

[55] Barrett AM, Oh-Park M, Chen P, Ifejika NL. Neurorehabilitation: Five new things. Neurology: Clinical Practice. 2013;**3**(6):484-492

[56] Michielsen M, Vaughan-Graham J, Holland A, Magri A, Suzuki M. The Bobath concept—A model to illustrate clinical practice. Disability and Rehabilitation. 2019;**41**(17):2080-2092

[57] Graham JV, Eustace C, Brock K, Swain E, Irwin-Carruthers S. The Bobath concept in contemporary clinical practice. Topics in Stroke Rehabilitation. 2009;**16**(1):57-68

[58] Best KL, Ethans K, Craven BC, Noreau L, Hitzing S. Identifying and classifying quality of life tools for neurogenic bladder function after spinal cord injury: A systematic review. The Journal of Spinal Cord Medicine. 2017;**40**(5):505-529

[59] Al Taweel W, Seyam R. Neurogenic bladder in spinal cord injury patients. Research and Reports in Urology. 2015;**7**:85-99

[60] Francis K. Physiology and management of bladder and bowel continence following spinal cord injury. Ostomy/Wound Management. 2007;**53**(12):18-27

[61] Emmanuel A. Neurogenic bowel dysfunction. F1000Research. 2019;**8**:1-6

[62] Ong B, Wilson JR, Henzel MK. Management of the patient with chronic spinal cord injury. Medical Clinics of North America. 2019;**104**(2):263-278

[63] Biering-Sørensen I, Bølling Hansen R, Biering-Sørensen F. Sexual function in a traumatic spinal cord injured population 10-45 years after injury. Journal of Rehabilitation Medicine. 2012;**44**:926-931

[64] Kasum M, Oreskovic S, Kordic M, Cehic E, Hauptman D, Ejubovic E, et al. Improvement of sexual and reproductive function in men with spinal cord lesión. Acta Clinica Croatica. 2018;**57**(1):149-156

[65] De Paula Miranda E, Mendes Gomes C, De Bessa J, Najjar Abdo CH, Suzuki Bellucci CH, De Castre Filho JE, et al. Evaluation of sexual dysfunction in men with spinal cord injury using the male sexual quotient. Physical Medicine and Rehabilitation. 2016;**97**(6):947-952

[66] Maasoumi R, Zarei F, Merghati-Khoei E, Lawson T, Emami-Razavi SH. Development of a sexual needs rehabilitation framework in women post-spinal cord injury: A study from Iran. Physical Medicine and Rehabilitation. 2018;**99**(3):548-554

[67] D'Andrea S, Castellini C, Paladino V, Totaro M, Felzani G, Francavilla S, et al. Metabolic syndrome is the key determinant of impaired vaginal lubrication in women with chronic spinal cord injury. Journal of Endocrinological Investigation. 2020:1-7

[68] Stover SL, Hale AM, Buell AB. Skin complications other than pressure ulcers following spinal cord injury. Archives of Physical Medicine and Rehabilitation. 1994;**75**:987-993

[69] A-Han ZA, Choi JY, Ko YJ. Dermatological problems following spinal cord injury in Korean patients. The Journal of Spinal Cord Medicine. 2015;**38**(1):63-67

[70] Shabadi SS, Shabadi VS. Skin care in spinal cord injury patients: A practical and scientific approach to the devastating problem. International Journal of Advanced Research. 2017;**5**(2):1233-1243

[71] Kruger EA, Pires M, Ngann Y, Sterling M, Rubayi S. Comprehensive management of pressure ulcers in spinal cord injury: Current concepts and future trends. The Journal of Spinal Cord Medicine. 2013;**36**(6):572-585

[72] Khalil RE, Gorgey AS, Janisko M, Dolbow DR, Moore JR, Gater DR. The role of nutrition in health status after spinal cord injury. Aging and Disease. 2013;**4**(1):14-22

[73] Bigford G, Nash MS. Nutritional health considerations for persons with spinal cord injury. Topics in Spinal Cord Injury Rehabilitation. 2017;**23**(3):188-206

[74] Westie KS. Psychological aspects of spinal cord injury. Clinical Prosthetics & Orthotics. 1987;**11**(4):225-229

[75] McDonald JW, Becker D. Spinal cord injury: Promising interventions and realistic goals. American Journal of Physical Medicine & Rehabilitation. 2003;**82**(10 Suppl):S38-S49

Chapter 7

Psychological Sexual Health of People with Paraplegia

Stefano Federici, Francesco Artegiani, Daniele Diotallevi, Giovanna Caruso and Alessandra Castellani Mencarelli

Abstract

People with paraplegia have to fight their own and societal attitudes and stereotypes that reduce sexuality to the physiological functions of genitalia. These psychological and social limitations arise from cultural and disability models that focus sexual pleasure on phallocentric primacy, and sexual attractiveness of perfect bodies. In this chapter, we evaluate the impacts of a psychoeducational intervention in a personal growth group on the sexual life of two groups of people with spinal cord injury (SCI) and their partners, throughout their sexual interest and satisfaction, depression, and anxiety. In the first study, nonparametric statistical tests were used to compare pre- and post-outcome measures for all participants. In the second study, the grounded theory was used to explore dialogs and activities that were audiotaped during the group meetings. The participants in both groups were patients and their partners. The psychoeducational intervention was clearly effective in increasing sexual interest and satisfaction as well as the motivation and ability to enjoy sexuality. Anxiety was minimized for all participants, although it may not have been associated with the psychoeducational intervention. In addition, the intervention significantly improved the partner and patient group's opportunity and ability to enjoy sexuality.

Keywords: spinal cord injury, sexuality, sex stereotypes, biopsychosocial model, sexuality and disability, people with paraplegia

1. Introduction

When someone has experienced spinal cord injury (SCI), the first question they often ask is, "Doctor, will I ever walk again?" The thought soon after—sometimes never verbalized—emerges with equal urgency: "Will I be able to have sex?" This question is not answered easily, although the slogan of the American Consortium for Spinal Cord Medicine [1] exhorts to believe that "No injury, no matter how serious, can take away your ability to have a relationship, experience love, and experience the attraction between two people" (p. 3). People with SCI face many difficulties to regain confidence in themselves and their ability to experience intimacy and affection [2]. These challenges do not just emanate from the genital dysfunction caused by the injury, including alterations or loss of genital sensation, or erection, ejaculation, lubricate, and orgasm [3, 4]. They also arise because they must rediscover a new way of pleasure to themselves and others by learning to inhabit a body that in many ways is new and dissimilar and requires a different way of touching, caressing, and exploring themselves and their partner [4].

In addition to this difficult adjustment to changes, like many other people with disabilities, people with SCI have to battle with their own and societal attitudes and stereotypes that deny individuals with disabilities are sexual beings [4, 5]. Such attitudes and stereotypes are the results of two pervasive and interrelated misconceptions (myths), which very often influence human thinking and behavior: bodily perfection [6] and asexuality [7–10]. These two myths arise from a disability model that is often known as the medical model of disability [11, 12], whereby people are deemed disabled due to their medical condition or impairment [13, 14]. Therefore, disability is understood as an individual inability to conform to a standard of normality, namely when the abnormality occurs within the person [15], making him/her different from the majority of people [16].

According to this (medical) disability model, people with SCI have a disability in sexual relations due to the limitation or lack (resulting from the injury) of ability to conduct sexual activity in the manner that is considered normal or ideal [17]. Here, the interrelation between bodily perfection and sexual activity is closely and precisely related. 'Abled' people have to see the person with SCI as asexual because the injury obviously has affected the capacity to perform the so-called normal sexual activity. Conceiving sexual activity by a person with a disability for a 'normal' population would mean admitting to imagine an abnormal (monstrous) sexuality [8, 18].

The myths of bodily perfection and asexuality of disabled persons are not mere social constructions that influence attitudes and stereotypes. Every cultural context and historical period encompasses an ideal of bodily beauty and sexual behavioral norms [19]. Therefore, we should find such myths as universal human convictions [20, 21] that emerged from psychological mechanisms that evolved to solve long-enduring adaptive problems characteristic of the ancestral human environment [22]. Mating with someone who is unhealthy could pose a range of adaptive risks to our ancestors, including transmitting communicable diseases or viruses, impacting survival and reproduction, infecting children, and jeopardizing the children's chances of survival and reproduction [23, 24]. Hence, human survival was guaranteed by an evolved psychological mechanism to avoid contact and sexual intercourse with persons with visible deformity [25, 26]. Park et al. [27] found that individual differences in disease perception predict immediate cognitive responses that connect physical disability to disease (medical model) and also predict behavioral avoidance (disgust) of people with physical disabilities. Meloni et al. [28] also found a relationship between an evolved disease avoidance mechanism and contemporary prejudices that affect individuals with physical disabilities.

It should be noted that the field of psychiatry has a specific term for the sexual attraction to the body of a person with a disability: devotism. This concept is considered suspect and, to a certain extent, pathological; it is classified as a paraphilia in the Diagnostic and Statistical Manual of Mental Disorders, Fifth Edition [29].

Another signal that the medical disability model might act as an innate psychological mechanism below the two cultural constructs of bodily perfection and asexuality, as a cognitive constraint [30], is the occurrence of disability explanation compatible with the medical model early in childhood [31–33], independent of parents' disability representations and explanations [13].

Like the nondisabled, most people with SCI have grown up believing that disability is deviance and that bodily perfection is the standard [34]. As Susan Wendell wrote in her famous autobiography book *The Rejected Body* [19], to identify oneself as a disabled person requires a change in one's own personality and a radically new way of thinking about oneself. The SCI is almost always a devastating event with many life-changing consequences, all of which require a number of changes during their post-injury lives [35, 36]. Sexual adjustment to SCI is one of those problems that is closely related to body image [2], general psychological health, overall self-esteem [37, 38], and body attractiveness [10, 39].

In a male-centered patriarchal culture [40]—characterized by unequal relationships between men and women (polarization) and power distribution (androcentrism), and biological essentialism (i.e., gender and roles vary by nature) [41]—the sex most people get to know is totally phallocentric (penis centered). According to Freud [42], around the age of five, children become aware that they either possess a penis or do not possess a penis and that having a penis is "a proud possession" [43]. Conversely, for women, the absence of a penis makes them "victim to envy for the penis" [42]. The recognition that one has or does not have a particular set of genitals is, for Freud, tantamount to recognizing the gender to whom they belong. "I have a penis" means "I am a boy" and "I do not have a penis" means "I am a girl." In this system, the gender identity is a genital (penis-centered) identity. As Rubin [44] wrote,

> *"The alternative presented to the child [to have a penis or to be castrated] may be rephrased as an alternative between having, or not having, the phallus. [...] The presence or absence of the phallus carries the differences between two sexual statuses, 'man' and 'woman'."* (p. 191)

This penis orientation relates to the awareness that having and using erections has something to do with masculinity [45]. Therefore, "males are in constant danger of losing their manhood and their identities" [45] when the erectile functions are compromised. As testified by Tepper [9], a sexuality educator and counselor living with SCI, "[T]he man with erectile dysfunction, inhibited ejaculation, loss of sensation, or physical limitations might conclude that his sex life is over." (p. 45).

Extensive research on erectile functions and male sexuality has largely overlooked the female sexuality of women with SCI [39, 46, 47]. This phenomenon is not surprising within Judeo-Christian androcentrism that restricts the sexual role of a woman to a reproductive function within the family and the ability to stimulate and satisfy a man's own sexual appetite [41]. This view denies women the experience of sexual pleasure [48]. Given that SCI neither compromises the receptive function of female sexual organs nor a woman's reproductive capacity [1], the biggest issues for women after SCI is usually focused on the perceived attractiveness of their bodies [39], that is, as a function of male sexuality. In an androcentric, penis-centered sense of sexuality—that Tom Shakespeare [49] defined as the "fucking ideology": heterosexual and penetrative intercourse with a male on top of a female—characterizing Judeo-Christian androcentrism, loss of genital sensation does not compromise a woman's sexual role. The Austrian philosopher Otto Weininger, a Jew who converted to Christianity in 1902 and who became a real posthumous celebrity within the German-speaking cultural world of the early twentieth century and beyond, in his popular and influential book on sex and character [50] published in 1903, explained the difference between a mother and a prostitute, woman's polar attributes (*sic*), "The mother does not experience sexual intercourse any *less* than the prostitute, but *differently*. The mother's behaviour is mainly receptive and accepting, while the prostitute feels and savors the pleasure to the extreme" (p. 205; emphasis in the original). Far from it, the loss of genital sensation ensures the woman's virginal and chaste role [48] (see also the traditional practice of female genital mutilation in Islamic cultures that involves more than 200 million girls and women in 30 countries worldwide: https://www.unicef.org/media/files/FGMC_2016_brochure_final_UNICEF_SPREAD.pdf). Alexander and Rosen [51] and Komisaruk and Whipple [52] provided other evidence of a different focus on the sexuality of women with SCI compared to men. Women are oriented to giving rather than receiving pleasure. As both studies found, the major sexual concern of women is the diminishing opportunity and ability to give their partner sexual fulfillment because the disability disfigured the beauty of their body. Moreover, according to Kettl et al. [39],

> *"The biggest and most remarkable change [for women] after spinal cord injury in our study was the worsening in body image. This was far greater than any change in ratings of sexual practice or enjoyment."* (p. 294)

Given that the sexual role of a woman in patriarchal cultures is restricted to the attractiveness of their body as a function of male sexuality, in a reverse sense, this factor can also be their shame. In fact, a woman's attractiveness is perceived similarly to penis erection, that is, a sexual behavior: when a male finds an attractive body, then sex is allowed because the former is a function of the latter. As LaRocca and Kromrey [53] found, male students consider an event to be more harassing when the victim was unattractive (read, not sexually available) compared to when the victim was attractive (read, sexually available). This stereotype is certainly no less affecting in women's judgment, who consider an event as more harassing when the victim was attractive (if sexually available, why violence?) than when the victim was unattractive (because of sexual unavailability, male violence allowed). Thus, Golden reports [54] that an action by an attractive male directed toward an unattractive female is more likely to be identified as not harassing. From a recent survey conducted by the Italian National Institute of Statistics [55] on stereotypes on gender roles and the social image of sexual violence, the prejudice that blames the woman for their suffered sexual violence still persists. For instance, 23% (without gender differences) believe that women can cause sexual violence with their way of dressing (read, their attractiveness). Therefore, it is not surprising that the main sexual concern of women with SCI is to have a body that is no longer attractive, no longer capable, that is, of giving their partner the 'right' sexual pleasure, and run the risk of deserving violence. Still in a recent survey conducted in the United Kingdom, Thrussell et al. [56], in accordance with previous literature, reaffirm that for women with SCI.

> *"satisfaction with body image was reduced. To look 'sexy' was difficult […]. Lacking confidence and feeling sexually unattractive during rehabilitation was common; support and opportunities to improve self-confidence, self-esteem, body image and social skills were identified as essential."* (pp. 1088–1091)

The aim of this chapter is to provide data for the Love & Life project that was collected from two interventional studies led by two growth groups. The project was performed in the Unipolar Spinal Unit of the 'S. *Maria* della Misericordia' hospital in Perugia (USU-PG). This unit is one of the 22 spinal units that comprise the Italian National Health System, of which 9 are unipolar. Love & Life aims to enhance the psychological sexual health of USU-PG in- and outpatients and their partners. To achieve this goal, the project follows the biopsychosocial sexual health model of the World Health Organization [57, 58] and human functioning [59]. This positive, holistic, and comprehensive view states that sexual health is "a state of physical, emotional, mental, and social well-being in relation to sexuality; it is not merely the absence of disease, dysfunction, or infirmity" ([58], p. 3). This view implies overcoming the reduction of the medical model and its socio-cultural products (myths, attitudes, stereotypes, and prejudices), which restrict sexuality to the physiological function of genitalia, phallocentric primacy of sexual pleasure, and attractiveness of only bodily perfection. The Love & Life initiative facilitates a psychological (emotional and behavioral) change, which increases self- and sexual esteem and satisfaction. By promoting a psychoeducational personal growth group [60], people with SCI and their partners can experience, express, and rework thoughts, fantasies, desires, beliefs, attitudes, values, behaviors, roles, and relationships about sexuality [58].

This project was approved by the ethics committee of the Department of Philosophy, Social & Human Sciences, and Education, University of Perugia. The project information was disseminated both orally and in paper format. Written informed consent was recorded for each group member on a prepared form by participant signature.

2. Study 1

2.1 Setting

The inpatients were recruited from the USU-PG by the psychologist working in the unit between November and December 2017. All inpatients admitted to the USU-PG received a brochure with the goal of the Love & Life initiative, participation requirements, topics for the sessions on sexual life in the personal growth group, schedule of meetings, and leaders' names and phone numbers. The same content was also presented in a poster format in unit corridors and in other hospital departments. In the same time, IR also recruited outpatients from the USU-PG patient registry by phone. The personal growth group on sexual life met in the USU-PG wheelchair accessible rehabilitation room from December 2017 through May 2018.

2.2 Participants

The inclusion criteria for attending the Love & Life personal growth group on sexual life were the following:

- Age $\geq$ 18 years
- Provide voluntary written informed consent
- USU-PG in- and outpatients with a traumatic SCI (para- or tetraplegic), with or without a partner
- Current partner (wife, husband, or sexual partner) of in- and outpatients of USU-PG who attended the Love & Life personal growth group

We use 'participants' to refer to all those who attended the growth group on sexual life and 'patients' to refer to both inpatients and outpatients. Fourteen participants attended the growth group on sexual life from December 2017 to May 2018. Only 11 participants were included in the present study, as explained in Section 2.7 (the subsection 'Sample').

2.3 Measurements and procedures

A sociodemographic questionnaire and three outcome measures were self-administered (see below) by participants and their partners who had provided voluntary written informed consent during the recruitment process. The outcome measures were administered again at the end of the last group meeting.

Sociodemographic questionnaire. This form was developed *ad hoc* to collect data on participants' age, gender, sexual orientation, type of SCI (para- or tetraplegia), civil status, children, education, employment, citizenship, political orientation, and religious beliefs. The sexual orientation was rated on the Kinsey scale [61], also called the Heterosexual-Homosexual Rating Scale. It ranges from 0 to 6, with '0' indicating exclusively heterosexual/opposite sex behavior or attraction and '6' indicating exclusively homosexual/same-sex behavior or attraction. Ratings 1–5 are for those who report varying levels of attraction or sexual activity with either sex. The sociodemographic questionnaire was administered to all participants once, before the start of the first group meeting.

Sexual Interest and Satisfaction (SIS) scale. This measure is a six-item scale designed to measure sexual adjustment after SCI [62]. It is used to assess interest in and satisfaction with sexuality before and after injury [63]. Partners of the participants with SCI were instructed to answer the questions by making reference to before and after their partners' injury. Participants are asked to give answers on a scale of 0 (non-existent/very dissatisfying) to 3 (increased/very satisfying). This sexuality scale is one of the few that has been used within the SCI population [64]. Only one study [62] reported validity and reliability properties of the scale on a sample of 73 SCI subjects (60 male; mixed injury types; SCI duration >1 year). The SIS scale showed a high correlation with age at injury and moderate-to-high correlation with quality of life, and a high internal consistency (Cronbach's $\alpha = 0.96$).

Beck Depression Inventory-II (*BDI-II*). In its current version, the BDI-II is a 21-question multiple-choice self-report inventory that comprises items relating to symptoms of depression such as hopelessness and irritability, cognitions such as guilt or feelings of being punished, and physical symptoms such as fatigue, weight loss, and lack of interest in sex [65]. Scores for statements ranged from 0 (e.g., "I do not feel sad") to 3 (e.g., "I am so sad or unhappy that I can't stand it"). Higher total scores indicate more severe depressive symptoms. The reliability and validity of the BDI-II in the Italian population have been demonstrated [65].

Beck Anxiety Inventory (*BAI*). This measure was designed to differentiate anxiety from depression [66]. The respondents indicate how much they have been bothered by each of the 21 symptoms during the past week. Symptoms include the inability to relax and trembling hands. Respondents rated each symptom on a scale ranging from 'not at all' (0) to 'severely' (3). The reliability and validity of the Italian BAI have been demonstrated [67].

2.4 Structure, content, and techniques of the psychoeducational intervention

The personal growth group met every fortnight for a total of 12 meetings, each of which lasted for 2 h. The sessions were held by psychologists and psychotherapists with expertise in sexuality and disability. The group meetings were organized in two parts: informative and practical. The informative part covered six topics, each for two meetings: (i) Me and my new body, (ii) Affective-relational communication, (iii) Between identity and sexual orientation, (iv) Discovering pleasure, (v) Live sexual life, and (vi) Aids to pleasure. The contents were also transmitted through the projection of videos and sexually explicit images, starting from the assumption that observational learning has an informative and motivational function [68–71]. The interactive practical part—dedicated to personal growth and body awareness—utilized cognitive-behavioral therapy, Gestalt therapy, and emotion-focused therapy techniques. Through the cognitive-behavioral therapy techniques (e.g., problem management, role-playing, imagery, and modeling) [72], Participants were driven by the cycle of creating thoughts and emotions associated with their own sexuality to address stereotypes and derogatory beliefs about sexuality and disability, masturbation, orgasm, pleasure, sexual fantasy, sexual identity, and the beauty and attractiveness of the body. This process included the identification of possible dysfunctional patterns of self that negatively influenced the relationship with their partners. This effort meant overcoming the reductionist view that stems from both the disability medical model, which limits sexuality to the physiological functions of genitalia and genital sensation as the only possibility for sexual experience and heterosexism. Through Gestalt therapy [73] and emotion-focused therapy techniques [74], the emergence of a new sexual concept has been reinforced by increasing awareness on bodily feelings, stressing the relationship and the cycle of reflection on exciting emotions to create new meaning. For example, we used an empty chair and the imagination of the participants to develop and direct dialogs to help them reconcile contrasting aspects of their experience, pay attention to the body and verbal language, concentrate on emotions and the here and now of the relationship with the therapist or other group members. See the Supplementary Material to [63], where two topic guides are provided as an example of two group meetings on sexual life.

2.5 Apparatus

During the personal growth group meetings, a computer (Lenovo, ThinkPad T560), projector (Epson EB-S05), and wireless speaker (JBL Clip 2) were used to watch educational videos and images and perform some psychology exercises (e.g., visualization and relaxation exercises).

2.6 Data analysis

All data were processed using IBM SPSS Statistics for Windows, Version 25 (Armonk, NY). Due to the small sample size, nonparametric statistical tests were used. Specifically, the Wilcoxon test for paired samples was used to compare pre- and post-intervention scores on the SIS, BDI-II, and BAI for the complete sample (participants) and the two sub-groups (patients and partners).

To determine the effect size of the intervention, r was used, which was calculated by dividing the z value by the square root of N (number of cases used in the analysis). The interpretation of r values for effect size is relatively similar to Cohen's d [75]. It was considered negligible if it was less than 0.10, small from 0.10 to 0.30, medium between 0.30 and 0.50, and high if it was greater than 0.50. Although we used nonparametric statistics for the analyses, means and standard deviations of the variables (instead of the median) were reported whenever possible. An independent sample Kolmogorov-Smirnov test was also used to compare the patients and partners groups and consider possible gender effects.

2.7 Results

Sample. Three out of fourteen male participants who signed the informed consent and participated in the group meetings did not complete the complete sociodemographic questionnaire and/or outcome measures. Therefore, they have been excluded from data analysis. Of the remaining 11 participants (female: N = 6,

54.5%; male: $N = 5$, 45.5%), 4 males had complete paraplegia, 1 female had complete tetraplegia, and 1 female and male each had incomplete paraplegia. All of them were outpatients during the group activity. For all participants, the cause of SCI was traumatic (years from injury: $M = 38.1$; min = 26; max = 50; $SD = 9.44$). All four partners of the participants with SCI were females. The 11 group participants included 4 couples (8 individuals). One female participant with SCI reported not having a romantic or sexual partner.

Outcome measures. All participants ($N = 11$) improved significantly on SIS scale item 5 ("How are your opportunity and your ability to enjoy sexuality yourself?"; $z = -3$; $p < 0.01$), SIS scale total score ($z = -2.53$; $p < 0.05$), and BAI scores ($z = -1.99$; $p < 0.05$). The effect size was high in all cases ($r = 0.90$, $r = 0.76$, and $r = 0.60$, respectively). There was no difference in the scores for the SIS general satisfaction after injury or BDI.

A significant effect was found on SIS scale item 5 ("How are your opportunity and your ability to enjoy sexuality yourself?") for both patients ($N = 7$; $z = -2.24$; $p < 0.05$) and partners ($N = 4$; $z = -2$; $p < 0.05$) with a high effect size ($r = 0.84$ and $r = 1$, respectively). There were no effects for the total score or general satisfaction after injury for the SIS scale, BDI-II, or BAI. Further, there were no significant differences between genders or patients and partners. See [63] for more details on the pilot data of Study 1.

3. Study 2

3.1 Setting and participants

Recruitment procedures and eligibility criteria for participation were the same as in Study 1. The personal growth group on sexual life met from January to June 2019 in the rehabilitation room of the USU-PG; it is accessible to wheelchairs. Only 7 participants were included in the present study, as explained in the subsection "Sample."

3.2 Measurements, procedures, and apparatus

The self-administered sociodemographic questionnaire, outcome measures, procedures for administration, and structure, content, and techniques of the psychoeducational intervention were the same as in Study 1. A Sony ICD-PX312 audio recorder was added to the apparatuses described for Study 1 (Section 2.5) to record the dialogs of each meeting. The COnsolidated criteria for REporting Qualitative studies (COREQ) checklist was followed in reporting the results [76]. The COREQ checklist is available at [77].

3.3 Data analysis

Outcome measures. Nonparametric statistical tests were used due to the small sample size (Wilcoxon test for paired samples), and the r to determine the effect size of the intervention interpreted similarly to Cohen's d [75], as in Study 1.

Qualitative data. In grounded theory, data collection and analysis occur simultaneously [78]. The 12 meetings of the personal growth group were all audiotaped by two independent researchers (GC and ACM). All audio recordings from the 24 meetings were then transcribed, carefully read, and indexed according to the grounded theory coding procedure [78, 79]. To investigate the effects that the psychoeducational intervention has had on the participants' sexual health, the most significant verbal expressions were identified, and a code/index was assigned to each one through a three-phase-inductive logic procedure, by studying the topic within its context and using an emerging design. See the Supplementary Material, where the codebook and detailed qualitative data analysis of each meeting are reported [77].

The reliability of codes was evaluated through measuring intercoder agreement, assessing the degree of trustworthiness of each code assigned to the same portion of text by GC and ACM. The level of agreement between two researchers was assessed using Krippendorff's alpha for nominal items [80]; reliability was considered optimal if $\alpha \geq 0.800$, suboptimal with $\alpha \geq 0.667$, and non-optimal otherwise (**Table 1**).

The manual text analysis was transferred to Atlas.ti software (version 8.4) to measure intercoder agreement and calculate the occurrences of the categories and their relevance. Finally, through the software, the codes that emerged from the transcriptions of each meeting were compared to evaluate any differences in the theoretical construct that characterized them. By detecting how the codes developed with the progression of the meetings, it was possible to infer the effect of the psychoeducational intervention on the participants' sexual health.

3.4 Results

Sample. One male and one female (out of nine participants) who signed the informed consent and participated in the group meetings did not complete the entire sociodemographic questionnaire and/or the outcome measures. Therefore, they were excluded from data analyses. Of the remaining 7 participants (female: $N = 1$), 2 males had complete paraplegia, 2 males had complete tetraplegia, 1 male had incomplete paraplegia, and 1 male had incomplete tetraplegia. Five of them were outpatients during the group activity. For 5, the cause of SCI was traumatic (years from injury: $M = 8$; min = 0.75; max = 11; $SD = 3.03$). The participating female was the partner of a male with SCI, the only couple in the group. Three male participants with SCI reported not having a romantic or sexual partner.

Outcome measures. Although not significant, there was an increase in the raw values for all participants ($N = 7$) on SIS scale item 5 ("How are your opportunity and your ability to enjoy sexuality yourself?"; $M = 1.29–3.57$), SIS scale total score ($M = 10.86–13.14$), and SIS scale general satisfaction after injury score ($M = -1.57$ to -2). The effect size was medium in all cases ($r = 0.36$, $r = 0.46$, and $r = 0.60$, respectively). There were no significant differences in the scores for BDI-II and BAI and between genders or patients and partners.

Semantic domain	Krippendorff's Cu-α/cu-α	Krippendorff's c-α-binary
Efficacy of therapeutic intervention	0.822**	0.885**
Rehabilitation of sexuality	0.945**	0.793*
Difficulties from exercises	0.900**	0.818**
Disability experience	0.951**	0.832**
Sexuality experience	0.887**	0.796*
Relationship	1.0**	0.774*
Perceived support	1.0**	0.853**
Total	0.788*	0.951**

**Suboptimal agreement.*
***Optimal agreement.*

Table 1.
Level of agreement between the two independent evaluators, as scored using Krippendorff's alpha.

Qualitative analysis assisted by Atlas.ti. The findings resulted in the core category 'psychological sexual health after SCI' and identified the experience of evolving sexuality during the personal growth group. Three main themes were identified, supported by seven categories: (1) disabled sexuality, (2) influences of family and social environment, and (3) effects of psychoeducational intervention. As shown in the diagram below (**Figure 1**), the three themes can be assumed to represent three stages of the same process—each one inextricably influenced by the others—and resulting in the ultimate purpose of the intervention, namely to achieve sexual health after SCI.

Theme 1—Disabled sexuality: "I don't know how your body can react to my caress, it's not like before."

Participants expressed their experience of sexuality as influenced by their impaired body. They reported psychological experiences related to living with a disability or with a partner with a disability, a phenomenon that negatively influenced daily life and sexuality, compromised the possibility of giving and receiving sexual pleasure, and hampered the ability to experience intimacy and affection after SCI.

Disability was experienced as an element that leads to an imbalance in the life of the person with SCI and their family, causing anger, anxiety, depression, difficulties in self-regulation of emotional states, and caregivers' psychophysical exhaustion.

> *It was better that I hadn't been saved from the accident [...] I would have felt nothing, and 11 years would have passed, that the people who love me wouldn't. (DM).*

There was a constant focus on past life, which was valued more positively than present life, often due to encountering difficulties in accepting disability (one's own or her or his partner's), discomfort, and negative self-perception. In fact, physical changes in sexual function and masturbation emerged.

> *Initially, I had written only a couple of problems related to masturbation, which were those of lack of sensitivity, [...] of not achieving orgasm as before and therefore this created small desire and small excitement, so small desire to masturbate. (DP).*

> *I wouldn't feel pleasure if I touched myself or someone touched it [my penis]. (DM).*

> *It often happens to me that it [my penis] thinks the way it thinks, and I think different from it [...] I can't see if I can put this [my penis] and this [my head] in synergy. (SF).*

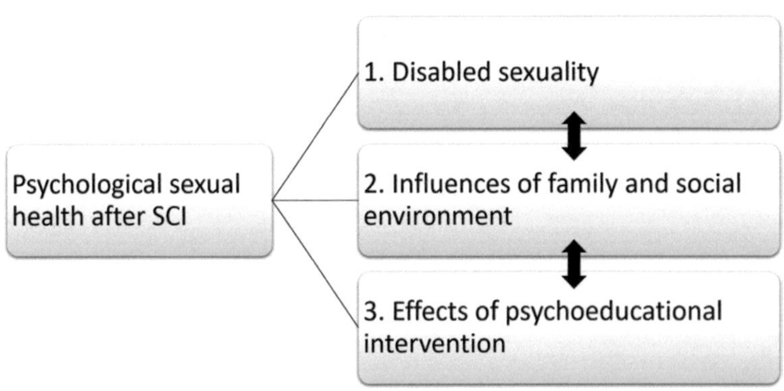

Figure 1.
Core categories resulted by the qualitative analysis assisted by Atlas.ti and their inter-relationship.

Related to masturbation before the accident and afterwards, it became almost completely absent for me, right? Because it doesn't give me, to this day, the same satisfaction that it did before. (DP).

Unfortunately, I haven't tried them [sensations] now, because I don't have the use of my hands and nothing, I can't even think about masturbating right now. (SA).

The participants presented common stereotypes about sexuality and consequent experiences with the topic: performance anxiety, sexual dissatisfaction, loss of interest, and perception of not being attractive.

I was the first one to call myself asexual or disabled (DP).

I can't... I couldn't, I mean, or I could more hardly woo a girl and then tell her to go get a pizza, and then I probably couldn't do what I was able to do when I was 30. (SP).

Finally, there were two opposing attitudes: sexual desire and fear.

I caress him (my partner with SCI) in the face and I feel something moving inside of me, but it doesn't go... it can't go any further. It can't... and then I think back to the past. And from there I get stuck. (GA).

Theme 2—Influences of family and social environment: "I've seen them look at me differently."

Familial, social, and professional relationships influenced sexual dialog with current or future partners. The participants expressed that there were changes in relational experiences and reflections on the perceived level of support.

The participants reported role changes within the family and conflicts in relationships.

At home I did everything, I was the fulcrum. (SA).

Now we talk to each other all the time with something... a little bit of anger, of... if he doesn't want to talk, shut up like he used to, and I'll raise my voice. (GA).

Furthermore, the participants expressed difficulties in finding a romantic/sexual partner, and disability was described as a cause of being discriminated.

I believe, from a purely subjective point of view, that not all, I speak of the female counterpart, have a detail, that is 'patience'. About knowing problems of who is in a wheelchair and then get to normal sexual intercourse, or... develop fantasies about being in a wheelchair and whatever else. (FC).

There was someone I haven't seen in a long time. When he saw me, I felt like I had the worst disease in the world from the look on his face. (SF).

Many people always see only the wheelchair; they don't see the person, the wheelchair as an inanimate object. I just need it to carry that person... not that person, that pile of muscle, bones and whatever else from point A to point B. (FC).

The participants also reported that they did not receive enough support (familial and institutional) in coping with the changes brought about by their disability. Others felt supported by family members and found the psychological support received in the rehabilitation process and in the personal growth group important.

I am working a lot, swimming pool, gym, all private clearly, because it is useless, after 3 years I have seen them all. (SA).

Even my children, they can't understand my anger. (GA).

[My partner] is sincerely facing this sexuality on her part, this sexuality [...] in general, she is facing this problem with extreme naturalness, tranquillity, and positivity. (SF).

Thanks to you, professionals, who have been supportive along the way. (FC)

Theme 3—Effects of psychoeducational intervention. "I have discovered that sexuality is not only physical, but there is also the more satisfying aspect, which is, really, that which goes beyond the physical part."

This theme includes the effects that the intervention had during personal growth. Starting from the expectations of the participants, there were moments in which the therapeutic environment proved to be effective in achieving its goals. At other moments, the group showed difficulties during the exercises.

The therapeutic environment was effective in changing the participants' state of activation. It provided relaxation and well-being and presented strategies and new perspectives that increased self-esteem.

I feel that there are a lot of things to do, and it has given me a line, a direction. I was really looking for it. (SA).

I did a good job. I also felt some emotions, perhaps crossing the eyes of SA., or FA... [...] and it made me feel good emotions. (SF).

Maybe more self-esteem? That is, if I was on a certain level of self-esteem and courage [...], the encounters have given back a bit of lymph in being able to deal face-to-face this kind of topic with a person. (FC).

The exercises stimulated insight and introspection. Sharing within the group was considered by the participants as a means of enrichment.

I realize [...] how limiting was my past way of doing. I understand very well the potential of the mind and how restricted was the vision of sexuality that I had before with respect to what could be or is. [DP].

The most encountered difficulties concerned the expression of personal experiences or those related to the intimate sphere, exercises of imagination, and auto analysis, the latter for members in whom the exercises evoked thoughts related to the traumatic event and past life.

When we started talking about sexology, my head went haywire. (GA).

By doing this, in quotes, experiment happiness took my breath away. (DM).

Finally, the intervention stimulated motivation to recover sexual health after SCI, with an emphasis on the relational component rather than the physical component of the sexual experience. The participants demonstrated that they understood the importance of exploring the body and resources, as well as the possibility of developing compensatory mechanisms and sexual assistance.

With my partner every little sign that approaches sexuality is amplified, every caress, every word, every gesture enters me with amplified power. (SF).

My new sexuality can be a caress, a kiss, a "thank you", a word in need... this is sexuality for me now. The closeness, the awareness of being together and interacting, sometimes. Together. (GA).

To be aware that, sexuality is not something that just sits there. We talked about physicality, but it finds its own progression also through other... other forms of... sharing, of participation. (SP).

Let [the sexual assistant] help me or reveal some secrets, some little tricks so that I can interact with him. (GA).

4. Discussion

The two studies provided pilot data on the effectiveness of a psychoeducational intervention for the sexual life of two groups of in- and outpatients and their partners performed at the USU-PG. We would like to emphasize that the first noteworthy outcome of this project (Love & Life) was the realization of an initiative aimed at promoting the sexual life of people with SCI in an Italian public health facility. As far as we know, this project was the first in Italy to tackle the issue of improving sex life and not just treating sexual dysfunction of people with SCI. Given the novelty of the initiative, we have had to battle with deep psychological, cultural, and religious reluctance to accepting the treatment of sexuality as an inherent aspect of personal well-being that no trauma can eradicate. Breaking the resistance of people (disabled and non-disabled, patients and partners, health workers and laypeople) even to consider that people with SCI also have the capacity to have relationships, experience love, and experience sexual and romantic attraction was a big deal. Having said that, 23 people's involvement is already reflective of the effectiveness of our initiative.

4.1 Sex, education, religion, and other characteristics of the participants

Although the composition of the personal growth groups on sexual life was not defined in any way by the criterion of representativeness of the Italian population to the SCI, some of the characteristics of the sample tend to be compatible with the main SCI data. For instance, the prevalence of males with SCI in the group reflected the worldwide male-to-female ratio (4:1) [81, 82]. Only one participant (Study 2) has reached a master's degree level, only one a bachelor's degree (Study 1), and six a high school diploma (Studies 1 and 2). This finding is consistent with another key fact: SCI is associated with lower rates of school enrolment [83].

Except for one patient (Study 2), the cause of SCI was traumatic. The mean age when the traumatic event occurred was 37.2 years, data that are consistent with Pagliacci et al. [81] on the Italian SCI population (38.5 years). Ten participants declared that they were Roman Catholic, five from Study 1 and five from Study 2. Two of them (Study 1) were a lesbian couple with a civil union. The remaining participants declared themselves non-religious. In the two samples studied, the Catholic affiliation was lower than the national average—74.4% according to Ipsos Public Affairs [84]. Dealing with a sexually explicit topic seems to attract more people who do not have a religious affiliation or an orthodox view (e.g., lesbian couples in civil unions) because religions have specific sex teachings that can condemn masturbation or sexual relations outside of a heterosexual marriage [1, 19, 45, 49, 85–87].

4.2 Outcome measures and effect size

The effectiveness of the psychoeducational intervention was clearly apparent, denoted by a high (Study 1) or medium (Study 2) effect size in improving sexual interest and satisfaction as well as the opportunity and ability to enjoy sexuality. Anxiety was also reduced for all participants in Study 1 but not Study 2, although this outcome may not have been related to the psychoeducational intervention. Conversely, the intervention did not appear to significantly reduce levels of depression in patients or partners (Studies 1 and 2). This result might be clarified by the fact that the level of anxiety reported at the beginning of the first group meeting may be influenced by the context of novelty and sensitivity of the topic. When the re-test was carried out at the conclusion of the last group meeting, the climate was more friendly and the issue of sexuality less concerning. Hence, the decreased levels of anxiety could be more due to an intervening variable (anxiogenic context) than to treatment effectiveness. This potential fact could also explain why there has been no improvement in the levels of depression, which usually tends to positively correlate with anxiety [66, 88]. Indeed, the personal growth group on sexual life was primarily focused on improving awareness of sexuality conveyed by sexually explicit videos and therapy techniques focused on feelings and social relationships. Anxiety and depression might be determined by many other factors [88] that affect the quality of life of the patients and, consequently, their partners, besides sexual function, interest, and satisfaction. In addition, an efficacious psychotherapeutic treatment for observing reduced anxiety and depression might require more than 12 meetings over a period of 3 months [89, 90]. However, our findings correspond to the study by Harrison et al. [91] in which anxiety and depression were experienced by the same individuals, and anxiety—but not depression—was related to the sexual dysfunction of a woman with SCI.

4.3 Qualitative data (study 2)

The effectiveness of the psychoeducational intervention also clearly emerged from the qualitative analysis because it has promoted a path of self-confidence ("The encounters have given back a bit of lymph in being able to deal face-to-face this kind of topic") and it shattered prejudices about sexuality ("I understand very well the potential of the mind and how restricted was the vision of sexuality that I had before").

The three themes that emerged from the qualitative analysis are consistent with those elements highlighted in the Introduction. Sexuality emerged as closely linked to one's own and other's perception of the functioning and image of the body. A disabled body has disabled sexuality [92]. Recovering sexual health involves regaining the image of one's body and confidence that one can still give and receive pleasure [2, 4].

It is also clear from the qualitative analysis that stereotypes do not only concern nondisabled people toward people with disability; they also affect the people with disability themselves ("I was the first one to call myself asexual or disabled") [4, 5]. Finally, the adjustments that every person with SCI must tackle to regain their sexual health inevitably pass from the quality of social relationships ("Many people always see only the wheelchair"), ranging from the recovery of intimacy with the partner to trust in their own attractiveness.

5. Conclusions

Several studies [5, 9, 93–96] and guides [1, 4, 68] urge that adequate education [96] and psychological support [97] be provided to people with SCI in order to facilitate successful participation in sexual activities. These studies also highlight the need to involve intimate partners in discussions related to sexuality during the rehabilitative process [96] in an inclusive approach that gives women—in the same way as for males—the opportunity to talk with peers with SCI about sexual health during the initial rehabilitation and after returning home [98]. The first and greatest achievement of the Love & Life project was to develop, in Italy, an environment where a psychoeducational intervention could meet the needs of people with SCI, provide adequate education and psychological support, include partners, and create a space for peer-to-peer interaction. The intervention effectiveness also offers strong, clear evidence of the validity of the accepted biopsychosocial model that overcomes a reductionist view that restricts sexuality to the function/dysfunction of genitalia, phallocentric primacy of sexual pleasure, and attractiveness of only perfect body. We do not believe we have solved the complexity of the sexual lives of women [99] and men with SCI and their partners, but we hope that the Love & Life initiative will lead to a new way forward to address this complexity.

Conflict of interest

The authors declare that the research was conducted in the absence of any commercial or financial relationships that could be construed as a potential conflict of interest.

Author details

Stefano Federici[1,2*], Francesco Artegiani[3], Daniele Diotallevi[4], Giovanna Caruso[1] and Alessandra Castellani Mencarelli[1]

1 Department of Philosophy, Social and Human Sciences and Education, University of Perugia, Perugia, Italy

2 Myèsis, Research and Development Company, Rome, Italy

3 MenteCorpo, Clinical Center of Psychology and Sexology, Perugia, Italy

4 Independent Professional, Perugia, Italy

*Address all correspondence to: stefano.federici@unipg.it

References

[1] Consortium for Spinal Cord Medicine. Sexuality and Reproductive Health in Adults with Spinal Cord Injury: What You Should Know. A Guide for People with Spinal Cord Injury. Washington, DC: Paralyzed Veterans of America; 2011

[2] Taleporos G, McCabe MP. The impact of physical disability on body esteem. Sexuality and Disability. 2001;**19**(4):293-308. DOI: 10.1023/A:1017909526508

[3] Chhabra HS, editor. ISCoS Textbook on Comprehensive Management of Spinal Cord Injuries. Philadelphia, PA: Lippincott; 2015

[4] Hammond MC, Burns SC. Yes, You Can! A Guide to Self-Care for Persons with Spinal Cord Injury. 4th ed. Paralyzed Veterans of America: Washington, DC; 2009

[5] Tepper MS. Becoming sexually able: Education for adolescents and young adults with disabilities. Contemporary Sexuality. 2005;**39**(9):i-vii

[6] Stone SD. The myth of bodily perfection. Disability & Society. 1995;**10**(4):413-424. DOI: 10.1080/09687599550023426

[7] Thompson SA, Bryson M, De Castell S. Prospects for identity formation for lesbian, gay, or bisexual persons with developmental disabilities. International Journal of Disability, Development and Education. 2001;**48**(1):53-65. DOI: 10.1080/10349120120036305

[8] Tremain S. We're here. We're disabled and queer. Get used to it. In: Tremain S, editor. Pushing the Limits: Disabled Dykes Produce Culture. Toronto, CA: Women's Press; 1996. pp. 15-24

[9] Tepper MS. Letting go of restrictive notions of manhood: Male sexuality, disability and chronic illness. Sexuality and Disability. 1999;**17**(1):37-52. DOI: 10.1023/a:1021451712988

[10] Milligan MS, Neufeldt AH. The myth of asexuality: A survey of social and empirical evidence. Sexuality and Disability. 2001;**19**(2):91-109. DOI: 10.1023/a:1010621705591

[11] Bickenbach JE. The international classification of functioning, disability and health and its relationship to disability studies. In: Watson N, Roulstone A, Thomas C, editors. Routledge Handbook of Disability Studies. London, UK: Routledge; 2012. pp. 51-66

[12] Altman BM. Disability definitions, models, classification schemes, and applications. In: Albrecht GL, Seelman KD, Bury M, editors. Handbook of Disability Studies. Thousand Oaks, CA: Sage; 2001. pp. 97-122. DOI: 10.4135/9781412976251

[13] Meloni F, Federici S, Dennis JL, et al. PLoS One. 2015;**10**(6):e0128876. DOI: 10.1371/journal.pone.0128876

[14] Federici S, Meloni F. Making decisions and judgments on disability: The disability representation of parents, teachers, and special needs educators. Journal on Systemics, Cybernetics and Informatics. 2009;**1**(3):20-26

[15] Nagi SZ. A study in the evaluation of disability and rehabilitation potential: Concepts, methods, and procedures. American Journal of Public Health and the Nation's Health. 1964;**54**(9):1568-1579. DOI: 10.2105/ajph.54.9.1568

[16] Friedman C, Owen AL. Defining disability: Understandings of and attitudes towards ableism and disability.

Disability Studies Quarterly. 2017;**37**(1). DOI: 10.18061/dsq.v37i1.5061

[17] Thomson RG. Extraordinary Bodies: Figuring Physical Disability in American Culture and Literature. New York, NY: Columbia University Press; 1997

[18] O'Toole CJ, Bregante JL. Lesbians with disabilities. Sexuality and Disability. 1992;**10**(3):163-172. DOI: 10.1007/BF01102282

[19] Wendell S. The Rejected Body: Feminist Philosophical Reflection on Disability. New York, NY: Routledge; 1996

[20] Brown DE. Human Universals. New York, NY: McGraw-Hill; 1991

[21] Ramachandran VS. The Tell-Tale Brain: A Neuroscientist's Quest for What Makes Us Human. W. W. Norton: New York, NY; 2011

[22] Tooby J, Cosmides L. The psychological foundation of culture. In: Barkow JH, Cosmides L, Tooby J, editors. The Adapted Mind: Evolutionary Psychology and the Generation of Culture. New York, NY: Oxford University Press; 1992. pp. 19-136

[23] Buss DM. Evolutionary Psychology: The New Science of the Mind. 4th ed. Pearson: Boston, NY; 2012

[24] Buss DM, editor. The Handbook of Evolutionary Psychology: Volume 1—Foundations. 2nd ed. New York, NY: Wiley; 2016

[25] Rozin P, Todd PM. The evolutionary psychology of food intake and choice. In: Buss DM, editor. The Handbook of Evolutionary Psychology: Volume 1—Foundations. 1. 2nd ed. New York, NY: Wiley; 2016. pp. 183-205

[26] Tybur JM, Lieberman D, Kurzban R, DeScioli P. Disgust: Evolved function and structure. Psychological Review. 2013;**120**(1):65-84. DOI: 10.1037/a0030778

[27] Park JH, Faulkner J, Schaller M. Evolved disease-avoidance processes and contemporary anti-social behavior: Prejudicial attitudes and avoidance of people with physical disabilities. Journal of Nonverbal Behavior. 2003;**27**(2):65-87. DOI: 10.1023/A:1023910408854

[28] Meloni F, Federici S, Bracalenti M. A cognitive approach to the functioning of the disability models. In: 17th International Association of Psychology & Psychiatry for Adults & Children Conference: APPAC '12; 2012 May 15-18; Athens, GR: MEDIMOND. 2012

[29] APA (American Psychiatric Association). Diagnostic and Statistical Manual of Mental Disorders. 5th ed. Arlington, VA: APA; 2013

[30] Boyer P. Cognitive constraints on cultural representations: Natural ontologies and religious ideas. In: Hirschfeld LA, Gelman SA, editors. Mapping the Mind: Domain Specificity in Cognition and Culture. Cambridge, NY: Cambridge University Press; 1994. pp. 391-411

[31] Federici S, Meloni F, Catarinella A, Mazzeschi C. Models of disability in children's pretend play: Measurement of cognitive representations and affective expression using the affect in play scale. Frontiers in Psychology. 2017;**8**(794): 1-8. DOI: 10.3389/fpsyg.2017.00794

[32] Smith LA, Williams JM. Children's understanding of the causal origins of disability. Journal of Cognition and Development. 2004;**5**(3):383-397. DOI: 10.1207/s15327647jcd0503_5

[33] Huckstadt LK, Shutts K. How young children evaluate people with and without disabilities. Journal of Social Issues. 2014;**70**(1):99-114. DOI: 10.1111/josi.12049

[34] Barnartt SN, editor. Disability As A Fluid State. Bingley, UK: Emerald; 2010

[35] Burns SM, Mahalik JR, Hough S, Greenwell AN. Adjustment to changes in sexual functioning following spinal cord injury: The contribution of men's adherence to scripts for sexual potency. Sexuality and Disability. 2008;**26**(4):197-205. DOI: 10.1007/s11195-008-9091-y

[36] Taleporos G, McCabe MP. Relationships, sexuality and adjustment among people with physical disability. Sexual and Relationship Therapy. 2003;**18**(1):25-43. DOI: 10.1080/1468199031000061245

[37] Romeo AJ, Wanlass R, Arenas S. A profile of psychosexual functioning in males following spinal cord injury. Sexuality and Disability. 1993;**11**(4): 269-276. DOI: 10.1007/bf01102171

[38] McCabe MP, Taleporos G, Dip G. Sexual esteem, sexual satisfaction, and sexual behavior among people with physical disability. Archives of Sexual Behavior. 2003;**32**(4):359-369. DOI: 10.1023/a:1024047100251

[39] Kettl P, Zarefoss S, Jacoby K, Garman C, Hulse C, Rowley F, et al. Female sexuality after spinal cord injury. Sexuality and Disability. 1991;**9**(4):287-295. DOI: 10.1007/bf01102017

[40] Code L, editor. Encyclopedia of Feminist Theories. London, UK: Taylor and Francis; 2002

[41] Bem SL. The Lenses of Gender: Transforming the Debate on Sexual Inequality. New Haven, CT: Yale University Press; 1993

[42] Freud S. Some psychological consequences of the anatomical distinction between the sexes. In: Jones E, editor. Sigmund Freud: Collected Papers. 5. New York, NY: Basic Books; 1925/1959. pp. 186-197

[43] Freud S. The passing of the Oedipus-complex. In: Jones E, editor. Sigmund Freud: Collected Papers. 2. New York, NY: Basic Books; 1924/1959. pp. 269-276

[44] Rubin G. The traffic in women: Notes on the "political economy" of sex. In: Reiter RR, editor. Toward an Anthropology of Women. New York, NY: Monthly Review Press; 1975. pp. 157-210

[45] Zilbergeld B. The New Male Sexuality: The Truth about Men, Sex, and Pleasure. Revised. New York, NY: Bantam Books; 2013

[46] Lombardi G, Del Popolo G, Macchiarella A, Mencarini M, Celso M. Sexual rehabilitation in women with spinal cord injury: A critical review of the literature. Spinal Cord. 2010;**48**(12):842-849. DOI: 10.1038/sc.2010.36

[47] Ferreiro-Velasco ME, Barca-Buyo A, Salvador de la Barrera S, Montoto-Marqués A, Miguéns Vázquez X, Rodríguez-Sotillo A. Sexual issues in a sample of women with spinal cord injury. Spinal Cord. 2004;**43**(1):51. DOI: 10.1038/sj.sc.3101657

[48] Ranke-Heinemann U. Eunuchen für das Himmelreich: Katholische Kirche und Sexualität. Hoffmann und Campe: Hamburg, DE; 1990

[49] Shakespeare T, Gillespie-Sells K, Davies D, editors. The Sexual Politics of Disability: Untold Desire. London, UK: Cassell; 1996

[50] Weininger O. Sex and Character: An Investigation of Fundamental Principles. Bloomington, Ind.: Indiana University Press; 2005

[51] Alexander M, Rosen RC. Spinal cord injuries and orgasm: A review. Journal of Sex & Marital Therapy. 2008;**34**(4):308-324. DOI: 10.1080/00926230802096341

[52] Komisaruk BR, Whipple B. Non-genital orgasms. Sexual and Relationship Therapy. 2011;**26**(4):356-372. DOI: 10.1080/14681994.2011.649252

[53] LaRocca MA, Kromrey JD. The perception of sexual harassment in higher education: Impact of gender and attractiveness. Sex Roles. 1999;**40**(11):921-940. DOI: 10.1023/a:1018829222894

[54] Golden JH, Johnson CA, Lopez RA. Sexual harassment in the workplace: Exploring the effects of attractiveness on perception of harassment. Sex Roles. 2001;**45**(11):767-784. DOI: 10.1023/a:1015688303023

[55] ISTAT (Istituto Nazionale di Statistica). Gli stereotipi sui ruoli di genere e l'immagine sociale della violenza sessuale: Anno 2018. ISTAT: Rome, IT; 2019

[56] Thrussell H, Coggrave M, Graham A, Gall A, Donald M, Kulshrestha R, et al. Women's experiences of sexuality after spinal cord injury: A UK perspective. Spinal Cord. 2018;**56**(11):1084-1094. DOI: 10.1038/s41393-018-0188-6

[57] WHO (World Health Organization). Defining Sexual Health: Report of a Technical Consultation on Sexual Health, 28-31 January 2002, Geneva. Geneva, CH: WHO; 2006

[58] WHO (World Health Organization). Developing Sexual Health programmes: A Framework for Action. Geneva, CH: WHO; 2010

[59] WHO (World Health Organization). ICF: International Classification of Functioning, Disability and Health. Geneva, CH: WHO; 2001

[60] Nugent PMS. Personal-Growth Group [Internet]: PsychologyDictionary.Org; 2013. Available from: https://psychologydictionary.org/personal-growth-group/ [Accessed: 15 January 2020]

[61] Kinsey AC, Pomeroy WB, Martin CE. Sexual Behavior in the Human Male. Philadelphia, PA: Saunders; 1948

[62] Siösteen A, Lundqvist C, Blomstrand C, Sullivan L, Sullivan M. Sexual ability, activity, attitudes and satisfaction as part of adjustment in spinal cord-injured subjects. Paraplegia. 1990;**28**(5):285-295. DOI: 10.1038/sc.1990.38

[63] Federici S, Artegiani F, Pigliautile M, Antonelli P, Diotallevi D, Ritacco I, et al. Enhancing psychological sexual health of people with spinal cord injury and their partners in an Italian unipolar spinal unit: A pilot data study. Frontiers in Psychology. 2019;**10**(754):1-12. DOI: 10.3389/fpsyg.2019.00754

[64] Abramson CE, McBride KE, Konnyu KJ, Elliott SL, Team SR. Sexual health outcome measures for individuals with a spinal cord injury: A systematic review. Spinal Cord. 2008;**46**(5):320-324. DOI: 10.1038/sj.sc.3102136

[65] Beck AT. BDI-II: Beck Depression Inventory—II. Florence, IT: Giunti O.S.; 2012

[66] Beck AT, Steer RA. Beck Anxiety Inventory Manual. PsychCorp/Pearson: San Antonio, TX; 1993

[67] Beck AT, Steer RA. BAI: Beck Anxiety Inventory. Manuale. Giunti O.S.: Florence, IT; 2007

[68] Tepper MS. Discussion guide for the sexually explicit educational video sexuality reborn: Sexuality following spinal cord injury. Sexuality and Disability. 1997;**15**(3):183-199. DOI: 10.1023/A:1024784819397

[69] Tepper MS. Use of sexually explicit films in spinal cord injury

rehabilitation programs. Sexuality and Disability. 1997;**15**(3):167-181. DOI: 10.1023/A:1024732802558

[70] Alexander CJ, Sipski ML. Sexuality Reborn: Sexuality Following Spinal Cord Injury. West Orange, NJ: Kessler Institute for Rehabilitation; 1993

[71] Bandura A. Social Foundations of Thought and Action: A Social Cognitive Theory. Upper Saddle River, NJ: Prentice-Hall; 1986

[72] Hollon SD, Cognitive BAT. Cognitive-behavioral therapies. In: Lambert MJ, editor. Bergin and Garfield's Handbook of Psychotherapy and Behavior Change. 6th ed. Hoboken, NJ: Wiley & Sons; 2013. pp. 393-394

[73] Perls FS, Hefferline RF, Goodman P. Gestalt Therapy: Excitement and Growth in the Human Personality. New York, NY: Julian Press; 1951

[74] Elliott R, Greenberg LS. Humanistic-experiential psychotherapy in practice: Emotion-focused therapy. In: Consoli AJ, Beutler LE, Bongar B, editors. Comprehensive Textbook of Psychotherapy: Theory and Practice. New York, NY: Oxford University Press; 2017. pp. 106-120

[75] Cohen J. A power primer. Psychological Bulletin. 1992;**112**(1):155-159. DOI: 10.1037/0033-2909.112.1.155

[76] O'Brien BC, Harris IB, Beckman TJ, Reed DA, Cook DA. Standards for reporting qualitative research: A synthesis of recommendations. Academic Medicine. 2014;**89**(9): 1245-1251. DOI: 10.1097/ACM.0000000000000388

[77] Federici S, Artegiani F, Diotallevi D, Caruso G, Castellani Mencarelli A. Supplementary materials to psychological sexual health of people with paraplegia. Reserchgatenet. 2020. DOI: 10.13140/RG.2.2.14481.38241

[78] Corbin JM, Strauss AL. Basics of Qualitative Research: Techniques and Procedures for Developing Grounded Theory. 4th ed. Thousand Oaks, CA: Sage; 2015

[79] Strauss AL, Corbin JM, editors. Basics of Qualitative Research: Techniques and Procedures for Developing Grounded Theory. 2nd ed. Thousand Oaks, CA: Sage; 1998

[80] Krippendorff K. Agreement and information in the reliability of coding. Communication Methods and Measures. 2011;**5**(2):93-112. DOI: 10.1080/19312458.2011.568376

[81] Pagliacci MC, Celani MG, Spizzichino L, Zampolini M, Aito S, Citterio A, et al. Spinal cord lesion management in Italy: A 2-year survey. Spinal Cord. 2003;**41**(11):620. DOI: 10.1038/sj.sc.3101521

[82] Singh A, Tetreault L, Kalsi-Ryan S, Nouri A, Fehlings MG. Global prevalence and incidence of traumatic spinal cord injury. Clinical Epidemiology. 2014;**6**:309-331. DOI: 10.2147/CLEP.S68889

[83] WHO (World Health Organization). Spinal Cord Injury. Geneva, CH: WHO; 2013. Available from: https://www.who.int/news-room/fact-sheets/detail/spinal-cord-injury [Accessed: 15 January 2020]

[84] Ipsos Public Affairs. I cattolici tra presenza nel sociale e nuove domande alla politica. 2017. Available from: https://web.archive.org/web/20180124122738/http://www.acli.it/wp-content/uploads/2017/11/Cattolici-e-politica-analisi-Ipsos-novembre-2017.pdf

[85] Abbott D, Howarth J, editors. Love—A human rights issue? The experiences of gay, lesbian, and bisexual people with intellectual disabilities. In: V IASSCS Biennial Conference: Sexual

Rights and Moral Panics; 2005 Jun 21-24. San Francisco State University, USA: Taylor & Francis; 2005. DOI: 10.1080/13691050410001680500

[86] Graham M. Homosexual rights versus religious freedom: Conflicts over sexual morality in the European Union. Culture, Health & Sexuality. 2005;7(Suppl 1):S34-SS5. DOI: 10.1080/13691050500166774

[87] Federici S. Sessualità alterabili. Indagine sulle influenze socioambientali nello sviluppo della sessualità di persone con disabilità in Italia. Roma, IT: Kappa; 2002. DOI: 10.13140/RG.2.1.3497.0644

[88] Beck AT, Emery G, Greenberg RL. Anxiety Disorders and Phobias: A Cognitive Perspective. New York, NY, USA: Basic Books; 1985

[89] Shedler J. The efficacy of psychodynamic psychotherapy. The American Psychologist. 2010;**65**(2):98-109. DOI: 10.1037/a0018378

[90] Hollon SD, Stewart MO, Strunk D. Enduring effects for cognitive behavior therapy in the treatment of depression and anxiety. Annual Review of Psychology. 2006;**57**:285-315. DOI: 10.1146/annurev.psych.57.102904.190044

[91] Harrison J, Glass CA, Owens RG, Soni BM. Factors associated with sexual functioning in women following spinal cord injury. Paraplegia. 1995;**33**(12): 687-692. DOI: 10.1038/sc.1995.144

[92] Shakespeare T. Disabled sexuality: Toward rights and recognition. Sexuality and Disability. 2000;**18**(3):159-166. DOI: 10.1023/a:1026409613684

[93] Celik EC, Akman Y, Kose P, Arioglu P, Karatas M, Erhan B. Sexual problems of women with spinal cord injury in Turkey. Spinal Cord. 2014;**52**(4):313-315. DOI: 10.1038/sc.2013.161

[94] Fisher TL, Laud PW, Byfield MG, Brown TT, Hayat MJ, Fiedler IG. Sexual health after spinal cord injury: A longitudinal study. Archives of Physical Medicine and Rehabilitation. 2002;**83**(8):1043-1051. DOI: 10.1053/apmr.2002.33654

[95] Mona LR. Sexual options for people with disabilities. Women & Therapy. 2003;**26**(3-4):211-221. DOI: 10.1300/J015v26n03_03

[96] Eglseder K, Demchick B. Sexuality and spinal cord injury: The lived experiences of intimate partners. OTJR. 2017;**37**(3):125-131. DOI: 10.1177/1539449217701394

[97] Tepper MS. Providing comprehensive sexual health care in spinal cord injury rehabilitation: Implementation and evaluation of a new curriculum for health care professionals. Sexuality and Disability. 1997;**15**(3):131-165. DOI: 10.1023/A:1024780718488

[98] Kreuter M, Siösteen A, Biering-Sørensen F. Sexuality and sexual life in women with spinal cord injury: A controlled study. Journal of Rehabilitation Medicine. 2008;**40**(1): 61-69. DOI: 10.2340/16501977-0128

[99] Mona LR, Cameron R, Goldwaser G, Miller A, Syme M, Fraley S. Prescription for pleasure: Exploring sex-positive approaches in women with spinal cord injury. Topics in Spinal Cord Injury Rehabilitation. 2009;**15**(1):15-28. DOI: 10.1310/sci1501-15

Chapter 8

Beyond the Quality of Life in Bowel Dysfunction after Spinal Cord Injury: Approaches to the Consequences in Motility, Immune System, and Microbiome

Estefanía de la Cruz-Castillo and Elisa García-Vences

Abstract

Spinal cord injury (SCI) is a harmful event that involves several repercussions on sensory and motor function that affects the quality of life (QoL) of patients. After SCI, many damage mechanisms are activated that impact on both autonomous extrinsic and intrinsic innervation toward the gut, and these changes modify the gut motility causing bowel dysfunction (BD), an entity that affects 40% of patients with SCI, being the second comorbidity after loss of mobility with no recognized cure. The severity of complications is ruled by the level and severity of injury, having a worse prognosis with an injury that is the most proximal to the brain. In the last 5 years, some experiments have tried to elucidate the consequences of dysbiosis in the gut and aggregated proinflammatory processes. The goal of this chapter is to establish the importance of bacterial composition and immune system repercussions in bowel dysfunction after SCI and how could it give rise to new therapies.

Keywords: neurogenic bowel dysfunction, autonomic dysreflexia, gut microbiota, spinal cord injury

1. Introduction

Spinal cord injury (SCI) refers to the traumatic damage to the spinal cord and represents a harmful event that involves several repercussions on sensory and motor function that affects the quality of life (QoL) of patients (Furlan, Global incidence and prevalence of traumatic spinal cord injury) [1].

The most severe consequences of SCI are partial or complete loss of sensory function or motor control of arms, legs, and/or body, followed by the neurogenic bowel and bladder dysfunction, and other autonomic dysreflexia (AD) signs [1, 2].

In addition, if that was not enough, due to several comorbidities, patients have 1.29-fold increased risk of depression or anxiety [3].

1.1 Epidemiology and public health

SCI is a worldwide disease; prevalence is estimated in 1298 per million, while the global incidence varies depending on the geographical region, so it has been calculated between 8 and up to 246 cases per million per year [2, 4, 5].

In the last 30 years, these data have been increasing [6–8], and most frequent etiology is traumatic, representing 90% of cases [8]; vehicle accidents are the main cause [9], followed by injury due to falls in elderly population.

Males are most at risk, corresponding to the 80% of those affected, with a male to female ratio of 3.2:1 [4, 10] aged between 16 and 35 years [6, 11].

SCI represents a public health problem as it affects the working age population, with a mortality risk two to five times more likely to die prematurely than healthy people; several studies report a mortality rate during the first year after trauma of about 15% [12].

Also, this disease demands financial resources from patients, their families, and the government [13]. Annually, the economic waste associated to SCI in the United States amounts up to approximately 21.5 billion dollars, while in other health systems, such as Canada, an investment of up to 2.67 billion dollars is estimated, considering direct and indirect costs, which range from posttraumatic infections, medical consultations, caregiver services and rehabilitation, etc. [14].

2. Systemic complications induced by SCI

These acute and chronic changes arise and are worsened by the gradual multiple organ dysfunction that in combination with an increasingly sedentary lifestyle leads the SCI patient to metabolic syndrome (trunk fat, low HDL levels, and high triglyceride levels), which affects more than a half of SCI patients [15], implying threefold increased risk of developing cardiovascular disease and fivefold increased risk of developing diabetes [16], as well as other systemic alterations like hematological (anemia in acute phase, thrombocytosis) and biochemical [low concentrations of albumin and globulins and high concentration of aspartate aminotransferase (AST)] [17], decreased immune function (spinal cord injury-induced immune deficiency syndrome SCI-IDS) [18], bowel dysfunction, and gut dysbiosis [19], perhaps, the last three caused by autonomic dysreflexia [20].

2.1 Is autonomic dysreflexia responsible for other comorbidities in SCI?

Clinically, patients with SCI have several comorbidities associated to the level of injury; when the lesion is above the seventh thoracic vertebra, it usually produces sympathetic hyperactivity causing symptoms like systemic vasoconstriction and parasympathetic activity, below and above the site of injury, respectively; this set of alterations are called autonomic dysreflexia (AD) [21].

AD is defined as "episodic hypertension and concomitant baroreflex-mediated bradycardia initiated by unmodulated sympathetic reflexes in the decentralized cord" [22]. This ambiguous definition identifies the elevation in systolic blood pressure as the main sign; however, these diagnostic criteria are not well defined [23]; in addition, these patients can suffer other symptoms such as headache, sweating, anxiety, and arrhythmia [24].

AD incidence in patients with lesion at or above T6 segment is 92.8% and, in some cases, could be asymptomatic, up to 42.9% [25] depending on intensity, level, and time elapsed since SCI. It is important because it represents the principal cause of mortality and must be diagnosed timely to prevent severe complications like cardiac arrest, stroke, and seizures [22].

The impaired visceral or somatic stimulation of the sympathetic preganglionic neurons (SPN), due to colon and bladder overdistension (most frequent), skin lacerations, and pressure sores, results in a massive sympathetic reflex as a result from three things: (1) the maladaptive plasticity of neural network, (2) the imbalance between excitatory and inhibitory neurotransmitters, and (3) the enhanced peripheral adrenergic sensitivity, which is predominantly established in chronic phase, 3–6 months after injury [21].

In addition, other less recognized alteration is in the immunomodulatory response, described as the SCI-IDS, characterized by decreased lymphocyte activity with poor proliferation of hematopoietic progenitor cells and spleen (secondary lymphoid organ) atrophy due to the loss of negative feedback on releasing catecholamines causing poor maturation of T and B lymphocytes [26].

Is well-known that the disruption of the parasympathetic nervous system (PNS) also affects cell proliferation [27, 28], and recent findings had confirmed that parasympathetic activity is linked to cell proliferation and cell cycle-related gene expression above the neurological level of injury rather than below it; in which case, the main neurotransmitter involved is the acetylcholine in the upregulation of some genes that participate in the chromosomal instability [29].

This suggests that SCI goes beyond the patient's locomotor impairment explaining the increased risk of cancer in these patients and the severe repercussions to the gastrointestinal tract conditioning BD (gastric ulcers, paralytic ileus, anal incontinence, anal fissures, and hemorrhoids) [22], a complex phenomenon secondary to hypoxia caused by the massive sympathetic discharge.

3. Bowel dysfunction

Bowel dysfunction (BD) is one of the most frequent complications in patients with SCI, with a frequency of 25–41% of cases [30–32].

In BD, there are changes in the extrinsic autonomous innervation that goes to the gut, resulting in impaired motility (constipation in 46% and anal/fecal incontinence in 41%), sphincter control (31% of cases), and abdominal cramps (18%) [32, 33].

On the other hand, intrinsic enteric innervation remains intact, but over time, it may lose its integrity due to changes in the extrinsic system [34].

3.1 Effect of neurogenic bowel dysfunction in quality of life following spinal cord injury

Most of the time, paraplegic patients receive special attention for the treatment of movement limitations instead of managing the patient like a whole entity setting aside another secondary health conditions and most importantly, quality of life.

In accordance to A. Donabedian, the Committee on Quality Health Care in America published "Crossing the Quality Chasm," focusing on six fundamental concepts, especially the third should be noted, as it points out to respectful patient-centered care in response to its values and necessities [35].

We must define QoL as the patient's perception of its own position in life, conditioned by its culture, value, goals, expectations, and concerns, and its importance is intimately associated with hospitalization, diminished social interaction, poor involvement in rehabilitation, and early death [36].

It is well-known that all comorbidities in SCI-reduced QoL patients injured at C5-T1 have the worst punctuation, being the most important causing pressure ulcers, respiratory complications, and BD [37]. BD is a major physical and psychological problem pointed out by several authors; constipation, gastrointestinal pain, and megacolon and fecal incontinence influence daily activities leading to social isolation [33].

There are about 13 questionnaires to determine objectively QoL in SCI like the Spinal Cord Independence Measure (SCIM III), a tool that indirectly evaluates some areas of self-care, respiration, sphincter control, and mobility. Another is the World Health Organization Quality of Life Assessment (WHOQOL-BREF), with four domains, physical and psychological health, social relationships, and environment [38], and the Short Form 36 (SF-36) that measures both physical and mental health component [39]. However, they have bad sensitivity in the identification of poor QoL dependent of BD, except the Health Utility Index Mark III (HUI-III) that additionally analyzes secondary health conditions with a good discrimination from patient with or without BD [40, 41].

Although there are a great variety of tools to evaluate QoL, it is not a usual practice in medical consultation, and in most cases, the problem is not properly addressed, only focusing on treating the symptoms until it is too late and an invasive procedure like colostomy is imminently required. The evidence has demonstrated the poor or null influence of this type of therapies in QoL [42], perhaps because they are not curative therapies.

Other authors suggest an individualized plan that includes diet and medication [43]; however, the lack of information about the pathophysiology has not allowed scientific advances in the development of strategies to restore intestinal motility and function.

3.2 How could BD in SCI patients be explained?

According to Mazzone and Farrugia, gastrointestinal motility is the property of the intestinal walls to contract and relax so that the contents of the intestine go from one place to another, allowing the proper absorption of nutrients [44].

First, we must remember that in this physiological process, three structures are involved: (a) the CNS, (b) enteric nervous system (ENS) [Meissner (submucosal) and Auerbach (myenteric) nerve plexus], and (c) autonomic nervous system (ANS) (sympathetic and parasympathetic).

The ENS connects with the CNS through afferent or sensory pathways (responsible for maintaining the reflexes and sensation of the visceral organs) and efferent or motor pathways (innervate all the smooth muscles of the body and glands) of the ANS. The ANS is organized into four ganglion groups: (a) paravertebral, (b) prevertebral, (c) paravisceral, and (d) intramural [45].

The paravertebral nodes are connected to each other and form two ganglionic or sympathetic chains, which connect to the spinal nerves through the communicating branches. The prevertebral nodes also connect with each other and form the abdominal plexus, consisting of the celiac and the superior mesenteric ganglion [46].

The paravisceral ganglion encompasses some viscera and highlights the cardiac and pelvic plexus. Meanwhile, the intramural ganglion is located in the wall of the gastrointestinal tract (GIT) and the bile duct [45].

In summary, paravertebral and prevertebral ganglia are the most important components of the sympathetic system (whose origins are in the thoracic and lumbar spinal cord segments) and the autonomic cranial ganglia of the parasympathetic system, which involves the vagus nerve and the pelvic plexus (sacral portion of the spinal cord), which also receives sympathetic innervation. Specifically, the intramural ganglion of the intestine is not considered sympathetic or parasympathetic because both pathways are interconnected, constituting the ENS [47].

The ENS has two main components, the Meissner plexus and the Auerbach plexus. The first is located between the inner layers of the circular and submucosal muscle layer, and its function is to regulate the function of digestion and absorption at the level of the mucosa and blood vessels, especially in the small intestine and colon. Meanwhile, the Auerbach is located between the circular and longitudinal muscular layer and is responsible for coordinating the contraction/relaxation of muscle layers along the entire GIT [46, 48].

Reaffirming, the consequences after SCI directly depend on the level of trauma, as well as intensity and type of injury, having a worse prognosis with lesions that are the most proximal to the brain. Classically, lesions can be divided by severity depending on the neurological level in (a) cervical, (b) thoracic, (c) lumbar, or (d) sacral. Based on this classification, the American Spinal Cord Injury Association (ASIA) designated the neurological standards of spinal cord injury [1].

The neurological level is defined as the most distal segment of the spinal cord with normal motor and sensory function on both sides of the body, while the severity is defined as complete/incomplete sensory and incomplete motor with preserved function in more than a half of the key muscles or incomplete motor with preserved function in at least half of the key muscles [49]. For example, those patients injured in segments C6–C8 will require additional care to avoid comorbidities caused by BD or neurogenic bladder (NB) [50].

These changes fail to explain the mechanisms of intestinal dysmotility [51, 52]; however, other explanations arise: the microbiota-gut-brain axis (MGBA), which communicates with each other via various routes, including endocrine, the vagus nerve, and immune signaling, whose main function is the monitoring and integration of intestinal function [53].

Other mechanisms of gut motility are the effect exerted by the substances generated at this level on the excitability of smooth muscle, peripheral enteric nerves, and central ones [54], as well as the direct action of microbial metabolites as signaling molecules in the brain [48].

3.2.1 What happens after spinal cord injury?

The SCI pathophysiology can be divided into two phases, primary and secondary. The primary injury occurs immediately, from seconds to minutes, causing cellular and extracellular damage induced by the mechanism of injury, whether mechanical or nonmechanical. This serves as the origin to trigger the secondary injury constituted by the mechanisms of damage, which involve vascular, cellular, and biochemical events that cause damage to the resident cells that survived the initial damage, which will take place in minutes to weeks [55].

Due to its temporality, the SCI is classified into three phases: the acute phase, the secondary or subacute phase, and the chronic phase. In each phase several groups of cells and molecules of the nervous, immune, and vascular system are involved [56, 57].

The acute phase occurs due to the direct damage of the trauma, causing cellular, physical, and biochemical alterations both locally and systemically. These reactions are triggered by hemorrhage, destruction of the blood spinal cord barrier, and infiltration of inflammatory cells causing systemic hypotension, spinal shock, vasospasm, ischemia, plasma membrane involvement, ionic homeostasis disorders, and neurotransmitter accumulation [58].

Subacute phase is carried out minutes after the injury, lasting for weeks or months. Further the ionic imbalance, edema and necrosis, and other events happen, such as the formation of free radicals, glutamate-induced delayed calcium (Ca^{2+}) entry, lipoperoxidation, demyelination, and cell death by apoptosis [56, 57]. These damage mechanisms establish an interconnected network characterized by an incessant feedback that self-propagates and perpetuates once the trauma has begun, promoting other secondary self-destructive mechanisms causing more damage to the neural tissue [59].

After this, the glial cells, which originally provided support to the neurons, will secrete cytokines in response to mechanical damage. The activation of astrocytes and pericytes and the recruitment of peripheral fibroblasts and Schwann cells [60] will result in the chronic phase, characterized by the formation of glial scar (cellular and fibrotic or acellular) and a cystic cavity around the epicenter of spinal cord injury within 28–42 days after the injury [60].

The scar is characterized in that the astrocytes, previously activated by TGF-β (in addition to the activation of microglia and macrophages and the deposition of fibronectin and laminin) [61], pericytes, and perivascular cells infiltrate within the nucleus of the lesion where they promote the secretion of extracellular matrix components (EMC; fibronectin, laminin, and collagen) [62]; meanwhile, peripheral Schwann cells infiltrate the epicenter where they upregulate fibroblast markers contributing to the addition of EMC components.

This process is aimed at neural regeneration (neurotrophin production, cell debris removal, repair of the blood spinal cord barrier, and sequestration of reactive species [63]); however, it is hindered by proliferative astrocytes and a cumulus of EMC superimposed around the lesion, which will become rigid, keeping up intact chronically, avoiding cell migration, and becoming a regulator of axonal growth and regeneration [60].

Each stage is well characterized by a group of inflammatory events that will determine the severity of sequelae in the patient.

These systemic changes also have an important impact in the gastrointestinal tract, and it has been proven that higher levels of tissue loss at the lesion epicenter are directly proportional to gastroparesis and delayed gastric emptying with a specific proinflammatory pattern, especially during the acute-subacute phase in which a mild inflammatory cascade produced by the mesenteric hypoperfusion takes place with macroscopic alterations as gastrointestinal atrophy, necrosis, phagocyte infiltration, serosa and submucosa fibrosis, and decreased villi in the duodenum at high lesion levels with absorption commitment [64].

3.2.2 From general to specific: the inflammatory response in BD after SCI

The immune response in the SCI begins in the acute phase, making cellular and molecular responses that lead to the development of the inflammatory response, which plays an important role in the cascade events caused by the secondary lesion [65].

Physiologically, the goal of any inflammatory process is to phagocyte cell debris at the site of injury; however, the CNS is considered an immune privileged organ; that is why an uncontrolled and exacerbated response is triggered, which causes damage to healthy tissue adjacent to the site of injury, so its role seems to be harmful rather than beneficial [65, 66].

In this inflammatory process, four categories of immune cells are mainly distinguished: neutrophils, monocytes, microglia, and T lymphocytes.

Neutrophils are the first to arrive at the site of injury, and their arrival is by recruitment of the circulatory system through the expression of adhesion molecules in their membranes, called chemokines. The neutrophils will be in charge to remove the remaining tissue; in addition, they will release cytokines, proteases, and free radicals. This activates other cells in the inflammatory cascade, triggering damage and neuronal death [67].

Shortly after the arrival of neutrophils, monocytes infiltrate the spinal cord, differentiating themselves into macrophages and acquiring a pro-inflammatory phenotype, contributing to the production of free radicals and pro-inflammatory cytokines such as interleukin (IL) 8, IL-1 beta (IL-1β), and tumor necrosis factor alpha (TNF-α) [66].

Free radicals and pro-inflammatory cytokines contribute to the expansion of the lesion, worsening the impact of the damage; this is because free radicals derived from nitrogen and oxygen can form highly neurotoxic compounds such as peroxynitrite and unchain the phenomenon of lipoperoxidation and subsequent axonal demyelination, losing electrical conductivity below the site of injury [66–68].

On the other hand, the microglia are the innate immune cells of the CNS, being the first cells to acquire an inflammatory phenotype, along with macrophages; when it is damaged, these produce IL-6 and nitric oxide and could activate lymphocytes in the injury site [69].

The role that lymphocytes play in SCI is controversial, because they can be activated by neural antigens such as the myelin basic protein and considered self-reactive T lymphocytes that have self-destructive and inflammatory properties, which together with all the inflammatory mechanism eventually promote demyelination, causing the loss of the function of the neuronal connections with the peripheral nervous system (PNS) [68].

All these alterations provoke the impairment of the ANS [70], therefore resulting in poor intestinal irrigation and BD with all its negative consequences, previously described. At the upper GIT, proinflammatory chemokines *Cc13*, *Cc12*, and *Icam1* are upregulated the first 3 days after trauma triggering an inflammatory response in the intestine causing an increased intestinal permeability that allows bacterial translocation, a vicious circle that maintains BD [64].

Recently, Pde4b [cAMP-specific, *Pde4* subfamily *b* (*Pde4b*)] enzyme activated in macrophages, in gut dysbiosis, has been associated in the induction of proinflammatory state in the CNS and the white matter loss after SCI through the production of LPS-induced TNF-α, IL-1, and nitric oxide contributing to neural damage [70].

3.3 The role of microbiome in bowel dysfunction after SCI

The GIT is the main interface of interaction and nutritional exchange between the inside of the individual and the outside of the world [71]. Around the 90% of the cells found in the human body are not human, but most have a *prokaryotic* origin, derived from at least 40,000 bacterial strains of 1800 different *genera*. During an average lifetime, about 60 tons of food passes through the human GIT, and with it are a large number of microorganisms from the environment [72].

The GIT is colonized by approximately 100 trillion of commensal microorganisms which is given the definition to gut microbiota that involves mostly *Archaea* and *Eukarya* bacteria, with up to 1000 species and more than 7000 strains [73].

The so-called microbiome encompasses the total microorganisms along with their genetic material, which corresponds to our genome 100 times larger.

Recent research has shown that at least 70% of the gut microbiota is integrated by two phylotypes, *Bacteroidetes* and *Firmicutes*, and in less quantity, *Proteobacteria, Actinobacteria, Fusobacteria*, and *Verrucomicrobia* [74].

Several factors, such as immune mechanisms, diet, and intestinal motility, as well as other stress mechanisms such as sepsis, burn, trauma, and infection, could modify bacterial composition [75]. However, there have been some studies that support the therapeutic restoration of the microbiota with the use of probiotics, prebiotics, or symbiotics.

The microbiota offers many benefits for the host by maintaining a symbiotic relationship, such as strengthening the integrity of the mucous barrier, which provides nutrients like vitamins and also protection against pathogens and immunomodulation [76]. Meanwhile, dysbiosis can alter the balance and induce disease [77].

In the last 10 years, there have been many researchers investigating the effects of these microorganisms and their metabolites at different levels with beneficial findings in the irritable bowel syndrome, visceral pain, psychiatric disorders, alterations in the memory, and traumatic injuries in the CNS such as stroke [71, 78].

Gut's bacteria, specifically those found at the ileocecal valve and colon, produce some carbohydrate-active enzymes, which gives them the ability to produce complex carbohydrates through anaerobic fermentation generating metabolites such as short-chain fatty acids (SCFA). Three SCFA are mainly recognized, propionate, butyrate, and acetate, typically found in the ratio 1:1:3. The SCFA are rapidly absorbed by colonocytes in order to participate in the cellular regulation processes such as gene expression, chemotaxis, differentiation, proliferation, and apoptosis [79].

Smaller monocarboxylic acids, with less than six carbon atoms, are participants in pleiotropic signaling [75].

Those involved in the microbiota-gut-brain axis (MGBA) develop in parallel, mostly being important in the first 3 years of life because the blood-brain barrier (BBB) is more permeable and could allow the intake of toxins into the brain when the patient is under stress, as in the case of inadequate bowel colonization, altering proliferation, myelination, and neuronal plasticity. This may worsen as an exacerbated response to stress carried out by the hypothalamic-pituitary-adrenal axis (HPA), which could also condition the development of the vagus nerve. Therefore, MGBA development must be considered especially important [80].

This axis is formed by the CNS, the neuroendocrine and neuroimmune system, branches of the sympathetic and parasympathetic ANS, the enteric nervous system, and the gut microbiota [81, 82].

In summary, signals are sent by the brain and could affect the motor, sensory, and secretory function of the bowel, while bidirectionally, visceral signals influence brain function [81].

Several routes of communication between the brain and gut have been described, such as the activation of afferent sensory fibers of the vagus nerve, neuroimmune pathways, neuroendocrine pathways, microbial metabolites such as SCFA, and microbiota-derived neurotransmitters, such as gamma-aminobutyric acid (GABA), serotonin, catecholamines, and acetylcholine [81, 83].

Both SCFA and gastrointestinal hormones and cytokines, whether pro-/anti-inflammatory, travel through the portal circulation and the meningeal lymphatic system to the CNS [81]. Its action mechanisms are carried out directly and indirectly; this means that it is not necessary for SCFA to get in the CNS; however, its transport through cell membranes is done with pH-dependent transporters, H^+-coupled, called monocarboxylate transporters (MCTs) and sodium-coupled (SMCTs) transporters [81]. These families transport pyruvate, lactate, and butyrate, as well as other ketone bodies [84].

MCTs and SMCTs are found at the apical surface of colonocytes, and their expression is regulated by lumen butyrate concentrations, through NF-κB signaling [85].

However, they are not only expressed in the intestine, they are also present in liver, kidney, intestinal dendritic cells [85, 86]. In the CNS, neurons have SMCT1, while astrocytes have a greater amount of MCT1 [84], although microglia [87] and oligodendrocytes also express them [88].

Meanwhile, in the blood-brain barrier (BBB), MCT1 is also expressed; its importance has been proven in experimental models with decreased butyrate levels where it is associated with loss of integrity and increased permeability. The ability of butyrate to cross the blood-brain barrier has been demonstrated in different studies where it has been administered orally and there is a dose-dependent increase in acetylation of histone H3 in neurons and glia [89].

The effects of SCFA can also be carried out by activating surface butyrate-related receptors [90]; there are four G protein-coupled receptors (GPCRs): free fatty acid receptor-2 (FFAR2), free fatty acid receptor-3 (FFAR3), hydroxycarboxylic acid receptor-2 (HCAR2), and olfactory receptor-51E1 (OR51E1) [91].

FFAR2, FFAR3, and OR51E1 are found in enteroendocrine cells; this is where the interaction between probiotics and prebiotics takes place, promoting the production of SCFA and catalyzing the release of hormones such as cholecystokinin (CCK), the tyrosine-tyrosine peptide (PYY), and the glucagon-like peptide type-1 (GLP-1). In the last one, prebiotics have greater effects than those of probiotics [92, 93].

Symbiotics promote the production of dopamine (DA), serotonin (5-HT), norepinephrine (NA), and GABA [94], which modulate the proximal synapse in the ENS, which in turn, will allow gut-brain communication when synapsing with the vagus nerve [95].

The regulation of the MGBA also has effects at the HPA axis level, by modifying the levels of the adrenocorticotropic hormone (ACTH) and/or corticosteroids (CORT) [96]. In addition, it can directly influence the biochemistry of the CNS by altering the levels of the brain-derived neurotrophic factor (BDNF) who plays an important role in the development and plasticity of the nervous system, memory, and learning. It has been reported that higher butyric acid levels, for example, by *Bifidobacterium breve* and *Clostridium butyricum*, in turn increases the levels of BDNF who inversely decreases the production of pro-inflammatory cytokines such as interleukin-1 beta (IL-1β) [97], c-Fos, and GABA [98].

As previously mentioned, the immune system is also influenced by regulating the production of limited pro-inflammatory cytokines which will consequently influence the CNS.

3.3.1 How does the microbiota influence the immune system?

Immune system is influenced by MGBA through the inhibition of histone deacetylase HDACs, a protein family capable to catalyze the removal of acetyl groups from lysine residues [57].

This type of intracellular signaling can modify the activation of transcriptional or posttranslational processes in more than 1700 proteins; more frequently, they are carried out in nucleosome where their acetylation provokes the activation of transcription [58].

The HDAC family is divided into five subclasses, and its function is triggered by endogenous products such as butyrate which inhibits HDAC I and IIa (more beneficial subtypes for the host). Through this activation/inactivation mechanism, butyrate has effects on the immune system by regulating the activity of T-regulatory cells (Tregs), T CD4+ and T CD8+, lymphocytes, and microglia. In addition, monitoring the gut microbiota is done when changes in butyrate levels are detected [55].

Inhibition of HDAC and activation of FFAR2 induce the differentiation of Tregs expressing FoxP3, producing anti-inflammatory cytokines such as transforming growth factor-beta (TGF-β) and IL-10, suppressing the production of IL-2 and interferon-gamma (IFN-γ), inhibiting the production of inducible nitric oxide synthase (iNOS), and inducing apoptosis of active or resting TCD4+ and TCD8 through HDAC inhibition [55].

Propionate is also capable of upregulating the Foxp3 and IL-10 production showing that SCFA work selectively [61].

Butyrate modulates the activity of microglia in non-inflammatory situations by interfering with their maturation, morphology, and functioning or inflammatory, by reducing NF-*κB* signaling and inducing neuroprotective effects [68].

3.4 Microbiota and SCI: a close relationship?

It is suspected that there are SCFA in the CNS due to the expression of transmembrane receptors and transporters in neurons; however, there is no evidence of physiological concentrations of butyrate in brain or cerebrospinal fluid; perhaps butyrate peaks that have not been measured in previous studies must be quantified. In in vitro studies, butyrate concentrations ranging from 0.4 to 0.7 mmol/L have been determined [83].

Under pathological circumstances, negative effects on microbiome have been described; particularly, SCI has negative effects on the gut microbiota as described by some authors (**Table 1**).

One more research that has not concluded is the multicenter, double-blind randomized placebo-controlled study that is ambitiously looking for better bowel

Experimental model	Outcome	Microbial composition identified	Reference
Fecal microbiota transplantation in one tetraplegic patient with severe recurrent *Clostridium difficile* infection	Patient recovered after transplantation and did not relapse from *C. difficile* infection until 12 weeks later	—	[99]
SCI-T9 mice	Bacterial translocation in the gut Increased gut epithelial permeability Increased activation of immune cells in the gut-associated lymphoid tissue (GALT) Gut dysbiosis results in a worse prognosis for locomotor recovery	Decreased relative abundance of *Bacteroidetes* and increased in *Firmicutes* (*Clostridium*)	[100]
Adult SCI patients [upper motor neuron (UMN); lower motor neuron(LMN)] vs. healthy adult patients	Decreased relative abundance of c members with differences between the different levels of injury (higher levels of injury provoke worse gut dysbiosis)	Decreased relative abundance of *Roseburia* and *Pseudobutyrivibrio* Genus associated with the increased production of butyrate is depleted	[13]
Thoracic SCI rat with antibiotic treatment	Significant differences in the gut microbiota beta diversity between SCI and healthy rats 35 OTUs were enriched Increased levels of proinflammatory cytokines (IL-12, MIP-2, and TNF-α) in the intestinal tissue	Increased relative abundance of *Lactobacillus intestinalis*, *Clostridium disporicum* and *Bifidobacterium choerinum* Depleted levels of *Clostridium saccharogumia*	[101]

Experimental model	Outcome	Microbial composition identified	Reference
Men with traumatic complete SCI (quadriplegics and paraplegics) vs. healthy patients	Significant differences in microbial composition Negative correlation with high-density lipoprotein cholesterol (cHDL) levels in the blood Increased gut epithelial permeability	Increased relative abundance of *Bacteroides* and *Bifidobacterium*	[102]
Adult male patients with traumatic cervical spinal cord injury vs. healthy male patients	Moderate bowel dysfunction in patients with SCI Decreased beta diversity of gut microbiota in SCI vs. healthy patients Decreased *Faecalibacterium* correlates with increased levels of triglycerides and cLDL Significantly decreased abundance of fatty acid metabolism in level 3 of the KEGG metabolic pathway hierarchy	Increased relative abundance of *Bacteroides* and *Blautia* Decreased levels of *Megamonas* and *Prevotella* correlate with lipid metabolism markers *Lactobacillus* positively correlates with serum glucose levels	[103]
Anxiety-like model in incomplete unilateral cervical SCI rats	Treatment with fecal transplant shows the reduction of anxiety-like behavior	112 OTUs (not specified) were found statistically different at day 3 post injury between SCI and healthy rats	[104]

Table 1.
Most important findings in the research field of SCI microbiota.

management and an increase in quality of life in SCI patients after their treatment with a multispecies probiotic [105].

In animal models, these results have been consistent, although in clinical studies it should be considered that there are confusing variables that cannot be controlled such as the intake of the same diet or the same level and intensity of injury, age of patients, diet intake, and administration of drugs that could modify the intestinal microbiota such as antibiotics.

4. Conclusion: what is next?

Spinal cord injury is a complex disease that involves several negative repercussions in the individual and society.

Its medical approach exclusively had been the treatment of movement impairment; however, in the last 14 years, the investigation is focusing on the treatment of other important comorbidities as the bowel dysfunction, which is responsible in decreasing the quality of life in patients with SCI that could worsen their health condition.

The answer apparently has been elucidated in the interaction between the individual and the gut microbiota.

Although, the study of the microbiota-gut-brain axis reveals with greater certainty the symbiotic dynamics that allow us to sustain homeostasis with our external environment; in this moment, the knowledge is still insufficient, with more reason in the SCI field.

Perhaps if the correct characterization of gut microbiota in this type of patients, considering their personalized features as the age, level, and severity of injury, is achieved, it could be possible to propose a targeted nutraceutical treatment aiming to restore the eubiosis and, with this, modulate the exacerbated inflammatory response in SCI at the spinal cord and the bowel hoping for neuroprotection and less damage.

Acknowledgements

We gratefully acknowledge the Universidad Anahuac México for their support for this project.

Author details

Estefanía de la Cruz-Castillo and Elisa García-Vences*
Centro de Investigación en Ciencias de la Salud (CICSA), Universidad Anáhuac México Campus Norte, Mexico

*Address all correspondence to: edna.garcia@anahuac.mx

References

[1] Kirshblum SC, Waring W, Biering-Sorensen F, Burns SP, Johansen M, Schmidt-Read M, et al. Reference for the 2011 revision of the international standards for neurological classification of spinal cord injury. The Journal of Spinal Cord Medicine. 2011;**34**(6):547-554

[2] Furlan JC, Sakakibara BM, Miller WC, Krassioukov AV. Global incidence and prevalence of traumatic spinal cord injury. The Canadian Journal of Neurological Sciences. 2013;**40**(4):456-464

[3] Lim S, Shiue Y, Ho C, Yu S, Kao P, Wang J, et al. Anxiety and depression in patients with traumatic spinal cord injury : A nationwide population-based cohort study. PLOS One. 2017;**12**(1):e0169623

[4] Cripps RA, Lee BB, Wing P, Weerts E, Mackay J, Brown D. A global map for traumatic spinal cord injury epidemiology: Towards a living data repository for injury prevention. Spinal Cord. 2011;**49**(4):493-501

[5] Ma VY, Chan L, Carruthers KJ. Incidence, prevalence, costs, and impact on disability of common conditions requiring rehabilitation in the United States: Stroke, spinal cord injury, traumatic brain injury, multiple sclerosis, osteoarthritis, rheumatoid arthritis, limb loss, and back pa. Archives of Physical Medicine and Rehabilitation. 2014;**95**(5):986.e1-995.e1

[6] Singh A, Tetreault L, Kalsi-Ryan S, Nouri A, Fehlings MG. Global prevalence and incidence of traumatic spinal cord injury. Clinical Epidemiology. 2014;**6**:309-331

[7] Wyndaele M, Wyndaele JJ. Incidence, prevalence and epidemiology of spinal cord injury: What learns a worldwide literature survey? Spinal Cord. 2006;**44**(9):523-529

[8] Lee BB, Cripps RA, Fitzharris M, Wing PC. The global map for traumatic spinal cord injury epidemiology: Update 2011, global incidence rate. Spinal Cord. 2014;**52**(2):110-116

[9] WHO. Spinal Cord Injury [Internet]. 2013. Available from: https://www.who.int/en/news-room/fact-sheets/detail/spinal-cord-injury [Accessed: 20 November 2019]

[10] Pérez R, Del Campo M, Renan S, Durán-Ortíz S. Aspectos epidemiológicos de la lesión medular de la población del Centro Nacional de Rehabilitación. Revista Mexicana de Medicina Física y Rehabilitación. 2008;**20**(3-4):74-82

[11] Pérez MD, Martínez CR, Zhurbenko R. Aspectos fundamentales sobre el género enterococcus como patógeno de elevada importancia en la actualidad. Revista Cubana de Higiene y Epidemiologia. 2010;**48**(2):147-161

[12] Azarhomayun A, Aghasi M, Mousavi N, Shokraneh F, Vaccaro AR, Haj Mirzaian A, et al. Mortality rate and predicting factors of traumatic thoracolumbar spinal cord injury; a systematic review and meta-analysis. Bulletin of Emergency and Trauma. 2018;**6**(3):181-194

[13] Gungor B, Adiguzel E, Gursel I, Yilmaz B, Gursel M. Intestinal microbiota in patients with spinal cord injury. PLOS One. 2016;**11**:e0145878

[14] Krueger H, Noonan VK, Trenaman LM, Joshi P, Rivers CS. The economic burden of traumatic spinal cord injury in Canada. Chronic Diseases and Injuries in Canada. 2013;**33**(3):113-122

[15] Nelson MD, Widman LM, Abresch RT, Stanhope K, Havel PJ, Styne DM, et al. Metabolic syndrome

in adolescents with spinal cord dysfunction. The Journal of Spinal Cord Medicine. 2007;**30**(Suppl 1):127-139

[16] Isomaa B, Almgren P, Tuom T. Cardiovascular morbidity and mortality. Diabetes Care. 2001;**24**(4):683-689

[17] Ibarra A, Ríos-Hoyo A, Suarez-Meade P, Malagon E, Colin-Rodríguez A. Influence of the level, severity and phase of spinal cord injury on hematological and biochemical parameters. Journal of Trauma & Treatment. 2014;**3**(4):2167-1222

[18] Brommer B, Engel O, Kopp MA, Watzlawick R, Müller S, Prüss H, et al. Spinal cord injury-induced immune deficiency syndrome enhances infection susceptibility dependent on lesion level. Brain. 2016;**139**:692-707

[19] Myers SA, Gobejishwili L, Saraswat Ohri S, Wilson CG, Andres KR, Riegler AS, et al. Following spinal cord injury, PDE4B drives an acute, local inflammatory response and a chronic, systemic response exacerbated by gut dysbiosis and endotoxemia. Neurobiology of Disease. 2019;**124**:353-363

[20] Wallin BG, Stjernberg L. Sympathetic activity in man after spinal cord injury: Outflow to skin below the lesion. Brain. 1984;**107**(1):183-198

[21] Eldahan KC, Rabchevsky AG. Autonomic dysreflexia after spinal cord injury. Autonomic Neuroscience. 2018;**209**:59-70

[22] Karlsson AK. Autonomic dysfunction in spinal cord injury: Clinical presentation of symptoms and signs. Progress in Brain Research. 2006;**152**:1-8

[23] Sharif H, Hou S. Autonomic dysreflexia: A cardiovascular disorder following spinal cord injury. Neural Regeneration Research. 2017;**12**(9):1390-1400

[24] Karlsson AK. Scientic review autonomic dysreflexia. Spinal Cord. 1999;**37**:383-391

[25] Lee ES, Joo MC. Prevalence of autonomic dysreflexia in patients with spinal cord injury above T6. BioMed Research International. 2017;**2017**:1-6

[26] Lucin KM, Sanders VM, Jones TB, Malarkey WB, Popovich PG. Impaired antibody synthesis after spinal cord injury is level-dependent and is due to sympathetic nervous system dysregulation. Experimental Neurology. 2007;**207**(1):75-84

[27] Pieper MP, Chaudhary NI, Park JE. Acetylcholine-induced proliferation of fibroblasts and myofibroblasts in vitro is inhibited by tiotropium bromide. Life Sciences. 2007;**80**:2270-2273

[28] Kurzen H, Henrich C, Booken D, Poenitz N, Gratchev A, Klemke CD, et al. Functional characterization of the epidermal cholinergic system in vitro. The Journal of Investigative Dermatology. 2006;**126**:2458-2472

[29] Baek A, Shin JC, Lee MY, Kim SH, Kim J, Cho SR. Parasympathetic effect induces cell cycle activation in upper limbs of paraplegic patients with spinal cord injury. International Journal of Molecular Sciences. 2019;**20**:5982

[30] Braddom R. Physical Medicine and Rehabilitation. 2nd ed. Philadelphia: WB Saunders Company; 2000. p. 1532

[31] Stone JM, Nino-Murcia M, Wolfe VA, Perkash I. Chronic gastrointestinal problems in spinal cord injury patients: A prospective analysis. The American Journal of Gastroenterology. 1990;**85**(9):1114-1119

[32] Glickman S, Kamm MA. Bowel dysfunction in spinal-cord-injury patients. Lancet. 1996;**347**(9016):1651-1653

[33] Lynch AC, Antony A, Dobbs BR, Frizelle FA. Bowel dysfunction

following spinal cord injury. Spinal Cord. 2001;**39**(4):193-203

[34] Levi R, Hultling C, Nash MS, Seiger A. The Stockholm spinal cord injury study: 1. Medical problems in a regional SCI population. Paraplegia. 1995;**33**(6):308-315

[35] Insua JT. Principialismo, bioética personalista y principios de acción en medicina y en servicios de salud. Persona y Bioética. 2018;**22**(2):223-246

[36] Whoqol Group. Development of the WHOQOL: Rationale and current status. International Journal of Mental Health. 1994;**23**(3):24-56

[37] Mashola MK, Mothabeng DJ. Associations between health behaviour, secondary health conditions and quality of life in people with spinal cord injury. African Journal of Disability. 2019;**8**:a463

[38] Catz A, Itzkovich M. Spinal cord Independence measure: Comprehensive ability rating scale for the spinal cord lesion patient. Journal of Rehabilitation Research and Development. 2007;**44**(1):65-68

[39] Ware JEJ, Sherbourne CD. The MOS 36-item short-form health survey (SF-36). I. Conceptual framework and item selection. Medical Care. 1992;**30**(6):473-483

[40] Craven C, Hitzig SL, Mittmann N. Impact of impairment and secondary health conditions on health preference among Canadians with chronic spinal cord injury. The Journal of Spinal Cord Medicine. 2012;**35**(5):361-370

[41] Choukou MA, Best KL, Craven BC, Hitzig SL. Identifying and classifying quality of life tools for assessing neurogenic bowel dysfunction after spinal cord injury. Topics in Spinal Cord Injury Rehabilitation. 2019;**25**(1):1-22

[42] Bølling Hansen R, Staun M, Kalhauge A, Langholz E, Biering-Sørensen F. Bowel function and quality of life after colostomy in individuals with spinal cord injury. The Journal of Spinal Cord Medicine. 2016;**39**(3):281-289

[43] Stone J, Wolfe V, Nino-Murcia M, Perkash I. Colostomy as treatment for complications of spinal cord injury. Archives of Physical Medicine and Rehabilitation. 1990;**71**(7):514-518

[44] Mazzone A, Farrugia G. Evolving concepts in the cellular control of gastrointestinal motility: Neurogastroenterology and enteric sciences. Gastroenterology Clinics of North America. 2007;**36**(3):499-513

[45] Gabella G. Autonomic nervous system. In: Paxinos G, editor. The Rat Nervous System. 3 ed. United States of America: Elsevier; 2004:77-109

[46] Navarro X. Fisiología del sistema nervioso autónomo. Revista de Neurologia. 2002;**35**:553-562

[47] Newgreen D, Young HM. Enteric nervous system: Development and developmental disturbances—Part 2. Pediatric and Developmental Pathology. 2002;**5**(4):329-349

[48] Romero-Trujillo JO, Frank-Márquez N, Cervantes-Bustamante R, Cadena-León JF, Montijo-Barrios E, Zárate-Mondragón F, et al. Sistema nervioso entérico y motilidad gastrointestinal. Acta Pediátrica de México. 2012;**33**(4):207-214

[49] Valles M, Mearin F. Alteraciones intestinales en pacientes con lesión medular. Gastroenterología y Hepatología. 2012;**35**(5):330-336

[50] Sekhon LH, Fehlings MG. Epidemiology, demographics, and pathophysiology of acute spinal cord injury. Spine (Phila Pa 1976). 2001;**26**(24 Suppl):S2-S12

[51] Longo WE, Ballantyne GH, Modlin IM. The colon, anorectum, and spinal cord patient. A review of the functional alterations of the denervated hindgut. Diseases of the Colon and Rectum. 1989;**32**(3):261-267

[52] Emmanuel A. Neurogenic bowel dysfunction. F1000Research. 2019;**8**(F1000 Faculty Rev):1800

[53] Emmanuel AV, Chung EA, Kamm MA, Middleton F. Relationship between gut-specific autonomic testing and bowel dysfunction in spinal cord injury patients. Spinal Cord. 2009;**47**(8):623-627

[54] Carabotti M, Scirocco A, Maselli MA, Severi C. The gut-brain axis: Interactions between enteric microbiota, central and enteric nervous systems. Annals of Gastroenterology. 2015;**28**(2):203-209

[55] Martin AR, Aleksanderek I, Fehlings MG. Diagnosis and acute management of spinal cord injury: Current best practices and emerging therapies. Current Trauma Reports. 2015;**1**(3):169-181

[56] Mataliotakis GI, Tsirikos AI. Spinal cord trauma: Pathophysiology, classification of spinal cord injury syndromes, treatment principles and controversies. Orthopaedics and Traumatology. 2016;**30**(5):440-449

[57] Oyinbo CA. Secondary injury mechanisms in traumatic spinal cord injury: A nugget of this multiply cascade. Acta Neurobiologiae Experimentalis. 2011;**71**(2):281-299

[58] Witiw CD, Fehlings MG. Acute spinal cord injury. Journal of Spinal Disorders & Techniques. 2015;**28**(6):202-210

[59] Tator CH, Fehlings MG. Review of the secondary injury theory of acute spinal cord trauma with emphasis on vascular mechanisms. Journal of Neurosurgery. 1991;**75**(1):15-26

[60] Orr MB, Gensel JC. Spinal cord injury scarring and inflammation: Therapies targeting glial and inflammatory responses. Neurotherapeutics. 2018;**15**(3):541-553

[61] Franze K, Janmey PA, Guck J. Mechanics in neuronal development and repair. Annual Review of Biomedical Engineering. 2013;**15**:227-251

[62] Wanner IB, Anderson MA, Song B, Levine J, Fernandez A, Gray-Thompson Z, et al. Glial scar borders are formed by newly proliferated, elongated astrocytes that interact to corral inflammatory and fibrotic cells via STAT3-dependent mechanisms after spinal cord injury. The Journal of Neuroscience. 2013;**33**(31):12870-12886

[63] Faulkner JR, Herrmann JE, Woo MJ, Tansey KE, Doan NB, Sofroniew MV. Reactive astrocytes protect tissue and preserve function after spinal cord injury. The Journal of Neuroscience. 2004;**24**(9):2143-2155

[64] Besecker EM, Deiter GM, Pironi N, Cooper TK, Holmes GM. Mesenteric vascular dysregulation and intestinal inflammation accompanies experimental spinal cord injury. American Physiological Society. 2017;**312**(1):R146-R156

[65] Tashiro S, Nakamura M, Okano H. The prospects of regenerative medicine combined with rehabilitative approaches for chronic spinal cord injury animal models. Neural Regeneration Research. 2017;**12**(1):43-46

[66] Gadani SP, Walsh JT, Lukens JR, Kipnis J. Dealing with danger in the CNS: The response of the immune system to injury. Neuron. 2015;**87**(1):47-62

[67] Carlson SL, Parrish ME, Springer JE, Doty K, Dossett L. Acute inflammatory response in spinal cord following impact injury. Experimental Neurology. 1998;**151**(1):77-88

[68] Donnelly DJ, Popovich PG. Inflammation and its role in neuroprotection, axonal regeneration and functional recovery after spinal cord injury. Experimental Neurology. 2008;**209**(2):378-388

[69] Gartner L. In: Gartner L, Hiatt JL, editors. Texto Atlas de Histología. 2nd ed. China: McGraw-Hill; 2007. p. 539

[70] Kigerl KA, Mostacada K, Popovich PG. Gut microbiota are disease-modifying factors after traumatic spinal cord injury. Neurotherapeutics. 2018;**15**:60-67

[71] Stilling RM, Dinan TG, Cryan JF. Microbial genes, brain & behaviour—Epigenetic regulation of the gut-brain axis. Genes, Brain, and Behavior. 2014;**13**(1):69-86

[72] Vernocchi P, Del Chierico F, Putignani L. Gut microbiota profiling: Metabolomics based approach to unravel compounds affecting human health. Frontiers in Microbiology. 2016;**7**:1144

[73] Estrada-Mondaca S, Carreón-Rodríguez A, Parra-Cid MC, León CI, Velasquillo-Martínez C, Vacanti CA, et al. Spinal cord injury and regenerative medicine. Salud Pública de México. 2007;**49**(6):437-444

[74] Stilling RM, van de Wouw M, Clarke G, Stanton C, Dinan TG, Cryan JF. The neuropharmacology of butyrate: The bread and butter of the microbiota-gut-brain axis? Neurochemistry International. 2016;**99**:110-132

[75] Robles Alonso V, Guarner F. Linking the gut microbiota to human health. The British Journal of Nutrition. 2013;**109**(Suppl):S21-S26

[76] Thursby E, Juge N. Introduction to the human gut microbiota. The Biochemical Journal. 2017;**474**(11):1823-1836

[77] Wang H, Lee IS, Braun C, Enck P. Effect of probiotics on central nervous system functions in animals and humans: A systematic review. Journal of Neurogastroenterology & Motility. 2016;**22**(4):589-605

[78] Clark J, Coopersmith C. Intestinal crosstalk: A new paradigm for understanding the gut as the "motor" incomplete spinal cord injury: Comparison with patients with motor complete spinal cord injury. Diseases of the Colon and Rectum. 2009;**52**:1589-1597

[79] Corrêa-Oliveira R, Fachi JL, Vieira A, Sato FT, Vinolo MA. Regulation of immune cell function by short-chain fatty acids. Clinical & Translational Immunology. 2016;**5**(4):e73

[80] Wiley NC, Dinan TG, Ross RP, Stanton C, Clarke G, Cryan JF. The microbiota-gut-brain axis as a key regulator of neural function and the stress response: Implications for human and animal health. Journal of Animal Science. 2017;**95**(7):3225-3246

[81] Dinan TG, Cryan JF. Melancholic microbes: A link between gut microbiota and depression? Neurogastroenterology and Motility. 2013;**25**(9):713-719

[82] Sherwin E, Sandhu KV, Dinan TG, Cryan JF. May the force be with you: The light and dark sides of the microbiota-gut-brain axis in neuropsychiatry. CNS Drugs. 2016;**30**(11):1019-1041

[83] Cryan JF, O'Mahony SM. The microbiome-gut-brain axis: From bowel to behavior. Neurogastroenterology and Motility. 2011;**23**(3):187-192

[84] Vijay N, Morris M. Role of monocarboxylate transporters in drug delivery to the brain. Current Pharmaceutical Design. 2014;**20**(10):1487-1498

[85] Ganapathy V, Thangaraju M, Gopal E, Martin PM, Itagaki S, Miyauchi S, et al. Sodium-coupled monocarboxylate transporters in normal tissues and in cancer. The AAPS Journal. 2008;**10**(1):193

[86] Ho JS, Anzai N, Enomoto A, He X, Do KK, Endou H, et al. Novel liver-specific organic anion transporter OAT7 that operates the exchange of sulfate conjugates for short chain fatty acid butyrate. Hepatology. 2007;**45**(4):1046-1055

[87] Moreira TJTP, Pierre K, Maekawa F, Repond C, Cebere A, Liljequist S, et al. Enhanced cerebral expression of MCT1 and MCT2 in a rat ischemia model occurs in activated microglial cells. Journal of Cerebral Blood Flow and Metabolism. 2009;**29**(7):1273-1283

[88] Lee Y, Morrison BM, Li Y, Lengacher S, Farah MH, Hoffman PN, et al. Oligodendroglia metabolically support axons and contribute to neurodegeneration. Nature. 2012;**487**(7408):443-448

[89] Minamiyama M, Katsuno M, Adachi H, Waza M, Sang C, Kobayashi Y, et al. Sodium butyrate ameliorates phenotypic expression in a transgenic mouse model of spinal and bulbar muscular atrophy. Human Molecular Genetics. 2004;**13**(11):1183-1192

[90] Bolognini D, Tobin AB, Milligan G, Moss CE. The pharmacology and function of receptors for short-chain fatty acids. Molecular Pharmacology. 2016;**89**(3):388-398

[91] Singh N, Gurav A, Sivaprakasam S, Brady E, Padia R, Shi H, et al. Activation of Gpr109a, receptor for niacin and the commensal metabolite butyrate, suppresses colonic inflammation and carcinogenesis. Immunity. 2014;**40**(1):128-139

[92] Nøhr MK, Pedersen MH, Gille A, Egerod KL, Engelstoft MS, Husted AS, et al. GPR41/FFAR3 and GPR43/FFAR2 as cosensors for short-chain fatty acids in enteroendocrine cells vs FFAR3 in enteric neurons and FFAR2 in enteric leukocytes. Endocrinology. 2013;**154**(10):3552-3564

[93] Sarkar A, Lehto SM, Harty S, Dinan TG, Cryan JF, Burnet PWJ. Psychobiotics and the manipulation of bacteria–gut–brain signals. Trends in Neurosciences. 2016;**39**(11):763-781

[94] Liu YW, Liu WH, Wu CC, Juan YC, Wu YC, Tsai HP, et al. Psychotropic effects of *Lactobacillus plantarum* PS128 in early life-stressed and naïve adult mice. Brain Research. 1631;**2016**:1-12

[95] Bercik P, Park AJ, Sinclair D, Khoshdel A, Lu J, Huang X, et al. The anxiolytic effect of *Bifidobacterium longum* NCC3001 involves vagal pathways for gut-brain communication. Neurogastroenterology and Motility. 2011;**23**(12):1132-1139

[96] Liang S, Wang T, Hu X, Luo J, Li W, Wu X, et al. Administration of *Lactobacillus helveticus* NS8 improves behavioral, cognitive, and biochemical aberrations caused by chronic restraint stress. Neuroscience. 2015;**310**:561-577

[97] O'Sullivan E, Barrett E, Grenham S, Fitzgerald P, Stanton C, Ross RP, et al. BDNF expression in the hippocampus of maternally separated rats: Does *Bifidobacterium breve* 6330 alter BDNF levels? Beneficial Microbes. 2011;**2**(3):199-207

[98] Bravo JA, Forsythe P, Chew MV, Escaravage E, Savignac HM, Dinan TG,

et al. Ingestion of lactobacillus strain regulates emotional behavior and central GABA receptor expression in a mouse via the vagus nerve. Proceedings of the National Academy of Sciences of the United States of America. 2011;**108**(8):16050-16055

[99] Brechmann T, Swol J, Knop-Hammad V, Willert J, Aach M, Cruciger O, et al. Complicated fecal microbiota transplantation in a tetraplegic patient with severe *Clostridium difficile* infection. World Journal of Gastroenterology. 2015;**21**(12):3736-3740

[100] Kigerl KA, Hall JCE, Wang L, Mo X, Yu Z, Popovich PG. Gut dysbiosis impairs recovery after spinal cord injury. The Journal of Experimental Medicine. 2016;**213**(12):2603-2620

[101] O'Connor G, Jeffrey E, Madorma D, Marcillo A, Abreu MT, Deo SK, et al. Investigation of microbiota alterations and intestinal inflammation post-spinal cord injury in rat model. Journal of Neurotrauma. 2018;**35**(18):2159-2166

[102] Zhang C, Zhang W, Zhang J, Jing Y, Yang M, Du L, et al. Gut microbiota dysbiosis in male patients with chronic traumatic complete spinal cord injury. Journal of Translational Medicine. 2018;**16**:353

[103] Zhang C, Jing Y, Zhang W, Zhang J, Yang M, Du L, et al. Dysbiosis of gut microbiota is associated with serum lipid profiles in male patients with chronic traumatic cervical spinal cord injury. American Journal of Translational Research. 2019;**11**(8):4817-4834

[104] Schmidt EKA, Torres-Espin A, Raposo PJF, Madsen KL, Kigerl KA, Popovich PG, et al. Fecal transplant prevents gut dysbiosis and anxiety-like behaviour after spinal cord injury in rats. PLOS One. 2020;**15**(1):e0226128

[105] Faber WXM, Nachtegaal J, Stolwijk-Swuste JM, Achterberg-Warmer WJ, Koning CJM, Besseling-van der Vaart I, et al. Study protocol of a double-blind randomised placebo-controlled trial on the effect of a multispecies probiotic on the incidence of antibiotic-associated diarrhoea in persons with spinal cord injury. Spinal Cord. 2020;**58**:149-156

Section 4

Technological Approaches

Chapter 9

Development of an Intelligent Standing Wheelchair with Reclining Characteristics

Ignatio Madanhire, Tawanda Mushiri and Panganai Musariri

Abstract

The widespread of motor neurone weakness has become a major concern as a result of accidents, ageing, birth defects and other hereditary diseases. A huge number of paraplegics can barely do activities for themselves without assistance from helpers. This study seeks to develop an intelligent wheelchair that has an assistive lifting and multi-posture reclining mechanisms to help in elevating the user from sit to stand posture as well as recline the seat for angles between 90 and 180 degrees through use of hydraulic linear actuators. The design would incorporate strain gauge sensors on the lower back area of the seat to enable the user to stand by merely leaning forward; thereby decreasing the strain on the lower back seat to trigger the lift mechanism until the required height is attained. While pressing the sit button on the console would enable the lowering of the user to a sitting position. The wheelchair development would also enable intelligent mobility through use of ultrasonic sensors to detect obstacles and assist in the braking effort by the user. An economic analysis was done to assess the feasibility viability of the design for local production. Some user requirement validation was undertaken to establish the extent to which the design would satisfy the key requirements of the intended beneficiaries.

Keywords: paraplegics, sit to stand, multi-posture reclining, intelligent, hydraulic linear actuators, strain gauge sensor, stress sensor, ultrasonic sensors

1. Introduction

An estimated 15% of the global population experience significant physical challenges [1] which affect the lower limbs and thus make mobility problems for this group of people. Assistive mobility technologies have been invented to aid the physically challenged people in moving from one point to another and these include wheelchairs, lifting aids, exoskeletons, walking devices and other devices [2]. However, in most cases, the user requires assistance in operating the device including help in pushing the wheelchair, support in using the bathroom, assistance in getting off the wheelchair etc. People using wheelchairs are exposed to secondary diseases associated with being sedentary. It was established that people with disabilities are more prone to coronary diseases and other related secondary diseases associated with lack of exercises and sedentariness. Effects on patients also include physical and psychological factors due to the prolonged seated posture [3]. With only a few caregivers, there is great need for improved assistive devices to give more independence to the physically challenged. It is in this regard that this study to develop an artificially intelligent wheelchair to assists users in reclining and getting up to standing posture and seat with reduced effort. Thus, it would aid the users to perform more tasks such as standing, maintaining eye to eye contact during conversations, cooking, exercising/physiotherapy, and reaching a top shelf among other activities.

2. Modern wheelchair review

With differing levels and causes of mobility impairment, this calls for upgraded wheel chair functions that can assist the users in performing standard tasks independently while minimising risk of contracting secondary diseases to the users. There is an increasing need for intelligent wheelchairs to elevate the user from seated to standing posture and vice versa as well as providing better flexibility of the user through improved manoeuvrability and increasing number of degrees of freedom (DoF) in terms of inclination of the chair.

Reclining wheelchairs: Also known as tilt-in-space wheelchairs, have seating platforms that can be tilted through various angles as shown in **Figure 1**. It allows the user to relax through different posture angles allowing blood flow to the lower limbs.

Manually operated standing wheelchair: The wheelchair uses bicycle chains to transfer power from tank tread-like push bars to the wheels or the system that lifts the user. It consists of a unique hand drive mechanism that allows users to drive the wheels of the wheelchair while seated, standing or in the range of positions in between (**Figure 2**).

Smart wheelchair: This typically consists of either a standard power wheelchair to which a computer and some sensors have been added or a mobile robot base to which a seat has been attached. Smart wheelchairs have been designed to provide navigation assistance to the user in a number of different ways, such as assuring collision-free travel, aiding the performance of specific tasks (e.g. passing through doorways), and autonomously transporting the user between locations. To avoid

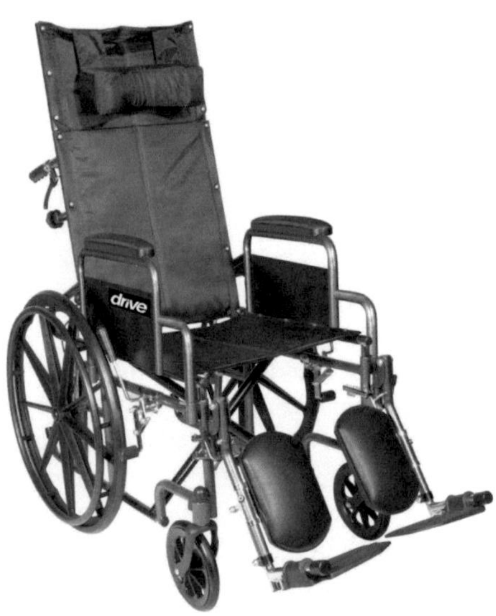

Figure 1.
Reclining wheelchair [4].

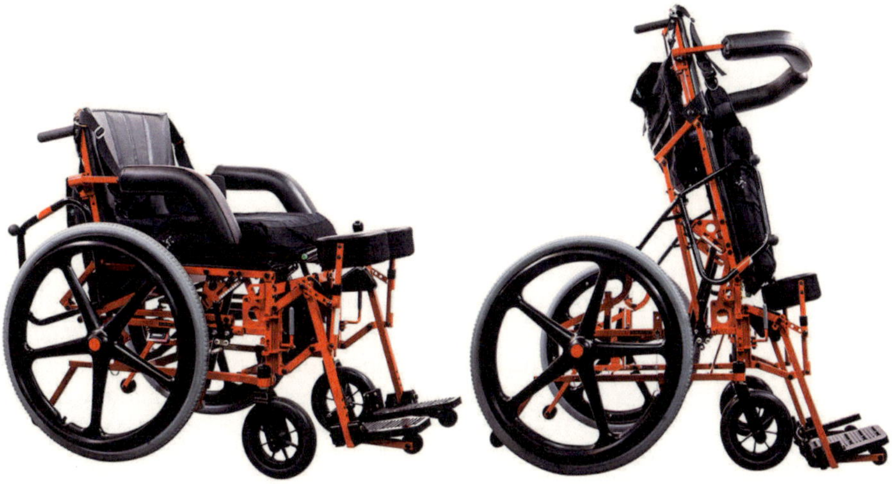

Figure 2.
Manually operated standing wheelchair [5].

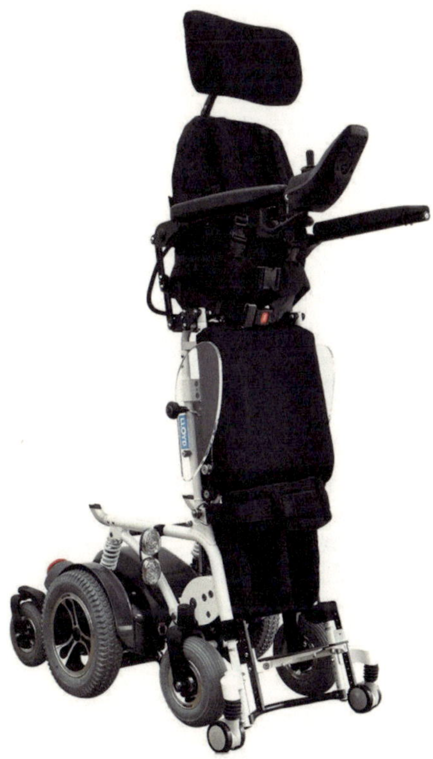

Figure 3.
Electric powered standing wheelchair [7].

obstacles, smart wheelchairs need sensors to perceive their surroundings. Proximity sensors are normally used to detect obstacles in the pathway of the wheelchair.

Powered standing wheelchair: This consists of an electric motor drive system powered by DC batteries mounted at the base of the frame. The speed of these motors is controlled by the remote control system to allow for forward, reverse and sideways propulsion of the wheelchair. On lifting the user, linear actuators and revolute motors (mounted at the back of the chair) are used to produce the required torque or control input signal from the remote control system to transform the shape of the wheelchair frame from seated to standing posture and vice versa [6]. The user is extended from a sitting position to a full standing position. The user's legs are locked and support the weight of the body at full extension. A hydraulic lift is used to complete the motion with elevation times ranging from 3 to 60 seconds (**Figure 3**).

2.1 Contemporary imitations of existing wheelchair designs

Most current designs use lots of expensive material and components, and this makes them unaffordable to the majority of the people who need them especially for communities in impoverished developing regions of the world. The wheelchair design in **Figure 3** requires the user to have legs that meet a minimum bone density to undergo this motion. Hence there is need for a design to accommodate all types of users with or without legs.

3. Materials and methods

The researchers conducted interviews with wheelchair users from local communities as well as visiting some patients at local health facilities such as Baines Physiotherapy & Rehabilitation Centre. The researchers managed to interpret the raw data in terms of customer needs and expectations into technical aspects thus helping in narrowing down the areas that needed improvement as per user needs as given in **Table 1**.

A network of contacts was developed to provide insight and guidance to refine the design output. These included members of the medical rehabilitation field, medical equipment suppliers as well as ergonomics and human motion experts in the field of physiotherapy.

In order to come up with the design mechanism for lifting the user from Sit to Stand (STS) and vice versa, it was crucial for the researchers to undertake a study in to the kinematics of standing up and sitting down from a chair. The next step was to analyse the joint movements (of the angles, knees and hips) for an individual as they stood up from a chair. It was important to follow this procedure (bio-mimicking human movements) so that the design would offer smooth operation as a physically unchallenged person.

Measurements of the individual formed the basis for determining wheelchair frame size, the need for adjustable ranges in component parts, and the need for customization to meet special needs. This was key in sizing the wheelchair for an

Wheelchair User Need	Technical Interpretation
Independence in operation	Automation & Intelligence
Multiple uses	Mechanisms (standing and reclining)
Balance	Safety and stability
Less cost	Economic
Comfortable ride	Suspension system and change of material
Adjustable	Functionality
Improved back rest design	Ergonomic design

Table 1.
Interpretation of user need.

average adult person. Appropriate size determinations of the wheelchair frame, seat, back, leg rests, and armrests based on measurements with an average bodied adult in an optimally seated position were taken and these built the foundation of the wheelchair design.

Three possible design concepts were generated, and the best option was selected using the Binary Dominance Matrix as the ideas were evaluated against the research objectives. Detailed engineering drawing designs were done using Solid Works and AutoCAD software. Special attention was also given to the actuation and sensory systems that were assembled in synergy to give the wheelchair autonomous and intelligent abilities.

The simulation process was carried out for both seated and standing postures. Calculations were done on the design to analyse it on the bending and torsional stresses acting on the components of the wheelchair under load in operation including deformation of stressed parts. The safety factor was obtained from these calculations and was compared against the standard safety factor. The researchers carried out the economic analysis to determine the costs of the parts and this was drafted in the Bill of Quantities to get the total cost of the components and their quantities.

4. Detailed design development

Table 2 gives the technical specifications of the intended wheel chair design.

4.1 Linear actuator and recliner concept

From the data gathered, the researchers came up with three possible solutions that were mainly different in the lift actuation mechanisms. Most of the attention of the drawings was paid to the working principle behind the lifting mechanism with the pros and cons for each concept discussed.

From the Binary Dominance Matrix (BDM), the concept on the Hydraulic Linear Actuator Lift and Recliner Mechanism (**Figure 4**) proved to be the optimal solution for the research design and was the most aligned with the requirements.

Eight selection criteria were considered and weighted for each of the design concepts; and each conceptual design was evaluated and scaled against a factor. The concept with the highest rating was considered the optimal solution for the design. The criterion factors considered included:

A. Ergonomics
B. Safety
C. Cost
D. Function
E. Simplicity of Mechanisms
F. Efficiency
G. Ease of Maintenance
H. Reliability

Figure 5 shows how the components that make up the mechanism are linked.

4.2 Linear actuator lift and recliner concept working principle

The mechanism consists of hydraulic linear actuators as the main source of power for the lifting and reclining mechanisms. When the command to lift the user is input, the battery powers the main hydraulic linear actuator to extend, pushing the wheelchair seat at an angle to the vertical. During this action, the

Specification	Measurement
Dimensions in mm	
1. Total Height (in seated posture)	1 200 mm
2. Total Height (in standing posture)	1 700 mm
3. Total length	1 280 mm
4. Armrest Height	$0 \leq h \leq 500\ mm$
5. Backrest tilt angle	90° – 180°
6. Seat Width	650 mm
7. Front Wheels	300 mm
8. Rear Wheels	600 mm
9. Footrest width	30 mm
Weights in kg	
10. Total Weight of chair	90 kg
11. Max User Weight	80 kg
12. Max Allowable Load	800 N
Features	
13. Power Source	24 V, 40 Ah
14. Max Driving Range with 40 Ah battery	30 km
15. Max Driving Speed	4.2 m/s
16. Max Safe Slope	15°
17.	

Table 2.
Technical specifications.

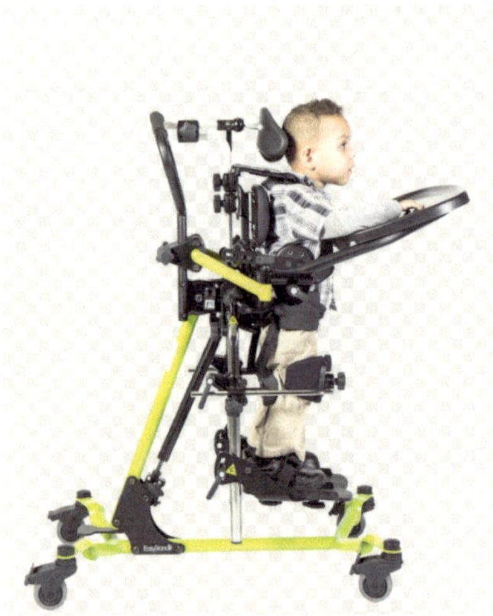

Figure 4.
Wheelchair in seated and standing posture showing max change in height $\Delta H_{max} = 0.5\,m$.

other actuators extend outwards and apply an upward force on the seat through the sliding assembly. The action of these actuators results in a resultant upward lift force that elevates and sustains the weight of the user as illustrated by **Figure 6** below.

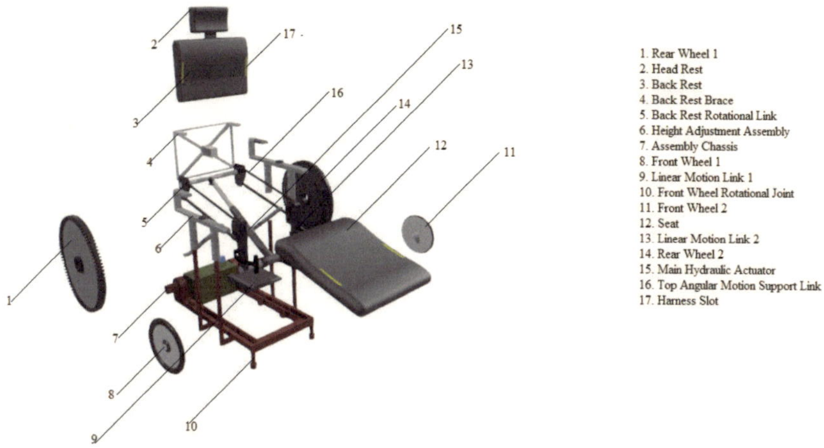

Figure 5.
Chosen concept exploded view.

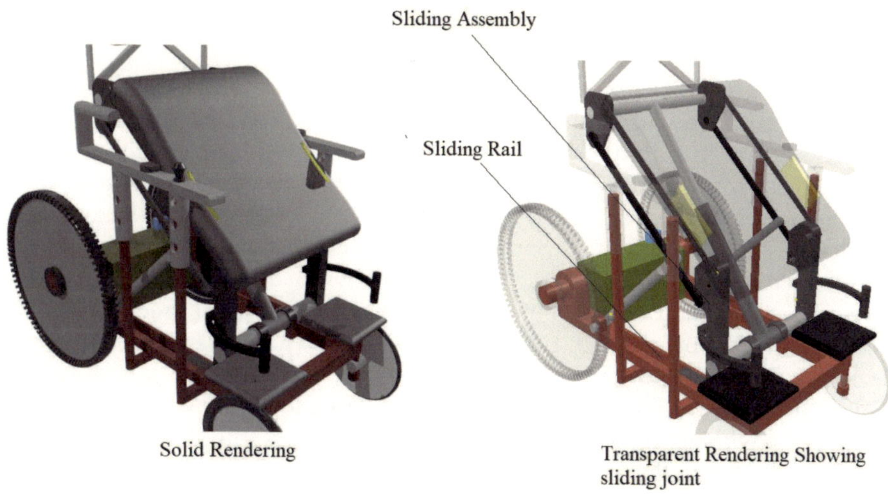

Figure 6.
Sliding joint mechanism providing lift for wheelchair.

The linear actuators used in this concept provide a smooth and stable movement of the wheelchair without delay, during height adjustment. The mechanism provides the possibility to design a better user control method for the convenience of most wheelchair users. However, application of this mechanism results in a relatively higher costs as costs of the linear actuators is higher as well as the other features that accompany it including power sources (batteries) (**Table 3**).

4.3 Autonomous drive control systems

The optimal design will consist of sensors and controls that to help in making it intelligent and providing autonomy. The wheelchair is driven by electronic speed differential motors that are directly coupled to the rear wheels of the chair. These motors provide the required torque for each wheel they are coupled to, and allow for different wheel speeds. This allows the motors to steer the wheelchair sideways when it is turning. The motors are powered by a 12 V lead acid battery connected to an Arduino microcontroller that receives input from the sensors and the joystick.

Wheelchair Operation	Left Rear Wheel	Right Rear Wheel	Wheel Speed V_W
Turn Left	Turns Backwards	Turns forward	$V_L < V_R$
Turn Right	Turns forward	Turns Backwards	$V_L > V_R$
Drive Forward	Turns forward	Turns forward	$V_L = V_R$
Reverse Drive	Turns Backwards	Turns Backwards	$V_L = V_R$
Brake/Stop	Stops	Stops	$V_L = V_R = 0$

Table 3.
Wheelchair controls.

The microcontroller is the central processing unit of the wheelchair. It receives input and gives commands according to the code embedded in it. The coding was done using MatLab and Python tools. According to the International Organisation for Standardisation (ISO), electrically powered wheelchairs intended to carry one person must have a maximum nominal speed not exceeding 15 km/h (4.2 m/s).

4.4 Proximity sensors

Ultrasonic proximity sensors are wired into the wheelchair drive system circuitry in order to assist the user in avoiding obstacles as well as in navigation. These sensors are crucial in assisting the user in preventing crashing into obstacles when they lose control of the wheelchair. The sensors convert electric signals into ultrasonic waves which are emitted towards the four sides of the wheelchair and are reflected back to the sensor upon encountering an obstacle. Measuring the time between sending and receiving the signal allows calculation of the distance between the wheelchair and the object and using a mathematical function model encoded in the microcontroller, they estimate the brake power required to stop the wheelchair. The brake power function is consists of an exponential decrease in the speed of the wheelchair as it is brought to a halt. This allows the wheelchair to make a smooth stop without agitating the user. For the sensors on the sides of the wheelchair, the microcontroller is coded to keep a safe constant distance from an obstacle thus helping the user from steering sideways into obstacles. These abilities make the wheelchair to be conscious of its surroundings when driving. The flow chart below summarises the algorithm followed on the decision making by the system (**Figure** 7).

4.5 Autonomous elevation control

The design incorporates intelligence in its elevating mechanism to detect when the user wants to stand. Strain gauge sensors are embedded on the lower back area of the wheelchair seat and when the user is seated, these sensors are in contact with the back area. They convert force, pressure, tension, weight, etc., into a change in electrical resistance which can then be measured. When external forces are applied to a stationary object, stress and strain are the result. The strain is defined as the displacement and deformation that occur. When the user needs to elevate to standing posture, they only need to bend their upper body, leaning forwards. This results in the displacement applied on the sensors (when greater than an average) and an electrical signal sent to the Arduino microcontroller which activates:

- The braking system of the wheelchair simply by covering the front ultrasonic sensor hence triggering the object avoidance system which cuts off power to the electric motors hence braking the wheelchair. Preventing the wheelchair from moving will aid to the stability of the user and reduce chances of falling over.

- The linear hydraulic actuators and hence the wheelchair lifts the user to a standing posture.

This is illustrated in the 5 steps shown in **Figure 8** below.

When the wheelchair reaches the maximum height, a signal is sent to the actuators to stop and remain bearing the weight of the user in standing posture. When the user needs to change from standing to seated posture, they can easily press the sit button on the joystick module. This reverses the direction of actuation of the lifting mechanism hence lowering the wheelchair back to its nominal position (**Figure 9**).

Figure 10 shows the algorithm followed in elevating the user to standing posture.

4.6 Autonomous reclining control

The design incorporates an autonomous intelligent reclining mechanism that is assisted by strain gauge sensors that are embedded on the top area of the wheelchair

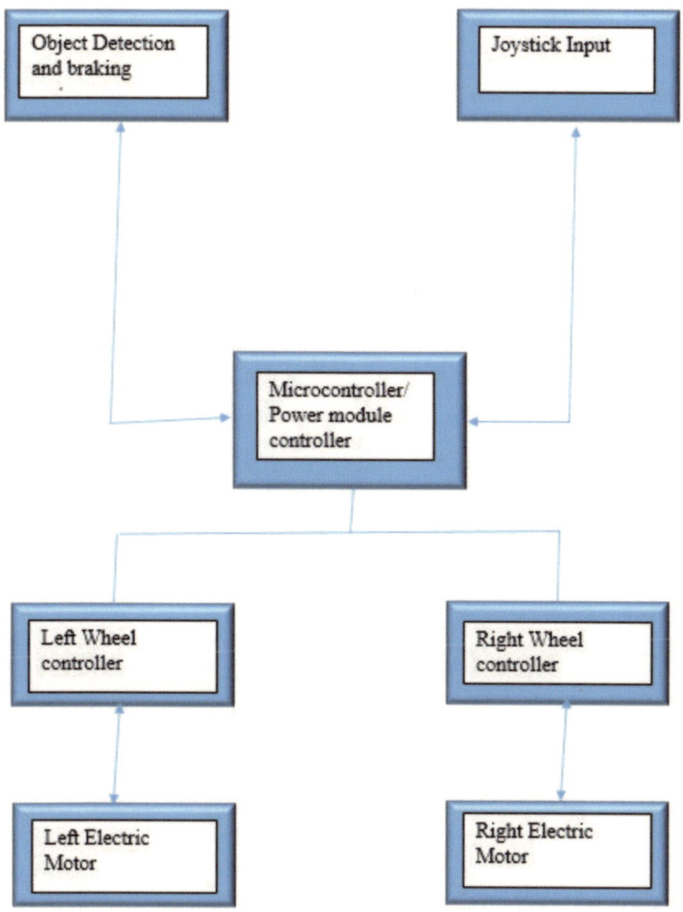

Figure 7.
Decision making algorithm flow.

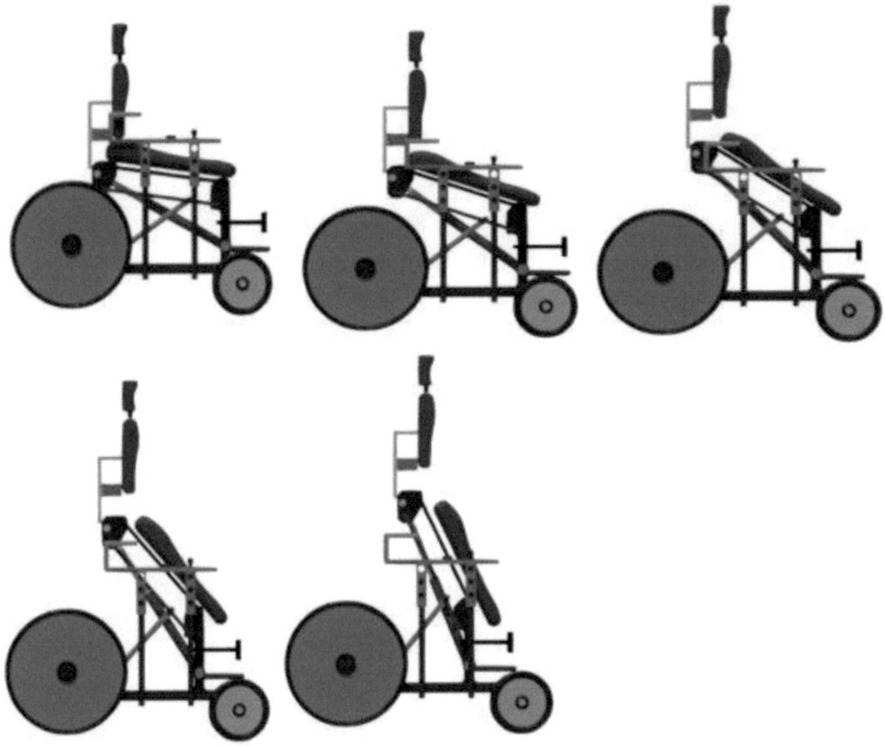

Figure 8.
Screenshots of simulation steps taken in lifting the user.

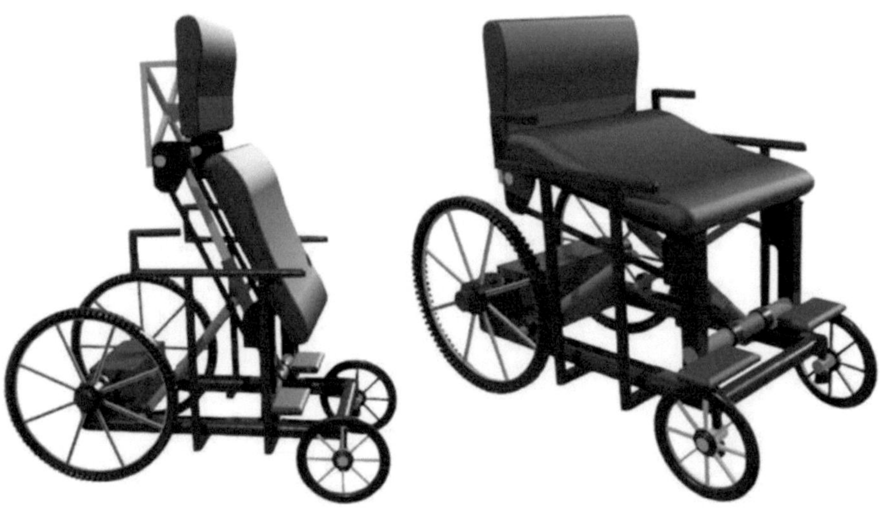

Figure 9.
Linear actuator lift and recliner concept in seated and standing posture.

head rest. When the user needs to recline the seat, they lay their head on the head rest and apply a minimum force (greater than 45 N the force applied by the weight of an average head) on the headrest (assuming the user condition allows them to do move their head). When the minimum head force is received by the stress sensors and converted to electric impulses which are sent to the control unit. This will unlock the wheelchair back rest and allow it to move backwards slowly (as

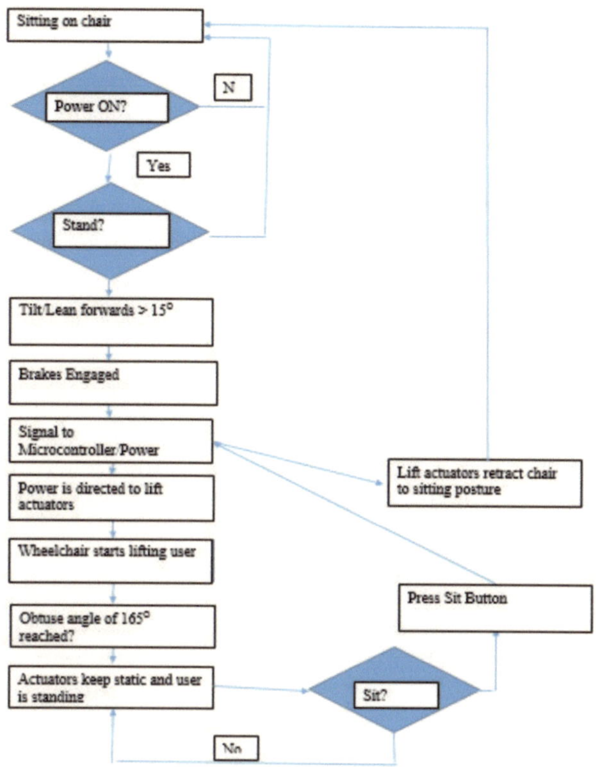

Figure 10.
Algorithm followed to elevated posture.

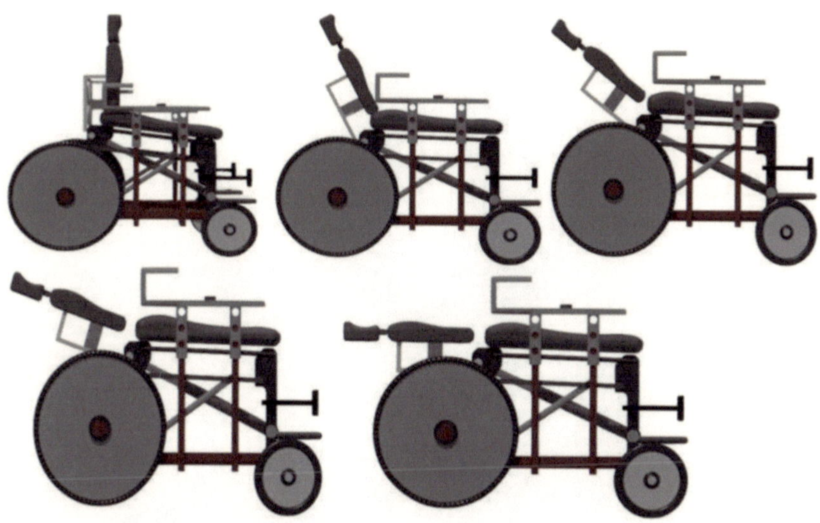

Figure 11.
Possible reclining angles.

permitted by the actuators) until it reaches an angle of tilt desired by the user. When this angle is reached, the user stops applying the force on the headrest and this sends signals to the control unit, commanding the actuators to stop reclining the seat and lock the mechanism (as the actuators will bear the load applied). The range of the reclining angles of tilt is shown in **Figure 11** shown below.

4.7 Height adjustable arm rests

The armrests are designed to be automatically adjustable up or down using a button input placed on the left arm rest of the wheelchair. The arm rests are actuated by telescoping arms that are placed in the tube of the wheelchair frame such that when they are activated, they protrude upwards, lifting the armrests to a desired height. Spiral lift telescoping arms are used for their ability to withstand the high the load exerted while projected at any height. These consist of threaded vertical profiles that move up or down inside a threaded cylinder bands that form a column. The bands are combined, separated and stored by an assembly with an electrical motor located at the base of the column and this is connected to the control unit while receiving input from the button pad on the arm rest. The desired height is determined by the duration on pressing the up/down button and on releasing the button, the armrest remain at their current height. They move simultaneously at a low constant speed that is safe for the user. When the user is in standing posture, the armrests automatically rise up for the sake of support and stability purposes.

4.8 Stability and suspension systems

The stability of the wheelchair is established by the use of four wheels instead of three and the user is supported in such a way that their centre of mass is lowered. This is also ensured by the dimensions of the wheelchair base as well as the weight and stress distribution exerted on the wheelchair. The wheelchair seat is also equipped with seatbelts/straps that help restrain the user from falling over during driving of when standing up by supporting the upper body weight of the user. The

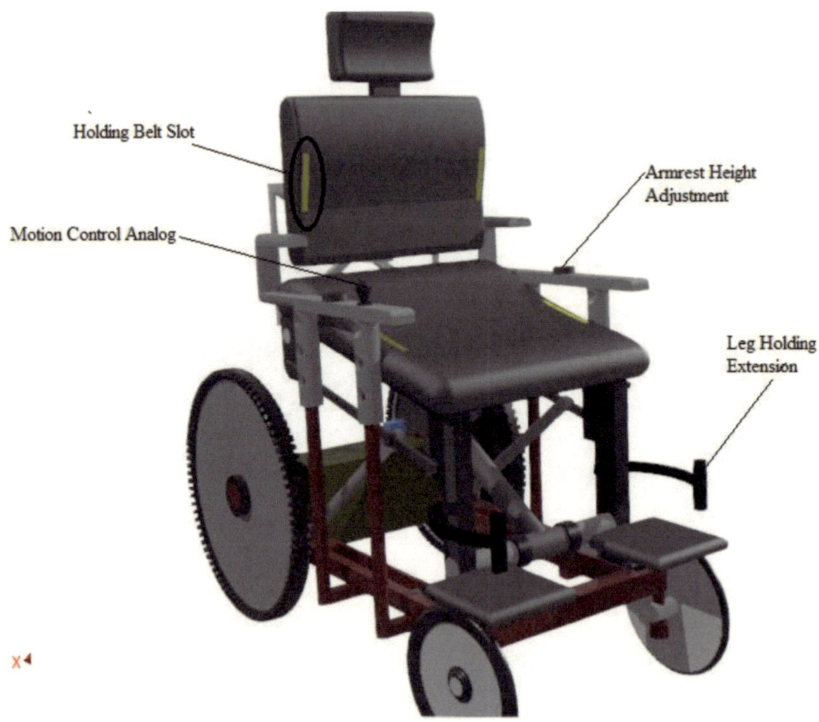

Figure 12.
Support mechanisms including seatbelt, arm rest and leg holding extension.

figure below shows the seatbelt slots on the wheelchair seat. A pair of leg holding extensions (shown in **Figure 12**) is mounted on the wheelchair in order to support the legs of the user hence aiding to the stability of the wheelchair.

The wheelchair hydraulic actuators absorb the vibrations during motion of the wheelchair along with the assistance of the wheels.

4.9 Component and materials selection

The wheelchair frame is made up of Aluminium because of its strength, light weight, corrosion resistance and resistance to shock loads that will be imposed on it during operation. Also the arm rests are also made of Aluminium as well as the spiral lift telescoping arm assembly. The leg rests are made of iron which is chosen for its high tensile strength as it will bear the body weight of the user when standing up. The seat, back and head rest are made up of silicone and are covered in foam cushion to enhance comfort to the user. While the wheels are made of rubber because of its excellent ability to absorb shock.

The joystick module which controls the power of wheelchair consists of command buttons and a knob. The module has 8 button commands namely:

- Power button-This switches the wheelchair system ON/OFF.
- Left- Steers left.
- Right – Steers right.
- Go- Moves the wheelchair forward.
- Back- Reverses the wheelchair.
- Stop- Brakes the wheelchair.
- Sit- Lowers the seat elevation system when the user needs to sit.
- Recline- Raises the seat recline back towards the initial seat angle of 90 degrees.

The joystick module is connected to the wheelchair's microcontroller/power module and these two communicate with each other using serial communication protocols. The speed and steering commands that are input by the user are converted to data packets by the internal processor of the joystick and then sent to the microcontroller via serial communication.

Finally the microcontroller module is the main system of whole wheelchair and it receives all commands from the joystick module and translates the commands into high current signals to the motors and mechanism actuators, receiving power from the 24 V battery power. Despite its small size, the power module is able to deliver a very high current per electrical motor and actuator.

4.10 Economic analysis

An effort was made to compile the cost and quantities of raw materials, and components as well as the cost of manufacturing a prototype. The grand total cost was about USD 1 511.

Part Name	Description	Cost per unit ($)	Quantity #	Total Cost ($)
Assembly Chassis	Hollow square steel tubes per meter	6.00	8	48.00
Wheelchair Frame	Aluminium Steel	9.00	6	54.00
Leg rest	Stainless Steel	6.50	2	13.00
Motion Links	Aluminium Steel	9.00	3	27.00
Leg Retainer	Aluminium Steel	9.00	2	18.00
Wheel Axle	Chrome molybdenum steel	8.00	2	16.00
Wheel bearings	Chrome Steel-SAE 52100	7.50	2	15.00
Wheel Shaft	SAE grade 41xx steel per meter	6.00	1	6.00
Arm rest props	Chrome Steel tubes per meter	8.50	4	34.00
	Total Material Cost			231.00
Electric motor	Speed differential electric motors coupled to wheel- 200 rpm, 2kw	79.00	2	158.00
Rear Wheel	Rear Rubber Wheel- 600 mm diameter	48.00	2	96.00
Front Wheel	Front Rubber Wheel-300 mm diameter	32.00	2	64.00
Head Rest, Seat Cushion, Back Rest	Foam rubber and leather covering per square meter	8.00	3	24.00
Linear Actuator	Hydraulic Linear Actuator	22.00	3	66.00
Ultrasonic Sensors	Ultrasonic Distance Sensor Module-HC-SR04	7.00	4	28.00
Strain gauge sensor	Load Cell transmitter with high accuracy	24.00	12	288.00
Joystick	Electric wheelchair joystick controller 24 V Anderson connector	80.00	1	80.00
Microcontroller	Arduino microcontroller A000079 Motor Shield, R3, 5 V–12 V	50.00	1	50.00
Battery	12 V Lead-Acid battery	60.00	2	120.00
Telescoping arm	Low noise waterproof 1500 mm Stroke 12 V/24 V telescoping linear actuator	19.00	2	38.00
Seat belt	Polyester and Nylon Seat belt straps- 900 mm	11.00	1	11.00
Connecting wires	Solid wire kit-6 different coloured spool per meter	3.00	4	12
	Total Component Cost			1 035.00
Manufacturing Process		Total $		
Welding		70.00		
Machining and Milling		80.00		
Riveting		20.00		
Miscellaneous		75.00		
TOTAL MNFNG COST OVERALL COST		245.00 USD 1 511		

Table 4.
Bill of quantities (BOQ).

From the costing analysis and evaluation carried out above, the wheelchair design proved to be relatively affordable compared to other wheelchairs on the market that can operate similarly.

4.11 Design validation summary

The evaluation of the design against the customer requirements as summarised by the **Table 4** below.

The design is fully automated with the drive, lift and recline mechanisms being controlled autonomously. It assists the user in elevating and reclining easily with use of sensors and intelligent awareness that prevents accidents and collisions. The design mechanism takes about 10 seconds in elevating to max height which makes it safe and efficient in handling the user with delicacy. The wheelchair allows the user to move around easily as well as perform more activities independently with the assistance of the wheelchair intelligence system. The design also includes a charging port to charge the battery (**Table 5**).

5. Recommendations

One key area of improvement is on the aspect of enhanced wheelchair comfort. Most wheelchairs should suit personalised seat dimensions and leg rest sizes. This could easily be incorporated into the wheelchair design.

A deeper ergonomic analysis should be conducted to improve the shapes of parts the user interacts with such as the armrests and the seating so that they provide enough comfort for long hours.

Leg supports can be added to assist in holding the user in standing posture so that they do not fall over. Also comfortable cushion material could be used for the seat and armrests such as foam padding. This can also be added to the leg supports so that the user is comfortable when standing up. The seat height at lowest elevation could be reduced to accommodate smaller body sized users.

Some considerations could be considered to change tubular material to reduce the weight of the chair. Titanium could be a good alternative to aluminium due

Criteria	Customer Requirement
Safety	Stable
	No harm to user
Mechanism Functionality	Autonomous
	Durable
	Minimum effort in operating wheelchair
	Same personal mobility as standard wheelchair
Wheelchair Functionality	Easy to move around
Geometry	Comfortable
	Cater for average user height
	Dimensioning to allow for manoeuvring.
Cost	Affordable

Table 5.
Validation of customer requirements with the design.

to its very high material strength with relatively lower weight. This change would increase the cost of the chair however and must be considered in the design.

To assist users who cannot use the remote control, future work can be done to use voice input commands to operate the wheelchair. Also some work can be done to link the wheelchair to the internet so that it can show locations, routes and report functionality levels of all parts thereby making it easy for maintenance of the wheelchair to be undertaken.

6. Conclusion

A study was done on the wheelchairs currently on the market as the basis to assess the extent to which existing mechanisms address the needs of the users. Some effort was made to gather relevant information from physically challenged wheelchair users, physiotherapists, doctors and wheelchair equipment supplying companies to establish areas of possible improvement with regards to ergonomic aspects of the wheelchair. Hydraulic linear actuator lift and recliner design concept was found to be the optimal design solution, and it was developed to come up with wheelchair characteristics, specifications, control systems and choice of construction materials. Engineering analysis and simulation were carried out to confirm the feasibility of the design. Also recommendations for future work were made on the areas that were not perfected by the design of this project, such as the need for voice input commands in the control of the wheelchair.

Acknowledgements

We would like to thank the Baines Avenue Clinic staff for allowing the researchers to interact with wheel chairs users and for the insight into health requirement for users. The Baines Physio Clinic gave us a detailed preview of how the wheel chair could contribute to the patient's physical wellbeing. Also the team from Wheelchairs Zimbabwe Company allowed us to appreciate the current wheel chair trends on the market and customer preferences.

Author details

Ignatio Madanhire*, Tawanda Mushiri and Panganai Musariri
University of Zimbabwe, Harare, Zimbabwe

*Address all correspondence to: imadanhire@gmail.com

References

[1] World Health Organisation. (2011). World report on disability. Malta: WHO Press. Torque Sensor Free Power Assisted19Wheelchair - Scientific Figure on ResearchGate. Available from: https://www.researchgate.net/figure/1-Schematic-example-of-the-joystick-controlled-wheelchairs-control-hardware_fig10_4310411 [accessed 5 Feb, 2020]

[2] Hemmingsson, H. &. (2009, October 24). Use of Assistive Technology Devices in Mainstream Schools: Students' Perspective. The American journal of occupational therapy, 463-72. Retrieved from National Institute of Child Health and Human Development: https://www.nichd.nih.gov/health/topics/rehabtech/conditioninfo/device

[3] Alicia A.Thorp, N. M. (2011). Sedentary Behaviors and Subsequent Health Outcomes in Adults: A Systematic Review of Longitudinal Studies, 1996-2011. American Journal of Preventive Medicine, 207-215.

[4] Devine Medical. (2019, August 21). Mediline Excel Reclining Wheelchair. Retrieved from Devine Medical: https://www.devinemedical.com/Medline-MDS808650-Excel-Reclining-Wheelchair-22-p/med-mds808650.htm

[5] Shirley Ryan AbilityLab. (2017, May 24). Manual Standing Wheelchair Lets Users Control It Whether Sitting or Upright. Retrieved from Medgadget: https://www.medgadget.com/2017/05/manual-standing-wheelchair-lets-users-control-whether-sitting-upright.html

[6] N. M. Abdul Ghani, M. O. (2016). Sit-to-Stand and Stand-to-Sit Control Mechanisms of Two-Wheeled Wheelchair. Biomechanical Engineering, 13.

[7] Karman Healthcare. (2019, July 22). Karman Healthcare. Retrieved from Karman: karmanhealthcare.com

Chapter 10

The Role of Supraspinal Structures for Recovery after SCI: From Motor Dysfunction to Mental Health

Braniff de la Torre-Valdovinos, Laura Paulina Osuna-Carrasco and Carlos Alberto Cuellar Ramos

Abstract

Neural circuitry controlling limbed locomotion is located in the spinal cord, known as Central Pattern Generators (CPGs). After a traumatic Spinal Cord Injury (SCI), ascending and descending tracts are damaged, interrupting the communication between CPGs and supraspinal structures that are fundamental to initiate, control and adapt movement to the environment. Although low vertebrates and some mammals regain some physiological functions after a spinal insult, the capacity to recover in hominids is rather limited. The consequences after SCI include physiological (sensory, autonomic and motor) and mental dysfunctions, which causes a profound impact in social and economic aspects of patients and their relatives Despite the recent progress in the development of therapeutic strategies for SCI, there is no satisfactory agreement for choosing the best treatment that restores the affected functions of people suffering the devastating consequences after SCI. Studies have described that patients with chronic SCI can achieve some degree of neurorestoration with strategies that include physical rehabilitation, neuroprosthesis, electrical stimulation or cell therapies. Particularly in the human, the contribution of supraspinal structures to the clinical manifestations of gait deficits in people with SCI and its potential role as therapeutic targets is not well known. Additionally, mental health is considered fundamental as it represents the first step to overcome daily adversities and to face progression of this unfortunate condition. This chapter focuses on the consequences of spinal cord disconnection from supraspinal structures, from motor dysfunction to mental health. Recent advancements on the study of supraspinal structures and combination of different approaches to promote recovery after SCI are discussed. Promising strategies are used alone or in combination and include drugs, physical exercise, robotic devices, and electrical stimulation.

Keywords: spinal cord injury, supraspinal, therapy, motor dysfunction, mental health

1. Introduction

Supraspinal circuits related to motor function have a complex neuronal organization which physiological function is highly conserved in most of the vertebrate species. Those have an important role in the neural control of locomotion and other complex motor tasks [1]. Enormous effort has been made to discover a therapeutic strategy aiming descending pathways to recover movement after SCI, but there are still no effective results promoting recovery [2]. The loss of specific descending tracts is related to the levels of motor dysfunction after SCI. For example, the corticospinal tract is an important pathway for achieving fine adjustments during locomotion, thus, restoring its connectivity may partially contribute to recover some locomotor functions after injury [3]. Additionally, several studies have described the role of the red nucleus and rubrospinal tracts in the activation of the flexor phase within the gait locomotion [4, 5]. The reticulospinal neurons of the pons and the medulla activating the flexor phase during stepping provide position information related to the motor response. The reticular formation provides control of the posture during locomotors tasks [6].

Seminal studies made by Russian researchers in the last century described a region in the cat within the mesencephalon (midbrain) which was named as mesencephalic locomotor region (MLR) [7]. They concluded that electrical stimulation to the MLR elicits coordinated locomotion. This circuit accesses descending spinal neurons from the reticular formation to transmit locomotion signals [8]. Today, this region is considered a target for electrical stimulation following a SCI because there is proof that homologous areas in the brainstem of humans can be identified as a MLR with some differences due to the possible adaptation to bipedalism [9].

It has been well documented that the above mentioned supraspinal circuits can contribute to remodel the spinal cord and promote in some extent, recovery after incomplete SCI [10]. The neural circuits within the spinal cord can exhibit a degree of plasticity at cellular level [11], therefore, these newly connections would allow the formation of new pathways that may contribute to functional sensorimotor recovery.

Although the neurologic classification of the AIS-ASIA (The American Spinal Injury Association Impairment Scale) as A represents total motor and sensory loss below the injury level, a complete section of the spinal cord is not frequently observed in the clinic. In a postmortem study, it was found that around 75% of subjects diagnosed with complete SCI, some portions of the spinal cord in the site of injury were preserved, representing "continuity" across tissue [12]. In 1998, Dimitrijevic and colleagues [13] described that some subjects AIS-ASIA A were able to produce voluntary motor activation in some muscles during epidural stimulation. It was evident that some spared fibers across injury were still functional, suggesting the term "discomplete" to describe this observation. This concept opened new questions regarding potential rehabilitation strategies developed in animal models. Unfortunately, translation into the clinic has not succeeded so far. Anatomical and physiological aspects are among the differences between animal models and humans [14]. However, in the last decade, new approaches have shown promising results in subjects with complete and incomplete SCI.

1.1 Neuroplasticity

Afferent inputs integrate sensory information that modulates the process of movement and theproprioception phenomena, cutaneous stimulation promotes the increase of spinal cord excitability and promotes plastic changes within the locomotor apparatus in humans [15]. Proprioceptive feedback contributes substantially to the posture maintenance phase of extensor activity as described in cats during treadmill locomotion [16, 17] and in humans [18], as well as improving motor functions with physical exercises designed to stimulate cortical and subcortical neural circuits [19] When SCI occurs, the supraspinal elements such as the corticospinal tracts often decreases its connectivity to its direct or indirect targets (i.e. lumbar CPGs); interestingly, the terminal territory of the motor cortex do not change significantly as compared to the somatosensory cortex, while the afferents fibers exhibit aberrant connections into deafferented regions of the spinal cord as described in monkeys [20]. In addition, proprioceptive neurons are relevant in the process of recovery within SCI, for example, it has been suggested that the neurons receiving feedback signals can help to reorganize motor circuits [21, 22].

The process for mediating remodeling of supraspinal circuits requires the specific selection for synaptic reconnection between supraspinal circuits and the deafferented spinal cord regions. Bradley et al. [23] proved that cyclic AMP response element-binding protein and NMDA receptors have a significant role in the process of reconnection since those promote the and reinforce the connections of relay neurons to the spinal cord in the mouse.

As mentioned above, many supraspinal circuits contribute to activate locomotor tasks. Strategies involving a combination of clinical treatments have been developed with the aim to predict restoration based on early clinical symptoms. Most of these methods correlated variables that indirectly influence supraspinal centers in the production of walking in humans [24].

After an SCI, the reaction of the glial tissue ends in the formation of a scar. There is great therapeutic potential in the ability to modulate the healing of glial cells in response to damage in the CNS. *In vivo* and *in vitro* studies, although relatively limited, have shown improvement in axonal regeneration and functional recovery after specific constituent's inhibition of the glial scar. Enzymatic digestion of GAG's (Glycosaminoglycans) chains of CSPGs (chondroitin sulfate and keratane proteoglycans), for example, stimulates axonal regeneration at the site of damage or injury [25, 26]. Axons chronically damaged in the SC can regenerate through implants of peripheral nerve grafts after 4 weeks of injury [27]. Even in lesions of one year of progression, regeneration of the rubrospinal tracts in adult animals has been described. This can be achieved with cells that are treated with the application of BDNF, allowing the normal conditions of the soma to be restored [28]. In the last decade, combined treatments with Chondroitinase ABC, or with novel forms to release and integrate this enzyme in the tissue has also been developing to improve plasticity and reconnection of the cells found at the injury site [29–32]. Therefore, biochemical and pharmacological management is important to reduce the glial scar and facilitate axonal regeneration and neuronal reconnection.

2. Motor pathways reorganization after SCI

To develop key strategies for functional improvement of injured spinal cord, the knowledge of the central nervous system organization under physiologic and pathophysiologic conditions is essential.

Premotor spinal oscillators (alternating flexor and extensor activity in neuronal spinal cord circuits) exhibit neuronal network organization based on their firing patterns and driving afferents. This oscillatory activity is also observed by firing patterns recorded in muscles, thus making possible to follow up therapeutic interventions in patients with SCI based on the activity of the muscles during flexor and extensor phases of locomotion. At the same time, it is possible to assess the abnormal firing patterns and dysfunction in spinal reflexes.

The concept of re-organization and pattern formation in imbalanced systems is associated to the firing patterns of groups of identified neurons in the spinal motor networks was extensively developed by Schalow and Zach [33]. Human CNS has integrative functions for learning, re-learning, storing and recalling, being all these necessary elements contributing to plasticity following injuries. Thus, understanding the Central Nervous System (CNS) reorganization in the short and the long-term memory process during a therapeutic intervention as an approach for re-learning adequate motor behavior is fundamental to achieve functional motor improvements. This intervention consists in the training of innate automatisms like creeping, crawling, up-righting, walking, and running. Moreover, the training of rhythmic, dynamic, stereotyped and movements could substantially be improved by applying different protocols of coordinate on dynamic therapy [33, 34]. Among therapeutic goals during coordination dynamic therapy are to induce cell proliferation and neurogenesis, so this could contribute to promote structural changes during the reconnection process in the injured tissue. New training paradigms are being created as a tool for retraining the spinal cord looking to engage the innate locomotor circuitry with appropriate afferent input to avoid lasting maladaptive sensory and motor effects, such as central pain and spasticity [35]. For accurate motor control, proprioceptive information from the body and environment has to be integrated and transformed into an appropriate motor command under physiological conditions [36, 37]. The inherent neural transmission and integration for motor output and the perception of limb position activated in the cortical areas during kinesthetic sensations are based on proprioceptive information [38]. This lead the notion that the activation of the propriospinal pathways in its different configurations may help activating supraspinal areas such as cortical regions where senses involved in modulating motor control are processed, and these can be used to take advantage of strategies for motor recovery from a SCI.

Interestingly, depending on the severity of the SCI, humans and animal models in most cases presentsome degree of spontaneous functional recovery during the first months after injury [39–43]. This outcome has been attributed to spared descendent axons bypassing the site of injury, although precise mechanisms underlying this phenomenon are not known. Courtine and collaborators investigated the spontaneous recovery in a spatially and temporally separated lateral hemisections in a mouse model, using kinematic, physiological and anatomical approaches. Their findings suggest that functional recovery can occur after severe SCI facilitated by the reorganization of descending and propriospinal connections [44]. Interventions headed for enhancing the remodeling of spread connections are important to explore in the various novel therapeutic strategies to reconnect spared tissue and restore function after SCI.

Neurorehabilitation must be in accordance with the re-organization of neuronal networks. Movement patterns re-learned by pattern formation and coordination dynamic therapy progress by cooperative and competitive interaction between intrinsic and extrinsic therapeutic inputs (afferent input) [45].

3. Combination of exercise and therapeutic strategies

Physical exercise provides important benefits after SCI both in clinical studies and in animal models [1, 46]. Specifically, studies in animal models have emphasized the importance of exercise and combined strategies to boost motor recovery. However, the functional recovery of locomotion has so far been limited, preventing its translation into the clinic.

Exercise and physical training demand adaptation in a wide range of movements and locomotion in upper, lower limbs and trunk, promoting interaction between CPG's, propriospinal neurons and supraspinal structures. Plastic changes induced by activity and sensory entry can take place both in the spinal cord and other supraspinal regions in the brain.

Studies have given evidence supporting the notion that exercise produces "motor learning" in the spinal motor circuits. One hypothesis is that the complex network of components of the extracellular matrix, inhibits the remodeling or reconnection [47]. Therefore, exercise induces the plasticity in the SCI circuitry, which could produce an interneuronal network reorganization [48]. For example, training intervention in a treadmill (20-minute protocol, 5 days a week for 3 weeks, after the complete injury) improved locomotion performance with a reversal in the asymmetric alternating movements that had occurred after a hemisection in a cat SCI model. The untrained group maintained the hemisection-induced asymmetry after the recovery period [49]. Increased excitability and the recruitment of motoneuronal populations drive limb coordination during gait and restores symmetry in a hemisection model of adult rats [50].

In other study in rats, a combination of Tamoxifen and treadmill exercise had a notorious improvement in the angular displacement kinematics after a hemisection SCI model. The untreated subjects remained considerable discrepancy in the hip and ankle joints. The drug tamoxifen presented neuroprotective effects as well as increased tissue integrity and inflammation reduction [51, 52] and the exercise exerted beneficial effects ameliorating the damage [48].

Complex network of the extracellular matrix components, which includes CSPGs, inhibits the axonal reconnection that exercise can induce, limiting plasticity in the damaged spinal circuitry. A Chondroitinase ABC treatment study was performed to see if it could enable plasticity in adult mice, combined with voluntary physical training on a rotating wheel. The results have not been positively conclusive [47]. It is necessary identifying an adequate protocol for pharmacological interventions as well as the type and amount of exercise. In 2016, another study with Chondroitinase ABC combined with intensive treadmill rehabilitation had a slight recovery, suggesting a beneficial role for chronic SCI in adult rats [32].

Physical training and elements such as the density of functional synapses, and the neurotrophic factors (NF) provide important clues to optimize recovery after injury [53]. Motoneurons and other ventral horn cells in sectioned rats synthesize BDNF in response to treadmill training, suggesting a support mechanism by which postsynaptic release of BDNF from motoneurons contribute to synaptic plasticity [54]. Moreover, BDNF levels had a significantly increase in the lumbar SC region in injured rats with training compared to the non-trained injured rats [55].

Exercise raise the levels of NT-3 and BDNF in the spinal cord, causing modulation of the NMDA receptor, which generates greater activation of the hindlimb muscles [53]. Neurotrophic factors, which include NT-3, NGF, and IGF, modulate neuronal growth, differentiation, and survival [56]. Endogenous NF higher levels can be better than exogenous administration. Exercise is also involved in the nervous system gene regulation, associated to apoptosis and cellular growth signaling pathways (PTEN, PDCD4, RAS mRNA and Bcl-2/Bax). This can produce axonal growth and reconnection improving injured SC morphology [57, 58].

Neurotrophic factors are fundamental for the normalization of spinal reflexes [59]. Limb spasms are phenomena of hyperreflexia that occur after SCI. AAV-NT3 gene therapy, exercise, and combination therapy all attenuated the frequency of spasms in the swimming test conducted at 6 weeks after SCI and increased rate-dependent depression of H-reflex in rats. Combination therapy was significantly superior to AAV-NT3 alone in protecting motoneurons and remodeling spinal cord circuits. Gene therapy and exercise can alleviate muscle spasm after spinal cord injury by altering the excitability of spinal interneurons and motoneurons, but adjusting the combined strategy is needed to get better results [60].

Exercise produces benefits such as improving strength and conduction to adaptations in skeletal muscle and nervous system [61]. In humans, with almost total loss of voluntary muscle activity in one or both lower extremities, free field gait rehabilitation can be performed [62]. Based on this, the improvement can be achieved by appropriate treadmill training due to the activity of the voluntary muscle [63].

The effectiveness of physiotherapy in people with SCI studied in randomized controlled trials give evidence that a small number of this interventions increase voluntary strength in muscles directly affected by SCI, comparing sham or no intervention, and different physiotherapy interventions [64]. Other randomized control trials studies provide outcomes of specific features of training interventions to improve both sitting and standing balance function in SCI indicate negligible effect sizes [65–70]. Given the importance of balance control underpinning all aspects of daily activities, there is a need for further research [71].

Passive cycling can be an alternative rehabilitation for patients who are too weak or medically unstable to repeatedly practice active movements. Experimental animal studies [72] revealed that passive cycling modulated spinal reflex, reduced spasticity and autonomic dysreflexia as well as elicited cardio-protective effects [73–76]. Also, increased BDNF mRNA levels, GDNF and NT-4 [77]. In contrast, human studies did not show an effect on spasticity reduction nor prevention of cardiovascular disease-related secondary complications [78, 79]. However, it is possible that passive cycling could provoke sensory inputs to induce cortical plasticity to improve lower limb motor performance, further wide perspectives are necessary in this direction [72].

In patients with chronic incomplete SCI, targeted physical exercises are designed to simultaneously stimulate cortical, and spared subcortical neural circuits. Participants of a study underwent 48 sessions each of weight-supported robotic-assisted treadmill training and a combination of balance and fine hand exercises. Multimodal training tended to increase short-interval H-reflex facilitation, whereas treadmill training tended to improve dynamic seated balance. The low number of participants who completed both phases was a limitation. However, it is important to address engagement of lower extremity motor cortex using skilled upper extremity exercises; and skill transfer from upright postural stability during multimodal training to seated dynamic balance. These multimodal approaches incorporating balance with skilled upper extremity exercises showed no benefit compared to an active control program of body weight-supported treadmill training. Thus, it is necessary to improve participant retention in long-term rehabilitation studies [19].

Criteria for exercise guidelines represent an important step for developing exercise policies and programs for people with SCI around the world. According to current guidelines, for cardiorespiratory fitness and muscle strength benefits, SCI patients should engage in at least 20 min of moderate to vigorous intensity aerobic exercise and strength exercises for each main functioning muscle group are a strong recommendation. For cardiometabolic health benefits, at least 30 min of moderate to vigorous intensity aerobic exercise 3 times per week are a conditional recommendation [80].

The study and analysis of exercise is a major issue for the developing of synergistic strategies in the SCI treatment with pharmacological treatments and stimulation of the damaged tissue (electrical or magnetic). Different combined treatments produce positive interaction that improve or optimize the results in functional motor recovery, and revealing the knowledge of which parameters work is fundamental, so it can be adjusted to the individual needs of people suffering from SCI.

3.1 Robotic exoskeletons

Mobility possibilities of SCI people in a wheelchair, are very limited. They usually adopt a sedentary lifestyle, with progressive physical deterioration and risk of musculoskeletal, cardiovascular and endocrine/metabolic morbidity and mortality increase [81]. Robotic exoskeletons can allow individuals with SCI with varying levels of injury to functionally walk or exercise and mitigate these potential negative health consequences. The aim of these powered exoskeletons devices is to improve the mobility for people with movement deficits by providing mechanical support and facilitate the gait training [82]. All long-term manual wheelchair users who participated in a robotic rehabilitation session, predominantly perceived improvements in their overall health status and felt motivated to engage in a regular physical activity program adapted to their condition [83].

Use of exoskeletons take advantage of spared fibers in incomplete injuries and involve the use of voluntary motor control as well as proprioception to promote recovery. Therapies with exoskeleton comprises 16 to 30 sessions [84, 85], during three 60-minute sessions a week [86]. Results indicate potential benefits on gait function and balance [87]. For example, a study measured walking progression, sitting balance, skin sensation, spasticity, and strength of the corticospinal tracts. Results indicate that about 45 sessions are needed to reach 80% of optimal performance. Functional improvements were reported, especially in people with incomplete injuries. Spasticity had mixed changes, suggesting differences between high versus low spasticity prior to training [88].

The sensory information in SCI subjects is missing below the level of lesion, which made difficult to control body posture and balancing with an exoskeleton making its use difficult according to another research group [89]. It is hypothesized that part of the missing sensory information can be provided to improve the control of an exoskeleton by delivering discrete vibrotactile stimulation [89]. Following a training robotic-based proprioception training protocol in people with chronic incomplete SCI, significant improvements in endpoint and knee joint position sense and in a precision stepping task performance were shown. These results suggest altering proprioceptive sense is possible in people with incomplete SCI using a passive proprioception training [90].

An autonomous wearable robot able to assist ankle during walking, utilizes a Neuromuscular Controller with assistance based on specific residual functional abilities of subjects. According to the study, 5 training sessions were necessary to significantly improve robot-aided gait speed on short paths and consequently to optimize the human-robot interaction [91].

Exoskeletons technology have different settings depending on the needs and requirements of protocols. Existent information and evidence must be integrated to optimize rehabilitation SCI therapies. Also, is important to fulfill main goals of exoskeletons as to define basic elements for restoring movement and sensitive functions in the people living with a SCI. Finally, the refinement of the robotic devices is highly desirable to assess the adjustment to individual cases and the application in conjunction with treatments focused on the spared tissue reconnection, as well as electrostimulation therapies.

3.2 Limitations

Exoskeleton control can be challenging for users and requires a long period of training [89]. Then, functional interaction subject-exoskeleton is a main factor to produce or increase walking abilities with interlimb coordinated movements [86]. The exoskeleton rehabilitation strategies transferring from laboratories to clinical settings and their effects remain uncertain due to the absence of large-scale clinical trials. Some researchers and clinicians call for developing pre-training rehabilitation programs to increase passive lower extremity range of motion and standing tolerance [84]. Future studies with larger sample size are needed to investigate the effectiveness and efficacy of exoskeleton-assisted gait training as single gait training and combined with other gait training strategies [92].

4. Electrical and magnetic stimulation strategies for evaluation of spinal and supraspinal circuits after SCI

Electrical and magnetic stimulation can be used to evaluate supraspinal and spinal structures and promote restoration of the motor function. These approaches consist of electrical or magnetic stimulation delivery into neural structures as therapy in motor, sensory and behavioral disorders such as chronic pain, Parkinson's disease, essential tremor, among others. Electrical stimulation can be invasive or noninvasive and complemented with imaging and electrophysiology to assess therapeutic strategies in subjects. At the same time, studying the mechanisms underlying electrical stimulation is essential to understand short- and long-term effects on neural tissue, explore novel approaches, and guarantee biosafety on implementation.

Electrical epidural stimulation (ES) was originally implemented for chronic pain in 1967 [93]. Later, it was evidenced that ES produced passive rhythmic activity in lower limbs in paraplegic subjects [13], initiating this seminal study a series of clinical investigations with the exploration of specific ES parameters in combination with physical therapy and locomotor training [94–97].

ES consist of the delivery of electrical current (typically square pulses) at different frequencies depending on the designed protocol (see below). An electrode composed of several contact leads (commonly 16) is placed on the dorsal midline of dura spanning the lumbar enlargement (T11-L1 vertebrae). Adequate positioning is monitored through electromyographic responses evoked by electrical pulses delivered at low frequencies (0.2 Hz). Implantation surgery and electrophysiology testing during surgery are described by Calvert et al. [98]. Once the subjects recovered from surgery, initial testing consists of monitoring motor activities (electromyography, EMG) produced by simple tasks during ES, including voluntary contractions on selected muscles and passive movements with suspended limbs [94, 95]. First sessions are essential to optimize parameters individually, for instance, intensities and frequencies to enable motor function in the upper [99, 100] and lower extremities [94–97]. After a couple of weeks, depending on the level and severity of SCI, subjects can be suspended on a treadmill using body weight support devices, allowing them to walk at low speeds (< 2 km/h). Even some subjects AIS-ASIA A can regain some steeping capabilities without using body weight support [94, 95]. The fact that ES enables voluntary motor activation even in subjects classified as AIS-ASIA A, suggests that some spare descending fibers can still be activated even at chronic SCI stages after several years [95, 96, 101, 102]. It is noteworthy to mention that in the absence of ES, the capacity to perform voluntary motor activities is somewhat limited, concluding that facilitation provided by ES should be continually administered in otherwise "dormant" spinal circuits. ES has shown improvements in motor function, and unexpectedly also in sensory and autonomic function [103–105]; however, a small number of highly selected subjects have been enrolled to date, making difficult to extrapolate results to general SCI population.

From animal [106–109] and human [110–113] studies, it is assumed that ES excites low threshold afferent fibers (posterior roots). Depending on the intensity of stimulation, anterior roots can also be activated, hence producing potentials (Motor Evoked Potentials, MEP) identified by their latencies. By producing MEP with known latencies, combination of other approaches such as Transcranial Magnetic Stimulation (TMS) and peripheral functional stimulation (FENS) allows the study of spinal and cortical plasticity as discussed below.

Transcranial magnetic stimulation (TMS) has also been used to stimulate muscles below the injury level in SCI subjects. Differences in latencies and thresholds of activation between controls and are widely described as well as emerging protocols to study plasticity in the spinal cord and cortex using TMS [65]. Changes in the motor cortex excitability have also been described [114–116].

Similarly, changes in cortical representations and events involving neural reorganization in rostral and caudal structures to lesion have been described after SCI [117–119]. Although precise mechanisms involving plasticity in cortices after trauma or SCI remains unanswered, animal models have provided valuable information [120].

In humans, targeting upper and lower limb muscles along with FENS has shown to promote spinal and cortical plasticity as partially explained by long-term potentiation mechanisms (LTP) [121]. Together, TMS and FENS are termed Paired Corticospinal-Motor Neuronal Stimulation (PCMS). For example, Jo and Perez [67] hypothesized that exercise promotes cortical plasticity in incomplete lesions. In the same study, the authors found that PCMS produced higher voltage amplitudes recorded in selected muscles. Performance during motor tests in upper and lower limbs also improved, although subjects not included in the "exercise plus PCMS group" also showed advancements. A conclusion is that TMS combined with other methods such as FENS and exercise, produces plasticity in spinal and supraspinal circuits (i.e., motor cortex), which benefits people suffering from SCI. Moreover, the effects on motor performance can last several months [67].

Yet some caveats remain unsolved. For instance, TMS technical aspects are not homogeneous across studies, for example, coils, motor tasks, and the number of muscles recorded [122]. Additionally, results obtained in small samples will be sustained in the heterogenous SCI spectrum, and potentially undesirable side effects should be discarded, as headaches are commonly reported during TMS [123]. Finally, technology advancements must overcome the high cost of TMS nowadays and to offer devices that can be used by patients and caregivers at home.

Noninvasive electrical stimulation techniques called transcutaneous electrical stimulation (tSCS) and transcranial or trans-spinal direct current stimulation (tDCS) have also been implemented as therapy for SCI. Both procedures include delivery of electrical current by surface electrodes placed on the back (as the cathode) and a pair of electrodes located over the iliac crest (as anodes). Like with ES, tSCS activates low threshold afferents, although higher stimulation intensities must be delivered as current must overcome high-resistance structures (skin, muscle, ligaments, and bones). For this reason, high intensities usually produce discomfort in subjects, perceived as painful abdominal muscle contractions. Recently, a strategy was proposed to mitigate pain and reduce current administered transpinally: a carrier frequency (10 KHz) and a lower frequency (40 Hz, for example) [124].

tSCS has shown that delivered electrical current excites large diameter fibers, thus evoking motor potentials with same characteristics (i.e., latencies) as previously demonstrated during ES [111, 125–128]. For this reason, research has explored this noninvasive technique recently as therapy for SCI subjects.

Spasticity appears after an insult to the central motor system compromises descending monoaminergic modulation of spinal circuitry [129]. Unfortunately, this sensory and motor disorder commonly develops in SCI subjects. In chronic, incomplete SCI subjects, Hofstoetter and colleagues applied tSCS over the T11 and T12 showed improvements in spasticity as measured by the Watenberg pendulum test, electromyography and 10 minutes walking. tSCS consisted of a single session of 30 min of stimulation at 50 Hz with subjects lying in supine position. The intensity of stimulation is an important parameter to consider. For example, tSCS is delivered at levels that produce paresthesia but below motor activation [130]. The involvement of brainstem inhibition seems to play a role in the activation of neural circuits through long-loop mechanisms, although the whole picture is not clear for now, as remaining fibers depending on the severity of the lesion may take part on results [131].

Additionally, spinal inhibitory circuitry could be transiently modified, decreasing exaggerated reflexes, such as during cutaneous stimulation on the foot's surface. Interestingly, motor incomplete SCI subjects increased their walking speed and voluntary control, making it less likely that reduced spasticity occurred as a diminished motor output [130, 132]. tSCS delivered tonically at 30 Hz, showed an immediate change in spinal circuitry, i.e., enabling motor output measured by EMG and kinematics [132] similarly as previously shown during ES (see above). At the same time, supraspinal and propriospinal circuitry could participate during steeping in incomplete injuries. For example, ES and tSCS are supposed to increase the excitatory drive necessary to activate central pattern generators [13]. However, tSCS is not feasible as a home-based therapy and carry-over effects are not easy to study. It was recently found in one subject with chronic SCI (AIS-D) that tSCS self-applied during 6 months improved spasticity as measured by several scales and functional tests and that beneficial effects lasted for seven days after cessation of tSCS [133].

Combining TMS and tSCS is possible to explore changes in cortical excitability before and after low frequency (0.2 Hz), continuous (52 m) tSCS after SCI. After 14 sessions of tSCS, paired TMS pulses on the left motor cortex delivered at different interstimulus intervals (ISI) in a range of 1–30 ms, evoked motor potentials that exhibited intracortical facilitation and inhibition that was related to a decrease in latencies and an increase in amplitudes recorded in right wrist flexor and extensor muscles [134]. Authors interpreted these results as changes in cortical map representations, bilateral connection strengthening, and increase in cortical drive, although plasticity in the spinal cord may also play an important role. Importantly, the subject enrolled in this study also reported improvements in autonomic and sensory functions below the lesion, as reported for ES (see above).

Few studies have used the transcutaneous spinal Direct Current Stimulation (tsDCS) technique to study motor activation in complete and incomplete SCI. Cathodal or anodal stimulation can be applied, and corticospinal excitability evaluated in recorded muscles by TMS [135] or spinal reflexes [136]. Although nonsignificant results have been reported, modifications in MEPs suggest differences in cathodal versus anodal stimulation, meaning lateralization in responses depending on the location of the reference electrode [135]. Cathodal tsDCS stimulation did not show differences in spinal reflexes compared to sham stimulation [136]. Overall, results with tsDCS must be taken cautiously as few SCI subjects have been enrolled, and motor outcomes are not readily comparable with healthy population.

4.1 Limitations

Although these findings may represent a new alternative to invasive methods to restore lost functions, limitations impede translation into the clinic. Research must be extended into the heterogeneity of injuries (extension, level, time after lesion, age, etc.). To date, a small sample of subjects have been included in trials, and carry-over effects have not been fully explored. It is important to mention that beneficial results during neurostimulation are immediate, observable, quantifiable, and self-perceived; however, after cessation of electrical stimulation, there is a notable reduction in the effects, being voluntary muscle contraction the most evident, although some improvements remain as described consistently, especially in incomplete SCI. In this context, evaluation of daily activities should be included in trials to assess patients' quality of life. Finally, long-term effects, especially adverse effects, must be appropriately assessed, being one of the barriers the difficulty of self-applied home-based therapy.

Spinal cord injury is a severe clinical issue that affects in the acute stage the body of the patient and in a chronic stage the mental health. As above mentioned, a cascade of phenomena occurs after a SCI such as: inflammatory response that lead to neurons and axon degeneration, muscular damage, cardiopathy process, etc. If a group of health practitioners give a proper clinical and or surgical management, its patient preserves his life but not his sensitivity and motor control (depending on the degree and location of the injury).

Therefore, patients tend to develop an important state of mental health problems that includes depression [137], chronic sadness states and mood changes [138], delirium [139], and suicidal thoughts [140]. Therefore, is important to address mental health management after SCI in a proper way to ensure an integral patient recovery.

5. Mental health after SCI

Mental good health is important for transitioning our life with equilibrium; however, a traumatic SCI can disrupt that equilibrium since it causes the loss of our ability to have motor independency. Although the life expectancy of SCI patients has improved in the last decade [141], unfortunately, this condition has no cure to date and therapeutic strategies are limited to physical rehabilitation and support groups.

Psychiatric professionals have studied the relation between depression and anxiety as a SCI sequel and found that one out of two patients share in common continuous anxiety outbreaks and depression with a profound suicidal desire [142]. In addition, there is a significant higher risk of suffering psychiatric disorder in patients with a SCI such as dementia, psychosis, bipolar disorder, sleep disorder and illicit drug use [143]. The previous statement reveals that retrieving a life with normal parameters of mental health represents a challenge for patients and the doctors involved in the recovery of such disease.

Among all the mental illness that patients with SCI can develop, depression prevails over all mental health disorders. A cross sectional survey revealed that over 30% of the patients had depressive disorder diagnosed [144].

Although the initial injury is only the first of many traumata in the life of these patients, there are other factors that are related to increase mental illness; intermittent catheterization, sphincterotomy, continuous bed shift among others insults that endure for the rest of their life [145]. Though these procedures are for the patients benefit, they often chose to protect themselves from being oppressed by these disruptions, some patients retrieve themselves into the conservation-withdrawal response until they become uncooperative, express of wanting to be left in loneliness and passively acquire depressive signs [146].

As previously mentioned, physical exercise has positive results at a systemic level in the rehabilitation therapies, this beneficial effects includes diminishing of depression in individuals with SCI. Mood data (POMS questionnaire) and analysis for inflammatory mediators resulted in a significant reduction in total mood disturbance pre to post-exercise, and pre to one-hour post-exercise and there was a significant decrease in TNF-α from pre to post-exercise. Thus, acute exercise can positively affect mood in SCI patients and exercise-induced changes in inflammation contribute to such improvements [147].

At last, is important to mention that pharmacological therapies may give the patients some relief but are not always sufficient to promote adaptability to such condition. Emotional assessment may play a role in long-term adjustment [148].

Neurobiological and psychiatric assessments for SCI have been evolving throughout the years and the results are promising, but social issues are important for the reinsertion of these patients to society. It has been documented that social necessities are as important as physical [149]. Lack of job opportunities, transportation, marriage, social relations are a few of a big list of the social outcomes followed by a SCI [150].

Several studies has demonstrated that a proper social assessment such a reintegration to the community, interaction with groups of SCI injured patients, sports and psychosocial treatment can improve the clinical health issues [151].

The family context is very important in order to achieve higher health scores within SCI patients. Family brings support and comprehension of the patient's situation. However, when family integration falls apart due to diver's socioeconomics, demographics and emotional variables the recuperation of the patients may be a challenge [152].

The economic weight of the health care systems and the family financial difficulties to deal with, are a great challenge. As it is, raising awareness for improve prevention to reduce occurrence of these types of injuries, and medical and technological advances management for medical care in the social resources allocation [153]. And socioeconomics impact that damage severely the life quality of the patients. However, since the life expectancy of these patients has improved in the last decade [141] these patients often present functional impairments in several areas of their life such as: psychological/psychiatric, organ dysfunction, sexuality, economics, family and social interactions [154].

6. Conclusions

SCI is a highly complex condition that affects several aspects of the patient's life. Physicians and society focus within this condition has been improving the physiology of the spinal cord *per se* and the indirect repercussions in the body. However, less is been done in terms of psychosocial issues that the patients are suffering. A better assessment to this terrible illness is to approach the patients in a more comprehensive way that includes physical, psychological and socioecomic methods. Mental health is vital for adaptation to dysfunctions and overcome challenging conditions in daily life after SCI.

An understanding of mechanisms following spinal cord injury to prevent extension of the damage and development of below-level pain aimed at a therapeutic approach. To improve outcomes and reduce morbidity in patients with SCI it is essential to work with an objective of supporting the standardization of precise protocols for the immediate care based on updated reports and international classification systems, and encouraging clinicians and patients to make evidence-informed decisions. Afterwards, the subsequent attention of the inflammatory and degenerative effects after the acute stage. For the long term, to establish rehabilitation strategies integrating the most current studies to restore autonomic, sensorimotor functions, pain management and psychological effects, having a clear picture of the sequelae. Finally, the improvement of the health system for priority care in these patients.

Author details

Braniff de la Torre-Valdovinos[1], Laura Paulina Osuna-Carrasco[1] and Carlos Alberto Cuellar Ramos[2]*

1 Centro Universitario de Ciencias Exactas e Ingenierías, Universidad de Guadalajara, México

2 School of Sport Sciences, Universidad Anáhuac México, Campus Norte Huixquilucan, Estado de México, México

*Address all correspondence to: carlos.cuellarra@anahuac.mx

References

[1] Edgerton, V. R., Tillakaratne, N. J., Bigbee, A. J., de Leon, R. D., & Roy, R. R. (2004). Plasticity of the spinal neural circuitry after injury. Annu Rev Neurosci, *27*, 145-167. doi:10.1146/annurev.neuro.27.070203.144308

[2] Wessels, M., Lucas, C., Eriks, I., & de Groot, S. (2010). Body weight-supported gait training for restoration of walking in people with an incomplete spinal cord injury: a systematic review. J Rehabil Med, *42*(6), 513-519. doi:10.2340/16501977-0525

[3] Grillner, S. (2003). The motor infrastructure: from ion channels to neuronal networks. Nat Rev Neurosci, *4*(7), 573-586. doi:10.1038/nrn1137

[4] Arshavsky, Y. I., Orlovsky, G. N., & Perret, C. (1988). Activity of rubrospinal neurons during locomotion and scratching in the cat. Behav Brain Res, *28*(1-2), 193-199. doi:10.1016/0166-4328(88)90096-4

[5] Tork, I. (1990). Anatomy of the serotonergic system. Ann N Y Acad Sci, *600*, 9-34; discussion 34-35. doi:10.1111/j.1749-6632.1990.tb16870.x

[6] Drew, T., Cabana, T., & Rossignol, S. (1996). Responses of medullary reticulospinal neurones to stimulation of cutaneous limb nerves during locomotion in intact cats. Exp Brain Res, *111*(2), 153-168. doi:10.1007/BF00227294

[7] Shik, M. L., & Orlovsky, G. N. (1976). Neurophysiology of locomotor automatism. Physiol Rev, *56*(3), 465-501. doi:10.1152/physrev.1976.56.3.465

[8] Shefchyk, S. J., Jell, R. M., & Jordan, L. M. (1984). Reversible cooling of the brainstem reveals areas required for mesencephalic locomotor region evoked treadmill locomotion. Exp Brain Res, *56*(2), 257-262. doi:10.1007/BF00236281

[9] Alam, M., Schwabe, K., & Krauss, J. K. (2011). The pedunculopontine nucleus area: critical evaluation of interspecies differences relevant for its use as a target for deep brain stimulation. Brain, *134*(Pt 1), 11-23. doi:10.1093/brain/awq322

[10] Presacco, A., Forrester, L. W., & Contreras-Vidal, J. L. (2012). Decoding intra-limb and inter-limb kinematics during treadmill walking from scalp electroencephalographic (EEG) signals. IEEE Trans Neural Syst Rehabil Eng, *20*(2), 212-219. doi:10.1109/TNSRE.2012.2188304

[11] van den Brand, R., Heutschi, J., Barraud, Q., DiGiovanna, J., Bartholdi, K., Huerlimann, M., . . . Courtine, G. (2012). Restoring voluntary control of locomotion after paralyzing spinal cord injury. Science, *336*(6085), 1182-1185. doi:10.1126/science.1217416

[12] Kakulas, A. (1988). The applied neurobiology of human spinal cord injury: a review. Paraplegia, *26*(6), 371-379. doi:10.1038/sc.1988.57

[13] Dimitrijevic, M. R., Gerasimenko, Y., & Pinter, M. M. (1998). Evidence for a spinal central pattern generator in humans. Ann N Y Acad Sci, *860*, 360-376. doi:10.1111/j.1749-6632.1998.tb09062.x

[14] Shah, P. K., & Lavrov, I. (2017). Spinal Epidural Stimulation Strategies: Clinical Implications of Locomotor Studies in Spinal Rats. Neuroscientist, *23*(6), 664-680. doi:10.1177/1073858417699554

[15] Pearcey, G. E. P. (2020). Exploiting evolutionarily conserved pathways to promote plasticity of human spinal circuits. Appl Physiol Nutr Metab, *45*(6), 686. doi:10.1139/apnm-2020-0093

[16] Donelan, J. M., & Pearson, K. G. (2004). Contribution of sensory

feedback to ongoing ankle extensor activity during the stance phase of walking. Can J Physiol Pharmacol, *82*(8-9), 589-598. doi:10.1139/y04-043

[17] Hiebert, G. W., & Pearson, K. G. (1999). Contribution of sensory feedback to the generation of extensor activity during walking in the decerebrate Cat. J Neurophysiol, *81*(2), 758-770. doi:10.1152/jn.1999.81.2.758

[18] Sinkjaer, T., Andersen, J. B., Ladouceur, M., Christensen, L. O., & Nielsen, J. B. (2000). Major role for sensory feedback in soleus EMG activity in the stance phase of walking in man. J Physiol, *523 Pt 3*, 817-827. doi:10.1111/j.1469-7793.2000.00817.x

[19] Martinez, S. A., Nguyen, N. D., Bailey, E., Doyle-Green, D., Hauser, H. A., Handrakis, J. P., . . . Harel, N. Y. (2018). Multimodal cortical and subcortical exercise compared with treadmill training for spinal cord injury. PLoS One, *13*(8), e0202130. doi:10.1371/journal.pone.0202130

[20] Darian-Smith, C., Lilak, A., & Alarcon, C. (2013). Corticospinal sprouting occurs selectively following dorsal rhizotomy in the macaque monkey. J Comp Neurol, *521*(10), 2359-2372. doi:10.1002/cne.23289

[21] Rossignol, S., Dubuc, R., & Gossard, J. P. (2006). Dynamic sensorimotor interactions in locomotion. Physiol Rev, *86*(1), 89-154. doi:10.1152/physrev.00028.2005

[22] Rossignol, S., & Frigon, A. (2011). Recovery of locomotion after spinal cord injury: some facts and mechanisms. Annu Rev Neurosci, *34*, 413-440. doi:10.1146/annurev-neuro-061010-113746

[23] Bradley, P. M., Denecke, C. K., Aljovic, A., Schmalz, A., Kerschensteiner, M., & Bareyre, F. M. (2019). Corticospinal circuit remodeling after central nervous system injury is dependent on neuronal activity. J Exp Med, *216*(11), 2503-2514. doi:10.1084/jem.20181406

[24] Field-Fote, E. C., Yang, J. F., Basso, D. M., & Gorassini, M. A. (2017). Supraspinal Control Predicts Locomotor Function and Forecasts Responsiveness to Training after Spinal Cord Injury. J Neurotrauma, *34*(9), 1813-1825. doi:10.1089/neu.2016.4565

[25] Fawcett, J. W., & Asher, R. A. (1999). The glial scar and central nervous system repair. Brain Res Bull, *49*(6), 377-391. doi:10.1016/s0361-9230(99)00072-6

[26] Smith-Thomas, L. C., Stevens, J., Fok-Seang, J., Faissner, A., Rogers, J. H., & Fawcett, J. W. (1995). Increased axon regeneration in astrocytes grown in the presence of proteoglycan synthesis inhibitors. J Cell Sci, *108 (Pt 3)*, 1307-1315.

[27] Houle, J. D. (1991). Demonstration of the potential for chronically injured neurons to regenerate axons into intraspinal peripheral nerve grafts. Exp Neurol, *113*(1), 1-9. doi:10.1016/0014-4886(91)90139-4

[28] Kobayashi, N. R., Fan, D. P., Giehl, K. M., Bedard, A. M., Wiegand, S. J., & Tetzlaff, W. (1997). BDNF and NT-4/5 prevent atrophy of rat rubrospinal neurons after cervical axotomy, stimulate GAP-43 and Talpha1-tubulin mRNA expression, and promote axonal regeneration. J Neurosci, *17*(24), 9583-9595.

[29] Jevans, B., James, N. D., Burnside, E., McCann, C. J., Thapar, N., Bradbury, E. J., & Burns, A. J. (2021). Combined treatment with enteric neural stem cells and chondroitinase ABC reduces spinal cord lesion pathology. Stem Cell Res Ther, *12*(1), 10. doi:10.1186/s13287-020-02031-9

[30] Muir, E., De Winter, F., Verhaagen, J., & Fawcett, J. (2019). Recent advances in the therapeutic uses of chondroitinase

ABC. Exp Neurol, *321*, 113032. doi:10.1016/j.expneurol.2019.113032

[31] Raspa, A., Carminati, L., Pugliese, R., Fontana, F., & Gelain, F. (2020). Self-assembling peptide hydrogels for the stabilization and sustained release of active Chondroitinase ABC in vitro and in spinal cord injuries. J Control Release. doi:10.1016/j.jconrel.2020.11.027

[32] Shinozaki, M., Iwanami, A., Fujiyoshi, K., Tashiro, S., Kitamura, K., Shibata, S., . . . Okano, H. (2016). Combined treatment with chondroitinase ABC and treadmill rehabilitation for chronic severe spinal cord injury in adult rats. Neurosci Res, *113*, 37-47. doi:10.1016/j.neures.2016.07.005

[33] Schalow, G., & Zach, G. A. (2000). Reorganization of the human central nervous system. Gen Physiol Biophys, *19 Suppl 1*, 11-240.

[34] Schalow, G., Jaigma, P., & Belle, V. K. (2009). Near-total functional recovery achieved in partial cervical spinal cord injury (50% injury) after 3 years of coordination dynamics therapy. Electromyogr Clin Neurophysiol, *49*(2-3), 67-91.

[35] Huie, J. R., Morioka, K., Haefeli, J., & Ferguson, A. R. (2017). What Is Being Trained? How Divergent Forms of Plasticity Compete To Shape Locomotor Recovery after Spinal Cord Injury. J Neurotrauma, *34*(10), 1831-1840. doi:10.1089/neu.2016.4562

[36] Davare, M., Zenon, A., Desmurget, M., & Olivier, E. (2015). Dissociable contribution of the parietal and frontal cortex to coding movement direction and amplitude. Front Hum Neurosci, *9*, 241. doi:10.3389/fnhum.2015.00241

[37] Reichenbach, A., Thielscher, A., Peer, A., Bulthoff, H. H., & Bresciani, J. P. (2014). A key region in the human parietal cortex for processing proprioceptive hand feedback during reaching movements. Neuroimage, *84*, 615-625. doi:10.1016/j.neuroimage.2013.09.024

[38] Suzuki, T., Suzuki, M., Kanemura, N., & Hamaguchi, T. (2019). Differential Effect of Visual and Proprioceptive Stimulation on Corticospinal Output for Reciprocal Muscles. Front Integr Neurosci, *13*, 63. doi:10.3389/fnint.2019.00063

[39] Ballermann, M., & Fouad, K. (2006). Spontaneous locomotor recovery in spinal cord injured rats is accompanied by anatomical plasticity of reticulospinal fibers. Eur J Neurosci, *23*(8), 1988-1996. doi:10.1111/j.1460-9568.2006.04726.x

[40] Bareyre, F. M., Kerschensteiner, M., Raineteau, O., Mettenleiter, T. C., Weinmann, O., & Schwab, M. E. (2004). The injured spinal cord spontaneously forms a new intraspinal circuit in adult rats. Nat Neurosci, *7*(3), 269-277. doi:10.1038/nn1195

[41] Dobkin, B., Barbeau, H., Deforge, D., Ditunno, J., Elashoff, R., Apple, D., . . . Spinal Cord Injury Locomotor Trial, G. (2007). The evolution of walking-related outcomes over the first 12 weeks of rehabilitation for incomplete traumatic spinal cord injury: the multicenter randomized Spinal Cord Injury Locomotor Trial. *Neurorehabil Neural Repair, 21*(1), 25-35. doi:10.1177/1545968306295556

[42] Fawcett, J. W., Curt, A., Steeves, J. D., Coleman, W. P., Tuszynski, M. H., Lammertse, D., . . . Short, D. (2007). Guidelines for the conduct of clinical trials for spinal cord injury as developed by the ICCP panel: spontaneous recovery after spinal cord injury and statistical power needed for therapeutic clinical trials. Spinal Cord, *45*(3), 190-205. doi:10.1038/sj.sc.3102007

[43] Weidner, N., Ner, A., Salimi, N., & Tuszynski, M. H. (2001). Spontaneous

corticospinal axonal plasticity and functional recovery after adult central nervous system injury. Proc Natl Acad Sci U S A, *98*(6), 3513-3518. doi:10.1073/pnas.051626798

[44] Courtine, G., Song, B., Roy, R. R., Zhong, H., Herrmann, J. E., Ao, Y., . . . Sofroniew, M. V. (2008). Recovery of supraspinal control of stepping via indirect propriospinal relay connections after spinal cord injury. Nat Med, *14*(1), 69-74. doi:10.1038/nm1682

[45] Wenger, N., Moraud, E. M., Gandar, J., Musienko, P., Capogrosso, M., Baud, L., . . . Courtine, G. (2016). Spatiotemporal neuromodulation therapies engaging muscle synergies improve motor control after spinal cord injury. Nat Med, *22*(2), 138-145. doi:10.1038/nm.4025

[46] Edgerton, V. R., Roy, R. R., Hodgson, J. A., Prober, R. J., de Guzman, C. P., & de Leon, R. (1991). A physiological basis for the development of rehabilitative strategies for spinally injured patients. J Am Paraplegia Soc, *14*(4), 150-157. doi: 10.1080/01952307.1991.11735848

[47] Jakeman, L. B., Hoschouer, E. L., & Basso, D. M. (2011). Injured mice at the gym: review, results and considerations for combining chondroitinase and locomotor exercise to enhance recovery after spinal cord injury. Brain Res Bull, *84*(4-5), 317-326. doi:10.1016/j.brainresbull.2010.06.002

[48] Osuna-Carrasco, L. P., Lopez-Ruiz, J. R., Mendizabal-Ruiz, E. G., De la Torre-Valdovinos, B., Banuelos-Pineda, J., Jimenez-Estrada, I., & Duenas-Jimenez, S. H. (2016). Quantitative analysis of hindlimbs locomotion kinematics in spinalized rats treated with Tamoxifen plus treadmill exercise. Neuroscience, *333*, 151-161. doi:10.1016/j.neuroscience.2016.07.023

[49] Martinez, M., Delivet-Mongrain, H., Leblond, H., & Rossignol, S. (2012). Effect of locomotor training in completely spinalized cats previously submitted to a spinal hemisection. J Neurosci, *32*(32), 10961-10970. doi:10.1523/JNEUROSCI.1578-12.2012

[50] Shah, P. K., Garcia-Alias, G., Choe, J., Gad, P., Gerasimenko, Y., Tillakaratne, N., . . . Edgerton, V. R. (2013). Use of quadrupedal step training to re-engage spinal interneuronal networks and improve locomotor function after spinal cord injury. Brain, *136*(Pt 11), 3362-3377. doi:10.1093/brain/awt265

[51] de la Torre Valdovinos, B., Duenas Jimenez, J. M., Estrada, I. J., Banuelos Pineda, J., Franco Rodriguez, N. E., Lopez Ruiz, J. R., . . . Duenas Jimenez, S. H. (2016). Tamoxifen Promotes Axonal Preservation and Gait Locomotion Recovery after Spinal Cord Injury in Cats. J Vet Med, *2016*, 9561968. doi:10.1155/2016/9561968

[52] Lopez Ruiz, J. R., Osuna Carrasco, L. P., Lopez Valenzuela, C. L., Franco Rodriguez, N. E., de la Torre Valdovinos, B., Jimenez Estrada, I., . . . Duenas Jimenez, S. H. (2015). The hippocampus participates in the control of locomotion speed. Neuroscience, *311*, 207-215. doi:10.1016/j.neuroscience.2015.10.034

[53] Petruska, J. C., Ichiyama, R. M., Jindrich, D. L., Crown, E. D., Tansey, K. E., Roy, R. R., . . . Mendell, L. M. (2007). Changes in motoneuron properties and synaptic inputs related to step training after spinal cord transection in rats. J Neurosci, *27*(16), 4460-4471. doi:10.1523/JNEUROSCI.2302-06.2007

[54] Joseph, M. S., Tillakaratne, N. J., & de Leon, R. D. (2012). Treadmill training stimulates brain-derived neurotrophic factor mRNA expression in motor neurons of the lumbar spinal cord in spinally transected rats. Neuroscience, *224*, 135-144. doi:10.1016/j.neuroscience.2012.08.024

[55] Beaumont, E., Kaloustian, S., Rousseau, G., & Cormery, B.

(2008). Training improves the electrophysiological properties of lumbar neurons and locomotion after thoracic spinal cord injury in rats. Neurosci Res, *62*(3), 147-154. doi:10.1016/j.neures.2008.07.003

[56] Hennigan, A., O'Callaghan, R. M., & Kelly, A. M. (2007). Neurotrophins and their receptors: roles in plasticity, neurodegeneration and neuroprotection. *Biochem Soc Trans, 35*(Pt 2), 424-427. doi:10.1042/BST0350424

[57] Liu, H., Skinner, R. D., Arfaj, A., Yates, C., Reese, N. B., Williams, K., & Garcia-Rill, E. (2010). L-Dopa effect on frequency-dependent depression of the H-reflex in adult rats with complete spinal cord transection. Brain Res Bull, *83*(5), 262-265. doi:10.1016/j.brainresbull.2010.07.005

[58] McCullough, M. J., Gyorkos, A. M., & Spitsbergen, J. M. (2013). Short-term exercise increases GDNF protein levels in the spinal cord of young and old rats. Neuroscience, *240*, 258-268. doi:10.1016/j.neuroscience.2013.02.063

[59] Cote, M. P., Azzam, G. A., Lemay, M. A., Zhukareva, V., & Houle, J. D. (2011). Activity-dependent increase in neurotrophic factors is associated with an enhanced modulation of spinal reflexes after spinal cord injury. J Neurotrauma, *28*(2), 299-309. doi:10.1089/neu.2010.1594

[60] Chang, Y. X., Zhao, Y., Pan, S., Qi, Z. P., Kong, W. J., Pan, Y. R., . . . Yang, X. Y. (2019). Intramuscular Injection of Adenoassociated Virus Encoding Human Neurotrophic Factor 3 and Exercise Intervention Contribute to Reduce Spasms after Spinal Cord Injury. Neural Plast, *2019*, 3017678. doi:10.1155/2019/3017678

[61] Park, S., Hong, Y., Lee, Y., Won, J., Chang, K. T., & Hong, Y. (2012). Differential expression of caveolins and myosin heavy chains in response to forced exercise in rats. Lab Anim Res, *28*(1), 1-9. doi:10.5625/lar.2012.28.1.1

[62] Wernig, A., & Muller, S. (1992). Laufband locomotion with body weight support improved walking in persons with severe spinal cord injuries. Paraplegia, *30*(4), 229-238. doi:10.1038/sc.1992.61

[63] Ziegler, M. D., Hsu, D., Takeoka, A., Zhong, H., Ramon-Cueto, A., Phelps, P. E., . . . Edgerton, V. R. (2011). Further evidence of olfactory ensheathing glia facilitating axonal regeneration after a complete spinal cord transection. Exp Neurol, *229*(1), 109-119. doi:10.1016/j.expneurol.2011.01.007

[64] Aravind, N., Harvey, L. A., & Glinsky, J. V. (2019). Physiotherapy interventions for increasing muscle strength in people with spinal cord injuries: a systematic review. Spinal Cord, *57*(6), 449-460. doi:10.1038/s41393-019-0242-z

[65] Christiansen, L., & Perez, M. A. (2018). Targeted-Plasticity in the Corticospinal Tract After Human Spinal Cord Injury. Neurotherapeutics, *15*(3), 618-627. doi:10.1007/s13311-018-0639-y

[66] de Araujo, A. V. L., Barbosa, V. R. N., Galdino, G. S., Fregni, F., Massetti, T., Fontes, S. L., . . . Magalhaes, F. H. (2017). Effects of high-frequency transcranial magnetic stimulation on functional performance in individuals with incomplete spinal cord injury: study protocol for a randomized controlled trial. *Trials, 18*(1), 522. doi:10.1186/s13063-017-2280-1

[67] Jo, H. J., & Perez, M. A. (2020). Corticospinal-motor neuronal plasticity promotes exercise-mediated recovery in humans with spinal cord injury. Brain, *143*(5), 1368-1382. doi:10.1093/brain/awaa052

[68] Mayr, W., Krenn, M., & Dimitrijevic, M. R. (2016). Motor Control of Human Spinal Cord Disconnected from the Brain and Under External Movement. Adv Exp Med Biol, *957*, 159-171. doi:10.1007/978-3-319-47313-0_9

[69] Raithatha, R., Carrico, C., Powell, E. S., Westgate, P. M., Chelette Ii, K. C., Lee, K., . . . Sawaki, L. (2016). Non-invasive brain stimulation and robot-assisted gait training after incomplete spinal cord injury: A randomized pilot study. NeuroRehabilitation, *38*(1), 15-25. doi:10.3233/NRE-151291

[70] Yozbatiran, N., Keser, Z., Davis, M., Stampas, A., O'Malley, M. K., Cooper-Hay, C., . . . Francisco, G. E. (2016). Transcranial direct current stimulation (tDCS) of the primary motor cortex and robot-assisted arm training in chronic incomplete cervical spinal cord injury: A proof of concept sham-randomized clinical study. NeuroRehabilitation, *39*(3), 401-411. doi:10.3233/NRE-161371

[71] Tse, C. M., Chisholm, A. E., Lam, T., Eng, J. J., & Team, S. R. (2018). A systematic review of the effectiveness of task-specific rehabilitation interventions for improving independent sitting and standing function in spinal cord injury. J Spinal Cord Med, *41*(3), 254-266. doi:10.1080/10790268.2017.1350340

[72] Nardone, R., Orioli, A., Golaszewski, S., Brigo, F., Sebastianelli, L., Holler, Y., . . . Trinka, E. (2017). Passive cycling in neurorehabilitation after spinal cord injury: A review. J Spinal Cord Med, *40*(1), 8-16. doi:10.1080/10790268.2016.1248524

[73] Chopek, J. W., MacDonell, C. W., Gardiner, K., & Gardiner, P. F. (2014). Daily passive cycling attenuates the hyperexcitability and restores the responsiveness of the extensor monosynaptic reflex to quipazine in the chronic spinally transected rat. J Neurotrauma, *31*(12), 1083-1087. doi:10.1089/neu.2013.3207

[74] Garrison, M. K., Yates, C. C., Reese, N. B., Skinner, R. D., & Garcia-Rill, E. (2011). Wind-up of stretch reflexes as a measure of spasticity in chronic spinalized rats: The effects of passive exercise and modafinil. Exp Neurol, *227*(1), 104-109. doi:10.1016/j.expneurol.2010.09.019

[75] West, C. R., Crawford, M. A., Laher, I., Ramer, M. S., & Krassioukov, A. V. (2016). Passive Hind-Limb Cycling Reduces the Severity of Autonomic Dysreflexia After Experimental Spinal Cord Injury. Neurorehabil Neural Repair, *30*(4), 317-327. doi:10.1177/1545968315593807

[76] West, C. R., Crawford, M. A., Poormasjedi-Meibod, M. S., Currie, K. D., Fallavollita, A., Yuen, V., . . . Krassioukov, A. V. (2014). Passive hind-limb cycling improves cardiac function and reduces cardiovascular disease risk in experimental spinal cord injury. J Physiol, *592*(8), 1771-1783. doi:10.1113/jphysiol.2013.268367

[77] Keeler, B. E., Liu, G., Siegfried, R. N., Zhukareva, V., Murray, M., & Houle, J. D. (2012). Acute and prolonged hindlimb exercise elicits different gene expression in motoneurons than sensory neurons after spinal cord injury. Brain Res, *1438*, 8-21. doi:10.1016/j.brainres.2011.12.015

[78] Johnston, T. E., Smith, B. T., Mulcahey, M. J., Betz, R. R., & Lauer, R. T. (2009). A randomized controlled trial on the effects of cycling with and without electrical stimulation on cardiorespiratory and vascular health in children with spinal cord injury. Arch Phys Med Rehabil, *90*(8), 1379-1388. doi:10.1016/j.apmr.2009.02.018

[79] Kakebeeke, T. H., Lechner, H. E., & Knapp, P. A. (2005). The effect of

passive cycling movements on spasticity after spinal cord injury: preliminary results. Spinal Cord, *43*(8), 483-488. doi:10.1038/sj.sc.3101747

[80] Martin Ginis, K. A., van der Scheer, J. W., Latimer-Cheung, A. E., Barrow, A., Bourne, C., Carruthers, P., . . . Goosey-Tolfrey, V. L. (2018). Evidence-based scientific exercise guidelines for adults with spinal cord injury: an update and a new guideline. Spinal Cord, *56*(4), 308-321. doi:10.1038/s41393-017-0017-3

[81] Escalona, M. J., Brosseau, R., Vermette, M., Comtois, A. S., Duclos, C., Aubertin-Leheudre, M., & Gagnon, D. H. (2018). Cardiorespiratory demand and rate of perceived exertion during overground walking with a robotic exoskeleton in long-term manual wheelchair users with chronic spinal cord injury: A cross-sectional study. Ann Phys Rehabil Med, *61*(4), 215-223. doi:10.1016/j.rehab.2017.12.008

[82] Wu, C. H., Mao, H. F., Hu, J. S., Wang, T. Y., Tsai, Y. J., & Hsu, W. L. (2018). The effects of gait training using powered lower limb exoskeleton robot on individuals with complete spinal cord injury. J Neuroeng Rehabil, *15*(1), 14. doi:10.1186/s12984-018-0355-1

[83] Gagnon, D. H., Vermette, M., Duclos, C., Aubertin-Leheudre, M., Ahmed, S., & Kairy, D. (2019). Satisfaction and perceptions of long-term manual wheelchair users with a spinal cord injury upon completion of a locomotor training program with an overground robotic exoskeleton. Disabil Rehabil Assist Technol, *14*(2), 138-145. doi:10.1080/17483107.2017.1413145

[84] Gagnon, D. H., Escalona, M. J., Vermette, M., Carvalho, L. P., Karelis, A. D., Duclos, C., & Aubertin-Leheudre, M. (2018). Locomotor training using an overground robotic exoskeleton in long-term manual wheelchair users with a chronic spinal cord injury living in the community: Lessons learned from a feasibility study in terms of recruitment, attendance, learnability, performance and safety. *J Neuroeng Rehabil, 15*(1), 12. doi:10.1186/s12984-018-0354-2

[85] Heinemann, A. W., Jayaraman, A., Mummidisetty, C. K., Spraggins, J., Pinto, D., Charlifue, S., . . . Field-Fote, E. C. (2018). Experience of Robotic Exoskeleton Use at Four Spinal Cord Injury Model Systems Centers. J Neurol Phys Ther, *42*(4), 256-267. doi:10.1097/NPT.0000000000000235

[86] Guanziroli, E., Cazzaniga, M., Colombo, L., Basilico, S., Legnani, G., & Molteni, F. (2019). Assistive powered exoskeleton for complete spinal cord injury: correlations between walking ability and exoskeleton control. Eur J Phys Rehabil Med, *55*(2), 209-216. doi:10.23736/S1973-9087.18.05308-X

[87] Bach Baunsgaard, C., Vig Nissen, U., Katrin Brust, A., Frotzler, A., Ribeill, C., Kalke, Y. B., . . . Biering-Sorensen, F. (2018). Gait training after spinal cord injury: safety, feasibility and gait function following 8 weeks of training with the exoskeletons from Ekso Bionics. Spinal Cord, *56*(2), 106-116. doi:10.1038/s41393-017-0013-7

[88] Khan, A. S., Livingstone, D. C., Hurd, C. L., Duchcherer, J., Misiaszek, J. E., Gorassini, M. A., . . . Yang, J. F. (2019). Retraining walking over ground in a powered exoskeleton after spinal cord injury: a prospective cohort study to examine functional gains and neuroplasticity. J Neuroeng Rehabil, *16*(1), 145. doi:10.1186/s12984-019-0585-x

[89] Muijzer-Witteveen, H., Sibum, N., van Dijsseldonk, R., Keijsers, N., & van Asseldonk, E. (2018). Questionnaire results of user experiences with wearable exoskeletons and their preferences for sensory feedback. J Neuroeng Rehabil, *15*(1), 112. doi:10.1186/s12984-018-0445-0

[90] Qaiser, T., Eginyan, G., Chan, F., & Lam, T. (2019). The sensorimotor effects of a lower limb proprioception training intervention in individuals with a spinal cord injury. J Neurophysiol, *122*(6), 2364-2371. doi:10.1152/jn.00842.2018

[91] Tamburella, F., Tagliamonte, N. L., Pisotta, I., Masciullo, M., Arquilla, M., van Asseldonk, E. H. F., . . . Molinari, M. (2020). Neuromuscular Controller Embedded in a Powered Ankle Exoskeleton: Effects on Gait, Clinical Features and Subjective Perspective of Incomplete Spinal Cord Injured Subjects. IEEE Trans Neural Syst Rehabil Eng, *28*(5), 1157-1167. doi:10.1109/TNSRE.2020.2984790

[92] Chang, S. H., Afzal, T., Group, T. S. C. E., Berliner, J., & Francisco, G. E. (2018). Exoskeleton-assisted gait training to improve gait in individuals with spinal cord injury: a pilot randomized study. Pilot Feasibility Stud, *4*, 62. doi:10.1186/s40814-018-0247-y

[93] Shealy, C. N., Mortimer, J. T., & Reswick, J. B. (1967). Electrical inhibition of pain by stimulation of the dorsal columns: preliminary clinical report. Anesth Analg, *46*(4), 489-491.

[94] Angeli, C. A., Edgerton, V. R., Gerasimenko, Y. P., & Harkema, S. J. (2014). Altering spinal cord excitability enables voluntary movements after chronic complete paralysis in humans. Brain, *137*(Pt 5), 1394-1409. doi:10.1093/brain/awu038

[95] Grahn, P. J., Lavrov, I. A., Sayenko, D. G., Van Straaten, M. G., Gill, M. L., Strommen, J. A., . . . Lee, K. H. (2017). Enabling Task-Specific Volitional Motor Functions via Spinal Cord Neuromodulation in a Human With Paraplegia. Mayo Clin Proc, *92*(4), 544-554. doi:10.1016/j.mayocp.2017.02.014

[96] Harkema, S., Gerasimenko, Y., Hodes, J., Burdick, J., Angeli, C., Chen, Y., . . . Edgerton, V. R. (2011). Effect of epidural stimulation of the lumbosacral spinal cord on voluntary movement, standing, and assisted stepping after motor complete paraplegia: a case study. Lancet, *377*(9781), 1938-1947. doi:10.1016/S0140-6736(11)60547-3

[97] Rejc, E., Angeli, C., & Harkema, S. (2015). Effects of Lumbosacral Spinal Cord Epidural Stimulation for Standing after Chronic Complete Paralysis in Humans. PLoS One, *10*(7), e0133998. doi:10.1371/journal.pone.0133998

[98] Calvert, J. S., Grahn, P. J., Strommen, J. A., Lavrov, I. A., Beck, L. A., Gill, M. L., . . . Lee, K. H. (2019). Electrophysiological Guidance of Epidural Electrode Array Implantation over the Human Lumbosacral Spinal Cord to Enable Motor Function after Chronic Paralysis. J Neurotrauma, *36*(9), 1451-1460. doi:10.1089/neu.2018.5921

[99] Inanici, F., Samejima, S., Gad, P., Edgerton, V. R., Hofstetter, C. P., & Moritz, C. T. (2018). Transcutaneous Electrical Spinal Stimulation Promotes Long-Term Recovery of Upper Extremity Function in Chronic Tetraplegia. IEEE Trans Neural Syst Rehabil Eng, *26*(6), 1272-1278. doi:10.1109/TNSRE.2018.2834339

[100] Lu, D. C., Edgerton, V. R., Modaber, M., AuYong, N., Morikawa, E., Zdunowski, S., . . . Gerasimenko, Y. (2016). Engaging Cervical Spinal Cord Networks to Reenable Volitional Control of Hand Function in Tetraplegic Patients. Neurorehabil Neural Repair, *30*(10), 951-962. doi:10.1177/1545968316644344

[101] Darrow, D., Balser, D., Netoff, T. I., Krassioukov, A., Phillips, A., Parr, A., & Samadani, U. (2019). Epidural Spinal Cord Stimulation Facilitates Immediate Restoration of Dormant Motor and Autonomic Supraspinal Pathways after Chronic Neurologically Complete Spinal

Cord Injury. J Neurotrauma, *36*(15), 2325-2336. doi:10.1089/neu.2018.6006

[102] Militskova, A., Mukhametova, E., Fatykhova, E., Sharifullin, S., Cuellar, C. A., Calvert, J. S., . . . Lavrov, I. (2020). Supraspinal and Afferent Signaling Facilitate Spinal Sensorimotor Network Excitability After Discomplete Spinal Cord Injury: A Case Report. Front Neurosci, *14*, 552. doi:10.3389/fnins.2020.00552

[103] Aslan, S. C., Legg Ditterline, B. E., Park, M. C., Angeli, C. A., Rejc, E., Chen, Y., . . . Harkema, S. J. (2018). Epidural Spinal Cord Stimulation of Lumbosacral Networks Modulates Arterial Blood Pressure in Individuals With Spinal Cord Injury-Induced Cardiovascular Deficits. Front Physiol, *9*, 565. doi:10.3389/fphys.2018.00565

[104] Harkema, S. J., Legg Ditterline, B., Wang, S., Aslan, S., Angeli, C. A., Ovechkin, A., & Hirsch, G. A. (2018). Epidural Spinal Cord Stimulation Training and Sustained Recovery of Cardiovascular Function in Individuals With Chronic Cervical Spinal Cord Injury. JAMA Neurol, *75*(12), 1569-1571. doi:10.1001/jamaneurol.2018.2617

[105] Herrity, A. N., Williams, C. S., Angeli, C. A., Harkema, S. J., & Hubscher, C. H. (2018). Lumbosacral spinal cord epidural stimulation improves voiding function after human spinal cord injury. Sci Rep, *8*(1), 8688. doi:10.1038/s41598-018-26602-2

[106] Capogrosso, M., Wenger, N., Raspopovic, S., Musienko, P., Beauparlant, J., Bassi Luciani, L., . . . Micera, S. (2013). A computational model for epidural electrical stimulation of spinal sensorimotor circuits. J Neurosci, *33*(49), 19326-19340. doi:10.1523/JNEUROSCI.1688-13.2013

[107] Gad, P., Lavrov, I., Shah, P., Zhong, H., Roy, R. R., Edgerton, V. R., & Gerasimenko, Y. (2013). Neuromodulation of motor-evoked potentials during stepping in spinal rats. J Neurophysiol, *110*(6), 1311-1322. doi:10.1152/jn.00169.2013

[108] Gerasimenko, Y. P., Lavrov, I. A., Courtine, G., Ichiyama, R. M., Dy, C. J., Zhong, H., . . . Edgerton, V. R. (2006). Spinal cord reflexes induced by epidural spinal cord stimulation in normal awake rats. J Neurosci Methods, *157*(2), 253-263. doi:10.1016/j.jneumeth.2006.05.004

[109] Lavrov, I., Dy, C. J., Fong, A. J., Gerasimenko, Y., Courtine, G., Zhong, H., . . . Edgerton, V. R. (2008). Epidural stimulation induced modulation of spinal locomotor networks in adult spinal rats. J Neurosci, *28*(23), 6022-6029. doi:10.1523/JNEUROSCI.0080-08.2008

[110] Courtine, G., Harkema, S. J., Dy, C. J., Gerasimenko, Y. P., & Dyhre-Poulsen, P. (2007). Modulation of multisegmental monosynaptic responses in a variety of leg muscles during walking and running in humans. J Physiol, *582*(Pt 3), 1125-1139. doi:10.1113/jphysiol.2007.128447

[111] Hofstoetter, U. S., Freundl, B., Binder, H., & Minassian, K. (2018). Common neural structures activated by epidural and transcutaneous lumbar spinal cord stimulation: Elicitation of posterior root-muscle reflexes. PLoS One, *13*(1), e0192013. doi:10.1371/journal.pone.0192013

[112] Minassian, K., Jilge, B., Rattay, F., Pinter, M. M., Binder, H., Gerstenbrand, F., & Dimitrijevic, M. R. (2004). Stepping-like movements in humans with complete spinal cord injury induced by epidural stimulation of the lumbar cord: electromyographic study of compound muscle action potentials. Spinal Cord, *42*(7), 401-416. doi:10.1038/sj.sc.3101615

[113] Sayenko, D. G., Angeli, C., Harkema, S. J., Edgerton, V. R., & Gerasimenko, Y. P. (2014). Neuromodulation of evoked

muscle potentials induced by epidural spinal-cord stimulation in paralyzed individuals. J Neurophysiol, *111*(5), 1088-1099. doi:10.1152/jn.00489.2013

[114] Davey, N. J., Smith, H. C., Wells, E., Maskill, D. W., Savic, G., Ellaway, P. H., & Frankel, H. L. (1998). Responses of thenar muscles to transcranial magnetic stimulation of the motor cortex in patients with incomplete spinal cord injury. J Neurol Neurosurg Psychiatry, *65*(1), 80-87. doi:10.1136/jnnp.65.1.80

[115] Roy, F. D., Zewdie, E. T., & Gorassini, M. A. (2011). Short-interval intracortical inhibition with incomplete spinal cord injury. Clin Neurophysiol, *122*(7), 1387-1395. doi:10.1016/j.clinph.2010.11.020

[116] Smith, H. C., Savic, G., Frankel, H. L., Ellaway, P. H., Maskill, D. W., Jamous, M. A., & Davey, N. J. (2000). Corticospinal function studied over time following incomplete spinal cord injury. Spinal Cord, *38*(5), 292-300. doi:10.1038/sj.sc.3100994

[117] Cortes, M., Thickbroom, G. W., Elder, J., Rykman, A., Valls-Sole, J., Pascual-Leone, A., & Edwards, D. J. (2017). The corticomotor projection to liminally-contractable forearm muscles in chronic spinal cord injury: a transcranial magnetic stimulation study. Spinal Cord, *55*(4), 362-366. doi:10.1038/sc.2016.161

[118] Freund, P., Rothwell, J., Craggs, M., Thompson, A. J., & Bestmann, S. (2011). Corticomotor representation to a human forearm muscle changes following cervical spinal cord injury. Eur J Neurosci, *34*(11), 1839-1846. doi:10.1111/j.1460-9568.2011.07895.x

[119] Topka, H., Cohen, L. G., Cole, R. A., & Hallett, M. (1991). Reorganization of corticospinal pathways following spinal cord injury. Neurology, *41*(8), 1276-1283. doi:10.1212/wnl.41.8.1276

[120] Brown, A. R., & Martinez, M. (2019). From cortex to cord: motor circuit plasticity after spinal cord injury. Neural Regen Res, *14*(12), 2054-2062. doi:10.4103/1673-5374.262572

[121] Donges, S. C., D'Amico, J. M., Butler, J. E., & Taylor, J. L. (2018). Involvement of N-methyl-d-aspartate receptors in plasticity induced by paired corticospinal-motoneuronal stimulation in humans. J Neurophysiol, *119*(2), 652-661. doi:10.1152/jn.00457.2017

[122] Squair, J. W., Bjerkefors, A., Inglis, J. T., Lam, T., & Carpenter, M. G. (2016). Cortical and vestibular stimulation reveal preserved descending motor pathways in individuals with motor-complete spinal cord injury. J Rehabil Med, *48*(7), 589-596. doi:10.2340/16501977-2101

[123] Taylor, R., Galvez, V., & Loo, C. (2018). Transcranial magnetic stimulation (TMS) safety: a practical guide for psychiatrists. Australas Psychiatry, *26*(2), 189-192. doi:10.1177/1039856217748249

[124] Gerasimenko, Y., Gorodnichev, R., Moshonkina, T., Sayenko, D., Gad, P., & Reggie Edgerton, V. (2015). Transcutaneous electrical spinal-cord stimulation in humans. Ann Phys Rehabil Med, *58*(4), 225-231. doi:10.1016/j.rehab.2015.05.003

[125] Danner, S. M., Hofstoetter, U. S., Ladenbauer, J., Rattay, F., & Minassian, K. (2011). Can the human lumbar posterior columns be stimulated by transcutaneous spinal cord stimulation? A modeling study. Artif Organs, *35*(3), 257-262. doi:10.1111/j.1525-1594.2011.01213.x

[126] Dy, C. J., Gerasimenko, Y. P., Edgerton, V. R., Dyhre-Poulsen, P., Courtine, G., & Harkema, S. J. (2010). Phase-dependent modulation of percutaneously elicited multisegmental muscle responses after spinal cord injury. J Neurophysiol, *103*(5), 2808-2820. doi:10.1152/jn.00316.2009

[127] Minassian, K., Persy, I., Rattay, F., Dimitrijevic, M. R., Hofer, C., & Kern, H. (2007). Posterior root-muscle reflexes elicited by transcutaneous stimulation of the human lumbosacral cord. Muscle Nerve, *35*(3), 327-336. doi:10.1002/mus.20700

[128] Sayenko, D. G., Atkinson, D. A., Floyd, T. C., Gorodnichev, R. M., Moshonkina, T. R., Harkema, S. J., . . . Gerasimenko, Y. P. (2015). Effects of paired transcutaneous electrical stimulation delivered at single and dual sites over lumbosacral spinal cord. Neurosci Lett, *609*, 229-234. doi:10.1016/j.neulet.2015.10.005

[129] Trompetto, C., Marinelli, L., Mori, L., Pelosin, E., Curra, A., Molfetta, L., & Abbruzzese, G. (2014). Pathophysiology of spasticity: implications for neurorehabilitation. Biomed Res Int, *2014*, 354906. doi:10.1155/2014/354906

[130] Hofstoetter, U. S., McKay, W. B., Tansey, K. E., Mayr, W., Kern, H., & Minassian, K. (2014). Modification of spasticity by transcutaneous spinal cord stimulation in individuals with incomplete spinal cord injury. J Spinal Cord Med, *37*(2), 202-211. doi:10.1179/2045772313Y.0000000149

[131] Gybels, J., & van Roost, D. (1987). Spinal cord stimulation for spasticity. Adv Tech Stand Neurosurg, *15*, 63-96. doi:10.1007/978-3-7091-6984-1_3

[132] Hofstoetter, U. S., Krenn, M., Danner, S. M., Hofer, C., Kern, H., McKay, W. B., . . . Minassian, K. (2015). Augmentation of Voluntary Locomotor Activity by Transcutaneous Spinal Cord Stimulation in Motor-Incomplete Spinal Cord-Injured Individuals. Artif Organs, *39*(10), E176–E186. doi:10.1111/aor.12615

[133] Hofstoetter, U. S., Freundl, B., Binder, H., & Minassian, K. (2019). Recovery cycles of posterior root-muscle reflexes evoked by transcutaneous spinal cord stimulation and of the H reflex in individuals with intact and injured spinal cord. PLoS One, *14*(12), e0227057. doi:10.1371/journal.pone.0227057

[134] Murray, L. M., & Knikou, M. (2017). Remodeling Brain Activity by Repetitive Cervicothoracic Transspinal Stimulation after Human Spinal Cord Injury. Front Neurol, *8*, 50. doi:10.3389/fneur.2017.00050

[135] Powell, E. S., Carrico, C., Salyers, E., Westgate, P. M., & Sawaki, L. (2018). The effect of transcutaneous spinal direct current stimulation on corticospinal excitability in chronic incomplete spinal cord injury. NeuroRehabilitation, *43*(2), 125-134. doi:10.3233/NRE-172369

[136] Hubli, M., Dietz, V., Schrafl-Altermatt, M., & Bolliger, M. (2013). Modulation of spinal neuronal excitability by spinal direct currents and locomotion after spinal cord injury. Clin Neurophysiol, *124*(6), 1187-1195. doi:10.1016/j.clinph.2012.11.021

[137] Capron, M., Stillman, M., & Bombardier, C. H. (2020). How do healthcare providers manage depression in people with spinal cord injury? Spinal Cord Ser Cases, *6*(1), 85. doi:10.1038/s41394-020-00333-x

[138] Cobos, P., Sanchez, M., Perez, N., & Vila, J. (2004). Brief report Effects of spinal cord injuries on the subjective component of emotions. Cogn Emot, *18*(2), 281-287. doi:10.1080/02699930244000471

[139] Torgauten, H. M., Sanaker, P. S., & Rekand, T. (2019). A man in his seventies with spinal cord injury, fever and delirium. *Tidsskr Nor Laegeforen, 139*(8). doi:10.4045/tidsskr.17.1104

[140] Poritz, J. M. P., Mignogna, J., Christie, A. J., Holmes, S. A., & Ames, H. (2018). The Patient Health Questionnaire depression screener in spinal cord injury. J Spinal Cord Med,

41(2), 238-244. doi:10.1080/10790268.2017.1294301

[141] Shavelle, R. M., Devivo, M. J., Paculdo, D. R., Vogel, L. C., & Strauss, D. J. (2007). Long-term survival after childhood spinal cord injury. J Spinal Cord Med, *30 Suppl 1*, S48–S54. doi:10.1080/10790268.2007.11753969

[142] Pakpour, A. H., Rahnama, P., Saberi, H., Saffari, M., Rahimi-Movaghar, V., Burri, A., & Hajiaghababaei, M. (2017). The relationship between anxiety, depression and religious coping strategies and erectile dysfunction in Iranian patients with spinal cord injury. Spinal Cord, *55*(7), 711. doi:10.1038/sc.2017.32

[143] Wan, F. J., Chien, W. C., Chung, C. H., Yang, Y. J., & Tzeng, N. S. (2020). Association between traumatic spinal cord injury and affective and other psychiatric disorders-A nationwide cohort study and effects of rehabilitation therapies. J Affect Disord, *265*, 381-388. doi:10.1016/j.jad.2020.01.063

[144] Ullrich, P. M., Smith, B. M., Blow, F. C., Valenstein, M., & Weaver, F. M. (2014). Depression, healthcare utilization, and comorbid psychiatric disorders after spinal cord injury. J Spinal Cord Med, *37*(1), 40-45. doi:10.1179/2045772313Y.0000000137

[145] Stewart, T. D. (1988). Psychiatric diagnosis and treatment following spinal cord injury. Psychosomatics, *29*(2), 214-220. doi:10.1016/S0033-3182(88)72400-7

[146] Weiner, M. F., & Lovitt, R. (1979). Conservation-withdrawal versus depression. Gen Hosp Psychiatry, *1*(4), 347-349. doi:10.1016/0163-8343(79)90012-4

[147] Donia, S. A., Allison, D. J., Gammage, K. L., & Ditor, D. S. (2019). The effects of acute aerobic exercise on mood and inflammation in individuals with multiple sclerosis and incomplete spinal cord injury. NeuroRehabilitation, *45*(1), 117-124. doi:10.3233/NRE-192773

[148] Harris, P., Patel, S. S., Greer, W., & Naughton, J. A. (1973). Psychological and social reactions to acute spinal paralysis. Paraplegia, *11*(2), 132-136. doi:10.1038/sc.1973.16

[149] Buckelew, S. P., Frank, R. G., Elliott, T. R., Chaney, J., & Hewett, J. (1991). Adjustment to spinal cord injury: stage theory revisited. Paraplegia, *29*(2), 125-130. doi:10.1038/sc.1991.17

[150] Khazaeipour, Z., Norouzi-Javidan, A., Kaveh, M., Khanzadeh Mehrabani, F., Kazazi, E., & Emami-Razavi, S. H. (2014). Psychosocial outcomes following spinal cord injury in Iran. J Spinal Cord Med, *37*(3), 338-345. doi:10.1179/2045772313Y.0000000174

[151] Zinman, A., Digout, N., Bain, P., Haycock, S., Hebert, D., & Hitzig, S. L. (2014). Evaluation of a community reintegration outpatient program service for community-dwelling persons with spinal cord injury. Rehabil Res Pract, *2014*, 989025. doi:10.1155/2014/989025

[152] Song, H. Y. (2005). Modeling social reintegration in persons with spinal cord injury. Disabil Rehabil, *27*(3), 131-141. doi:10.1080/09638280400007372

[153] Wyndaele, M., & Wyndaele, J. J. (2006). Incidence, prevalence and epidemiology of spinal cord injury: what learns a worldwide literature survey? Spinal Cord, *44*(9), 523-529. doi:10.1038/sj.sc.3101893

[154] Giardino, N. D., Jensen, M. P., Turner, J. A., Ehde, D. M., & Cardenas, D. D. (2003). Social environment moderates the association between catastrophizing and pain among persons with a spinal cord injury. Pain, *106*(1-2), 19-25. doi:10.1016/s0304-3959(03)00226-4

Chapter 11

Use of Exoskeletons in the Treatment and Rehabilitation of Paraplegia Patients

Susana Martiñón and Ricardo Hernández-Miramontes

Abstract

This chapter presents a review that includes five robotic exoskeletons used in the rehabilitation of paraplegic patients, highlighting the qualities of each one and offering the doctor and the rehabilitator a tool to select the exoskeleton that is most appropriate to the needs of their patient and a more satisfying and integral therapy. A systematic search was carried out in different platforms of scientific interest, the publications that met the inclusion criteria were selected. The information collected was classified and synthesized, resulting in a review that covers the five most relevant exoskeletons for the rehabilitation of paraplegic patients. Concluding with a tool that helps the therapist select the most appropriate exoskeleton for each patient.

Keywords: paraplegia, rehabilitation, exoskeleton

1. Introduction

Paraplegia is the paralysis of the lower half of the body, affecting both legs; it is usually the result of spinal cord trauma [1, 2], however, it can also be caused by diseases such as ischemic events [3, 4], multiple sclerosis and amyotrophic lateral sclerosis among other neurodegenerative diseases, including Parkinson's disease [1].

The care of the patient with paraplegia must be integral, including medical, surgical, psychological treatment and finally rehabilitation by physiotherapy [5].

At this last point, various therapies have been developed, including the use of exoskeletons. Studies have determined that the uses of exoskeletons include: increasing human performance, improving mobility of individuals with neurological pathologies, and providing assistive technology for people with disabilities [6]. In this chapter, different exoskeletons that are in use are presented for the rehabilitation of patients.

For this chapter, a review was carried out in the search engines *PubMed, Google Academics, Elsevier, Science Direct and Medline*, finding 15 scientific papers that met the inclusion criteria.

Inclusion criteria: Documents published between the years 2005 to 2020 were included. The search terms were: *exoskeleton device, rehabilitation and paraplegia*, in English; exoesqueletos, *paraplegia, lesión de médula espinal, rehabilitación*, in Spanish.

Subsequently, the electronic pages of the manufacturers were consulted.

IntechOpen

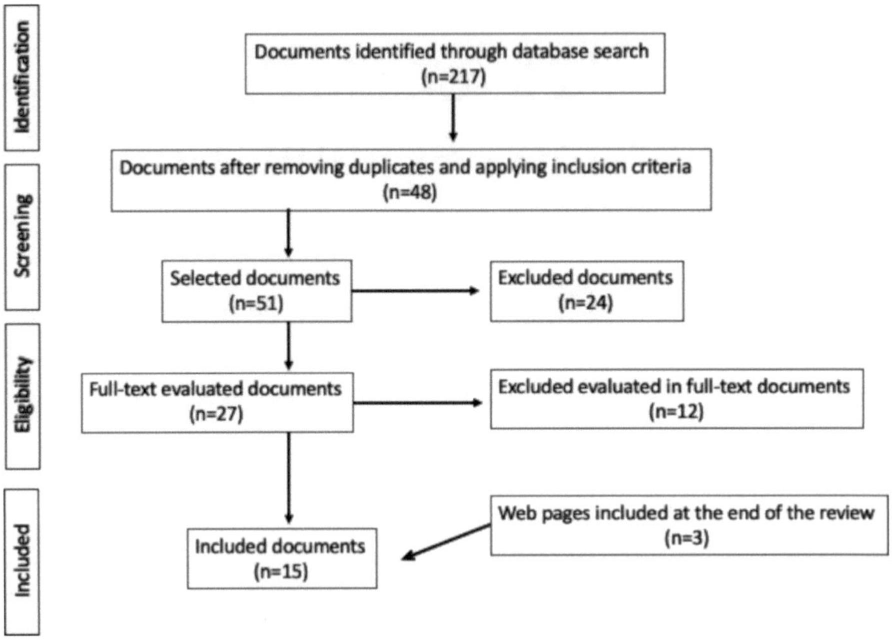

Figure 1.
Flow chart for the information selection.

Exclusion criteria: Studies published before 2005. Studies that did not include the search terms established in the inclusion criteria, incomplete or unavailable articles.

Figure 1 shows the flow diagram of the obtaining information process.

2. Exoskeletons

The operation of exoskeletons depends on a series of biometric sensors that are activated through nerve signals sent from the brain to different muscle groups so that an exact action is developed. For the creation of exoskeletons, electrical and computer patterns are used that will allow the adaptation and generation of movement in different degrees [1].

5 different models of exoskeletons were found, which are discussed below. Images of the exoskeletons are shown in **Figure 2**.

2.1 Exoskeleton Exo-H2®

It is an exoskeleton designed for the rehabilitation of adults, it is indicated for patients between 1.5 and 1.95 m in height, with a maximum body weight of 100 kg with neurological damage that prevents their motor skills [4].

It was developed by the CSIC Bioengineering Group, who granted an exclusive license to Technaid S.L. for the design, manufacture and commercial exploitation of the system.

H2 presents an open architectural design, which allows the integration with other stimulation systems, giving it an advantage over other exoskeleton models. It has motorized joints in the hips, knees and ankles, which are powered by rechargeable batteries, and it has sensors that allow a good control to perform the desired activity, whether it is walking, getting up or sitting [7].

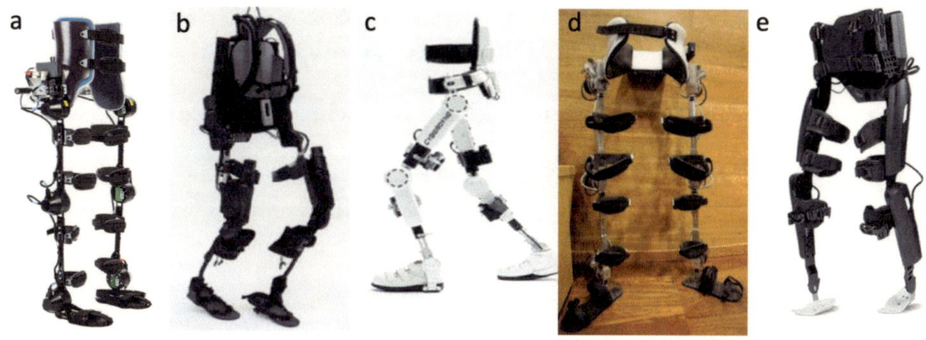

Figure 2.
Exoskeletons: a) H2, b) EKSO, c) HAL, d) KINESIS y e) ReWalk (images taken from Mardomingo-Medialdea, 2018 [7], and companies web pages).

This robotic system works through an interface that connects via Bluetooth to a smartphone; through a Wi-Fi connection, the kinetics and kinematics generated by the exoskeleton are captured and a database is formed that can be statistically analyzed [4].

The interaction between the user and the exoskeleton is very important for the comfort and safety of the users in a robotic device, as the sensors must be physically placed on the human limbs and due to several issues, specifically related to safety, comfort and reliability, placement must be taken into consideration.

The H2 exoskeleton is designed in such a way that there are no sensors physically attached to the human being, all the information indicates that the sensors placed on the exoskeleton are 6 potentiometers, 18 hall effect sensors and 4 foot switches that are used to determine parameters such as angular position and speed, and the force and interaction between the user's limb and the exoskeleton. The H2 exoskeleton is equipped with industrial precision, it includes a potentiometer used as an angular position sensor, that exhibits high linearity and long rotation life. Its gear is through a steel shaft that is coupled to a toothed pulley and a belt that is used to transmit the movement of the joint avoiding slipping and therefore an absolute loss of reference. The exoskeleton platform is equipped with two foot switches based on binary resistive sensors that allow detecting the contact between the subject's foot and the ground, these sensors are located under the heel and toe and their main objective is to detect the different phases during segmented motion [4].

The main controller is based on an H2-ARM electronic board specifically designed to control usage time. The H2-ARM plate's small size (56 x 44 mm) allows it to be placed on the exoskeleton reducing volume, as well as complexity and the difficulty of hiding wiring and connections, as well as eliminating the need for the user to carry a backpack that most lower limb exoskeletons have as a disadvantage.

During a pilot study, the H2 exoskeleton function was consistent during a clinical motion rehabilitation protocol. It was shown as a safe therapy without unwanted effects and with good tolerance by patients [8]. These results have opened the possibility of testing with a larger number of patients.

2.2 ReWalk exoskeleton

This robotic exoskeleton has the ability to use motion supports, which facilitates the autonomous movement of the patient. It was developed by ReWalk Robotics Inc [9]. Its use is designed for patients who have suffered a complete spinal cord injury between C7 and T12, which puts it at an advantage over other more limiting designs in their therapeutic applications [10].

It is an open architectural exoskeleton, which has a 28 V electric motor, located on the user's back and powered by lithium batteries with autonomy of up to three hours [9].

A novel feature of this exoskeleton is that it has inclination sensors and a wireless communicator for its control [9].

The control of the exoskeleton is given by the movements of the trunk and the movements of the center of gravity, that is, when the body moves forward, the system translates it as the beginning of the step [10].

2.3 EKSO exoskeleton

The EKSO exoskeleton, formerly known as the exoskeleton lower extremity motion system, eLEGS, was developed by Berkeley ExoWorks, a company that currently holds the name EKSO Bionics [11].

It is an open structure exoskeleton, open architectural exoskeletons make it easy to connect to other types of equipment that help with the monitoring of muscle activity [7].

This exoskeleton is designed to help people who have suffered strokes, multiple sclerosis, Parkinson's disease, or spinal cord injury below C7, limiting its use for patients with higher or invasive injuries [10].

Its operation depends on a single engine, which is located on the patient's back through a backpack, which makes it uncomfortable for some activities, however, the engine is highly efficient and favors motor skills, allowing the movement of 100% of the weight, lateral motion and squat position, a position not achieved with any other exoskeleton. It also allows the patient to sit up and return to the standing position. Among the advantages offered by this exoskeleton is that it favors the reduction of spasticity. Although the use of a backpack on the back is its greatest disadvantage because it makes it less comfortable than other models, it is still one of the most efficient and functional exoskeletons for patients with paraplegia caused by different diseases [10, 11].

2.4 HAL exoskeleton

The Hybrid Assistive Limb (HAL) exoskeleton has been developed by the Japanese company CYBERDINE Inc [12].

It is an exoskeleton with an open architectural structure.

It has electric engines located in the lateral part of the legs and arms, making this exoskeleton one of the most comfortable of those analyzed in this chapter.

The monitoring of the operation of the exoskeleton is carried out through bioelectric signal sensors located on the user's waist, connected to an interface that allows the monitoring of motor activity [5].

It is aimed at patients who have even lost all of the motor function of the lower limbs, which gives it a great advantage over other exoskeletons that are limited to the fact that the user has limited motility [10].

2.5 Kinesis exoskeleton

The Kinesis exoskeleton has been developed under the auspices of the Spanish Higher Council for Scientific Research [13].

Like the past reviewed exoskeletons, it is an open architectural exoskeleton.

This exoskeleton works with a 24 V electric engine, located on the back, a position that gives the user some discomfort, especially when changing from a standing to a sitting position [13].

NAME	EXO-H2	EKSO before eLEGS (Exoskeleton Lower Extremity Gait System)	HAL (Hybrid Assistive Limb)	KINESIS	ReWalk
DEVELOPER	CSIC Bioengineering Group, but currently the exclusive license is for Technaid S.L.	**EKSO BIONICS** before Berkeley ExoWorks	**CYBERDYNE inc.**	**CSIC** Spain	**ReWalk robotics Inc.**
TARGET POPULATION	Adults between 1.5 and 1.95 m in height, with a maximum weight of 100 kg, with neurological damage that inhibits motor skills.	It is aimed at those people with stroke, multiple sclerosis, Parkinson's or Spinal Cord Injury up to C7.	Aimed at people with walking problems due to neuromuscular pathologies such as Spinal Cord Injury.	It is aimed at people with incomplete Spinal Cord Injury capable of making short movements.	It is a lower limb exoskeleton for people with complete spinal cord injury from C7 to T12.
OPEN OR CLOSED STRUCTURE	OPEN	OPEN	OPEN	OPEN	OPEN
ENGINE AND LOCATION	Motorized joints in hips, knees and ankles	Electric engine located in the back.	Electric engine located on the side of the legs and arms, sensors on the waist. HAL-5.	24 V electric engine, located in the back.	28 V electric engine with lithium batteries with autonomy of 3 hours, located on the back.
USER-SKELETON INTERFACE	Interface that connects via Bluetooth to a smartphone.	Independent motor assistance.	Bioelectric signal sensor.	Functional electrical stimulation.	Tilt sensors. Wireless communicator.
ADVANTAGES AND DISADVANTAGES	Due to its open architecture, it can be used in combination with muscle function readers. It does not need the use of uncomfortable backpacks for the user. It can be used in patients whose paraplegia is caused by various pathologies.	Allows 100% weight shift, lateral movement and squatting position. Spasticity reduction.	It can be used even if the person has totally lost the motor function of the lower limbs.	Can effectively balance robotic performance and functional electrical stimulation during movements.	It is controlled thanks to the movement of the trunk and the movements of the center of gravity, when the body moves forward the system translates it as the beginning of the step.

Table 1.
Comparison among exoskeletons.

The user-exoskeleton interface is through functional electrical stimulation [14].

One of the great advantages of this exoskeleton is that it can effectively balance robotic performance and functional electrical stimulation during motion [10].

However, a major drawback is that it is intended almost exclusively for the usage with patients with an incomplete spinal cord injury, who are capable of short movements.

Table 1 offers a comparison of the most important characteristics of the five exoskeletons analyzed.

3. Discussion

The use of exoskeletons in the rehabilitation of patients with paraplegia shows promising results in the recovery of subjects with motor deficits [1].

There are several exoskeletons developed by different companies. These exoskeletons have evolved over time to help patients who suffer from paraplegia caused by different pathologies. To get the maximum benefit from using these devices, it is necessary for the therapist to carefully choose the appropriate device for each patient. The exoskeletons presented in this chapter have proven to be excellent aids in the partial recovery of motor skills and the improvement of spasticity, although not permanently yet, with minimal pain reported by patients who have used them. However, the cost of exoskeletons is very high, as it varies among $65,000.00 and $100,000.00, which makes it prohibitive for many patients who may require it. Clinical studies in patients have different degrees of advancement, for example: the Kinesis exoskeleton has significant potential to rehabilitate walking motion of patients with incomplete spinal cord injury. The results of tests carried out with KINESIS show that the operative controller adapted to the functional deficits of the patient as well as to voluntary actions during gait, through modulating stimulation and robotic assistance, which was the objective of the controller's design. Further developments should address the simultaneous modulation of robot stimulation and assistance based on explicit patient needs. This includes more robust methods of managing muscle fatigue. The creators foresee additional work related to various aspects of hybrid gait control: stimulation control based on estimating muscle activation, improved semi-automatic gait control, and improved muscle fatigue monitoring [15].

The EXO-H2 exoskeleton is a robust and safe exoskeleton useful for patients with partial leg weakness, while using assistive devices for the upper extremities or with the help of a healthcare professional. It can be used by patients after a stroke or traumatic injury that results in difficulties while walking. There is a preliminary study of EXO-H2 in three patients with stroke-related hemiparesis. The training was well tolerated and there were no adverse events. The authors suggest that Exo-H2 opens the opportunity to study ways to optimize a rehabilitation treatment that can be customized for each patient. These results are promising and encourage future rehabilitation training with a larger cohort of patients [9].

On the other hand, the HAL exoskeleton has been tested in eight patients recovering from hemiparetic strokes, in a study sponsored by the manufacturer and the Stockholm City Council, improving the ability to walk in the 10-meter walk test and in the categories of functional ambulation; it also improves torso posture and facilitates treadmill training, reporting the HAL exoskeleton as safe when used in conjunction with an inpatient rehabilitation program. In a current study between Dandeyd Hospital and the University of Tsukuba, the conventional gait training techniques are compared to the use of HAL in patients recovering from strokes, although the results are not conclusive yet.

The Ekso exoskeleton in its GT model is the first exoskeleton approved by the United States Food and Drug Administration (FDA). It is currently under evaluation in many centers in the United States and Europe.

The Kolakowsky-Hayner et al. [16] team found it safe to use with patients with complete thoracic spinal cord injury in a controlled environment.

The team of Kressler et al. found that people with chronic complete spinal cord injury who used the Ekso for ground walking training could achieve speeds and walking distances comparable to the averages of those with incomplete motor injuries, but there was little change in the activation of the leg muscles [17].

Ekso may help stroke patients stand longer and take more steps [9].

Finally, the ReWalk exoskeleton has proven to work well in patients with spinal cord injury. Outcomes of patients who have been able to walk independently have been documented. In the United States it began to be used in the middle of this decade; the United States Veterans Administration has implemented the use of ReWalk in veterans with paraplegia; and its use in patients recovering from cerebrovascular accidents and people with multiple sclerosis is currently under investigation [9].

4. Conclusions

The use of robotic technology as support for the rehabilitation of patients with paraplegia is a very important tool, which should be considered as part of recovery plans, improving the quality of life of users who require them. However, it is important to note that although it has great advantages for users, the cost of these exoskeletons is so high that it becomes difficult to be provided to all those patients who need them, besides there are also some models that are in early preliminary studies to be still considered for use in regular clinical practice.

4.1 Perspectives

In the next 10–15 years, another important area of development will be modular robotics, specifically exoskeletons made for unique joints such as the hip, knee or ankles, as well as the so-called "soft robotics" that use non-rigid materials, in custom positions to provide movement for people with different physical limitations that do not fit in the current rigid robots. An example of this type of modular robot is the Honda Strike Management Assist (SMA), which fits around a person's waist and thighs like a belt and provides assistance to people with weakened leg muscles. Weighing approximately 2.8 kg, the SMA is much smaller and lighter than other exoskeletons. It is designed to help users regulate their walking pace and lengthen their stride, particularly for people who can walk but have mild gait deficiencies due to aging or other medical conditions. Researchers at the Chicago Rehabilitation Institute are currently evaluating the use of SMA with task-specific training, comparing it to traditional physical therapy in the outpatient setting, for people who have suffered a stroke. Additionally, soft robotics, an emerging area focused on developing systems that are lighter and more flexible to help people with weakened upper or lower limbs, is also evolving. Currently, groups such as Harvard University [18], Yale University, and ETH Zurich are working on soft material technologies that are made up of polymers, gels, and soft microfluidic electronics that exhibit significant elasticity with the potential to enhance the utility of wearable robotics. Finally, systems that combine functional electrical stimulation, pattern recognition, and brain-machine interfaces are also likely to emerge. All of these technologies have the potential to work separately or synergistically with exoskeletons, depending on a person's level of injury and rehabilitation goals [9].

Acknowledgements

We thank the National Institute of Psychiatry Ramón de la Fuente, especially to Dr. Edgar Mixcoha; and Faculty of Health Sciences of Anahuac University.

Conflict of interest

The authors declare that there is no conflict of interest regarding the publication of this paper.

Author details

Susana Martiñón[1,2]* and Ricardo Hernández-Miramontes[1]

1 National Institute of Psychiatry Ramón de la Fuente, Mexico City, Mexico

2 Anáhuac University, A.C. Huixquilucan, Mexico State, Mexico

*Address all correspondence to: susimar2000@yahoo.com

References

[1] Alfonso-mantilla JI, Martínez-santa J. Tecnología De Asistencia : Exoesqueletos Robóticos En Rehabilitación Assistive Technology : Robotic Exoskeletons in Rehabilitation. 2016; 10: 83-90.

[2] Shimizu Y, Kadone H, Kubota S, et al. Voluntary ambulation using voluntary upper limb muscle activity and Hybrid Assistive Limb® (HAL®) in a patient with complete paraplegia due to chronic spinal cord injury: A case report. *J Spinal Cord Med* 2019; 42: 460-468.

[3] Yoshimoto T, Shimizu I, Hiroi Y, et al. Feasibility and efficacy of high-speed gait training with a voluntary driven exoskeleton robot for gait and balance dysfunction in patients with chronic stroke: Nonrandomized pilot study with concurrent control. *Int J Rehabil Res* 2015; 38: 338-343.

[4] Bortole M, Venkatakrishnan A, Zhu F, et al. The H2 robotic exoskeleton for gait rehabilitation after stroke: Early findings from a clinical study Wearable robotics in clinical testing. *J Neuroeng Rehabil* 2015; 12: 1-14.

[5] Jansen O, Grasmuecke D, Meindl RC, et al. Hybrid Assistive Limb Exoskeleton HAL in the Rehabilitation of Chronic Spinal Cord Injury: Proof of Concept; the Results in 21 Patients. *World Neurosurg* 2018; 110: e73–e78.

[6] Louie DR, Eng JJ. Powered robotic exoskeletons in post-stroke rehabilitation of gait: A scoping review. *J Neuroeng Rehabil* 2016; 13: 1-10.

[7] Mardomingo Medialdea H, Fernández González P, Molina Rueda F. Usabilidad y aceptabilidad de los exoesqueletos portables para el entrenamiento de la marcha en sujetos con lesión medular: revisión sistemática. *Rev Neurol* 2018; 66: 35.

[8] A. Gil-Agudo JLP. Robot therapy with the H2 exoskeleton for gait rehabilitation in patients with incomplete spinal cord injry. A clinical experience. *Rehabillitaciòn* 2020; 54: 87-95.

[9] Esquenazi A, Talaty M, Jayaraman A. Powered Exoskeletons for Walking Assistance in Persons with Central Nervous System Injuries: A Narrative Review. *PM R* 2017; 9: 46-62.

[10] Camina Paniagua C. Rehabilitación de la marcha con exoesqueleto HAL en lesionados medulares Autor.

[11] eksobionics.com.

[12] cyberdyne.com.

[13] del Ama AJ, Moreno JC, Gil-Agudo Á, et al. Hybrid FES-robot cooperative control of ambulatory gait rehabilitation exoskeleton for spinal cord injured users. *Biosyst Biorobotics* 2013; 1: 155-159.

[14] del-Ama AJ, Gil-Agudo Á, Pons JL, et al. Hybrid gait training with an overground robot for people with incomplete spinal cord injury: A pilot study. *Front Hum Neurosci* 2014; 8: 1-10.

[15] Del-Ama AJ, Gil-Agudo Á, Bravo-Esteban E, et al. Hybrid therapy of walking with Kinesis overground robot for persons with incomplete spinal cord injury: A feasibility study. *Rob Auton Syst* 2015; 73: 44-58.

[16] Kolakowsky-Hayner SA, Crew J, Moran S, Shah A. Safety and feasibility of using the EksoTM bionic exoskeleton to aid ambulation after spinal cord injury. J Spine. 2013 Sep; 4(3).

[17] Kressler J, Thomas CK, Field-Fote EC, et al. Understanding therapeutic benefits of overground

bionic ambulation: Exploratory case series in persons with chronic, complete spinal cord injury. *Arch Phys Med Rehabil* 2014; 95: 1878-1887.e4.

[18] Exosuits H seas. harvard. edu/ sof.-559.